Management of Strabismus and Amblyopia

A Practical Guide

Second Edition

John A. Pratt-Johnson, M.B., F.R.C.S.(C), F.R.C.S.(Edin)

Professor Emeritus, Department of Ophthalmology
University of British Columbia

Head, Department of Ophthalmology (1982–1992)
British Columbia's Children's Hospital
Vancouver, British Columbia, Canada

and

Geraldine Tillson, D.B.O.(T), O.C.(C)

Director, Orthoptic Training Programme
Department of Ophthalmology
British Columbia's Children's Hospital

Clinical Instructor, Department of Ophthalmology
University of British Columbia
Vancouver, British Columbia, Canada

2001
Thieme
New York • Stuttgart

Thieme New York
333 Seventh Avenue
New York, NY 10001

MANAGEMENT OF STRABISMUS AND AMBLYOPIA, 2ND EDITION
John A. Pratt-Johnson
Geraldine Tillson

Consulting Editor: Esther Gumpert
Editorial Assistant: Owen Zurhellen
Director, Production and Manufacturing: Anne Vinnicombe
Senior Production Editor: Eric L. Gladstone
Marketing Director: Phyllis Gold
Sales Manager: Ross Lumpkin
Chief Financial Officer: Peter van Woerden
President: Brian D. Scanlan
Cover Designer: Kevin Kall
Compositor: The PRD Group
Printer: Hamilton Printing Company

Library of Congress Cataloging-in-Publication Data

Pratt-Johnson, John A
   Management of strabismus and amblyopia : a practical guide / John A. Pratt-Johnson,
  Geraldine Tillson.—2nd ed.
     p. cm.
   Includes bibliographical references and index.
   ISBN 0-86577-992-9
   1. Strabismus. 2. Amblyopia. I. Tillson, Geraldine. II. Title.

RE771 .P73 2001
617.7'62—dc21   00-061561

Important note: Medical knowledge is ever-changing. As new research and clinical experience broaden our knowledge, changes in treatment and drug therapy may be required. The authors and editors of the material herein have consulted sources believed to be reliable in their efforts to provide information that is complete and in accord with the standards accepted at the time of publication. However, in view of the possibility of human error by the authors, editors, or publisher of the work herein, or changes in medical knowledge, neither the authors, editors, publisher, nor any other party who has been involved in the preparation of this work, warrants that the information contained herein is in every respect accurate or complete, and they are not responsible for any errors or omissions or for the results obtained from use of such information. Readers are encouraged to confirm the information contained herein with other sources. For example, readers are advised to check the product information sheet included in the package of each drug they plan to administer to be certain that the information contained in this publication is accurate and that changes have not been made in the recommended dose or in the contraindications for administration. This recommendation is of particular importance in connection with new or infrequently used drugs.

Some of the product names, patents, and registered designs referred to in this book are in fact registered trademarks or proprietary names even though specific reference to this fact is not always made in the text. Therefore, the appearance of a name without designation as proprietary is not to be construed as a representation by the publisher that it is in the public domain.

5 4 3 2 1

TNY ISBN 0-86577-992-9
GTV ISBN 3-13-117602-4

*This book is dedicated to all the ophthalmologists
and orthoptists in Vancouver, British Columbia, Canada,
as well as our many colleagues in other parts of the
world who have made our endeavors at managing
strabismus and amblyopia challenging, rewarding,
and enjoyable. We are also indebted to them for the
social fun and camaraderie that seem inseparable
from this type of practice.*

Table of Contents

Foreword to the First Edition

Individuals with great intellectual depth, organizational abilities, and practical skills are rare, but to have them share a lifetime of experience in strabismus is a special gift to the ophthalmic community. John Pratt-Johnson and Geraldine Tillson are such individuals and have privileged us with their experience in the field of strabismus at a time when most individual would not have the energy to do so. As a clinical ophthalmologist who has called upon this team on a number of occasions for advice on the management of complex strabismic disorders, I can assure you that the advice given was always thoughtful, practical, and specific. This clinical orientation is clearly carried over in the layout and context of this excellent guide to the management of strabismus.

An interesting thing about this book is that it demonstrates the intellectual framework necessary for understanding strabismus in the practical day-to-day clinical care of patients. One has a sense that in looking at the various problems outlined and their solutions, the authors sit in front of the patient. This patient-oriented approach will undoubtedly be of great use to the practicing ophthalmologist, ophthalmic technologist, or ophthalmic assistant. They have focused on the patient encounter, and it emerges as a theme that continually sets the stage and frames the questions and answers so clearly outlined in their text. The human side of the equation drives their endeavor and frames the entire context of their discussions. This book has a logical assembly and order of thought evolving from fundamental aspects of clinical examination, scientific knowledge, and experience in strabismus. The style of the text is precise, with excellent use of day-to-day examples.

One cannot help but note the number of references within this text that are obtained from original articles produced by these two individuals during their professional association. We ought to be grateful to be the beneficiaries of a critically analyzed experience within the context of a broadly based scientific and clinical understanding of strabismus. The Department of Ophthalmology at the University of British Columbia will certainly reflect well in the mirror of their experience.

Jack Rootman, M.D., F.R.C.S.(C)
Ocular Oncology and Orbital Disease
Professor of Ophthalmology and Pathology
Head, Department of Ophthalmology
University of British Columbia and
Vancouver General Hospital
Vancouver, British Columbia
Canada

Preface to the First Edition

We have written this book for the busy general ophthalmologist, orthoptist, ophthalmic technologist and assistant as well as the subspecialist in strabismus. It outlines the diagnostic and treatment methods that have produced the best results from our private practice as an ophthalmologist and an orthoptist who have worked together as a team for the past 17 years. It gives clear recommendations for consideration in treating patients.

We acknowledge that there are often several ways of dealing with a particular problem and many different surgical techniques, but we have presented only those of which we have considerable personal experience. Anatomical details are only included when they are essential to the proper understanding of a diagnosis or treatment, since the gross and microscopic anatomy of the eye and orbit are readily available in many excellent texts. Surgery cannot be learned from a book. However, presuming that the ophthalmologist is being, or has been, trained in eye surgery, some important and useful tips in specific procedures are given.

The detailed table of contents and comprehensive index that we have included are designed to allow the busy practitioner or student easy access to the information required to decide what is wrong and how best to correct it. A glossary of some terms, words, and phrases used in this book is included to minimize semantic confusion.

John A. Pratt-Johnson, M.B., F.R.C.S.(C), F.R.C.S.(Edin)
Geraldine Tillson, D.B.O.(T), O.C.(C)

Preface to the Second Edition

The Second Edition is completely updated and includes two new chapters. Special attention has been directed to the World Health Organization's initiative "Vision 20/20, The Right to Sight," which aims to rid the world of the preventable and treatable causes of blindness in the world by the year 2020, particularly as it relates to strabismus and amblyopia in developing nations. Attention also has been directed to the effect of refractive surgery and intraocular lenses on strabismus and amblyopia. Details of telemedicine and e-mail consultation concerning strabismus and amblyopia are included. Case reports illustrating common mistakes in the management of strabismus and amblyopia should be a useful addition.

John A. Pratt-Johnson, M.B., F.R.C.S.(C), F.R.C.S.(Edin)
Geraldine Tillson, D.B.O. (T), O.C.(C)

Acknowledgments

We are indebted to our peers and the generations of predecessors who have shared their knowledge in the field of strabismus and amblyopia. Little in our book is original, and although we have provided references, in some detail, it is likely that we have inadvertently omitted some references to those whose work has had some direct or indirect influence on us.

We express our gratitude to Drs. A.J. Elliot and S.M. Drance, past Chairmen of the Department of Ophthalmology, and the present Chairman, Dr. J. Rootman, for their wholehearted support of our academic and teaching program at the University of British Columbia.

Our weekly Motility Clinics have been a forum for the presentation of patient problems, always followed by considerable discussion. This has been a most stimulating and enjoyable highlight of our work and has helped formulate some of the material included in this book. In this regard, we wish to thank Drs. A. Cohen, A.Q. McCormick, W.B. Purcell, J.D.A. Carruthers, R.A. Kennedy, R.A. Cline, and A. Tischler, as well as Orthopists C.T. Lunn, A. Pop, and J. Jones for contributing so richly to this academic function which provided the stimulus for the First Edition.

We give our very special thanks to Betty Pratt-Johnson, author and publisher, for her constant advice, help, and encouragement; Jane Rowlands for all the art work; Nancy Mason, Executive Secretary of the practice for the past 27 years, for help with the production of this book, and the tireless repetitive typing of the manuscript; and Marc Strauss, Philip van Tongeren, and Kimberly Wright of Thieme Medical Publishers, Inc., for their most enthusiastic support and help with editing and producing the First Edition of this book.

We would also like to thank Don Johnson, who photographed Figures 4-1, 4-4, and 4-6 and Dale Northey, who photographed Figures 4-3, 5-6, 5-8, and 5-10. All of the remaining photographs in the book were taken by John A. Pratt Johnson.

We would also like to thank the following persons for their help with the Second Edition: Vicky Earl, medical artist for Figure 16-1D,E,F, and G and Figures 21-1 and 21-2, and Andrea Seils, Michelle Carini, and Anne Vinnicombe of Thieme for their advice and help. We are particularly grateful for the skill of the Senior

Production Editor, Eric L. Gladstone, for collating all the material needed to produce the Second Edition.

We gratefully acknowledge also the contributions of two pediatric anesthetists from British Columbia's Children's Hospital and The University of British Columbia: Dr. Michael Smith for his contribution on malignant hyperthermia in Chapter 17, and Dr. G.A.R. O'Connor for the section on ketamine anesthesia in Chapter 22.

Finally, as immigrants to this great country, we wish to express our joyful gratitude to Canada and all our Canadian friends for the fun and professional opportunity life has given us in our adopted land.

John A. Pratt-Johnson, M.B., F.R.C.S.(C), F.R.C.S.(Edin)
Geraldine Tillson, D.B.O.(T), O.C.(C)

The Development of Vision, Fusion, and Stereopsis

How Vision, Fusion, and Stereopsis Develop

Physiologic research has shown that different visual functions mature at different times. Visual acuity is approximately 6/30 at 6 months[3,27] and 6/6 at about 2 years of age.[6] Contrast sensitivity for lower spatial frequencies and motion detection has been shown to develop by 3 months and to be mature by 6 months of age.[21] Stable alignment of the visual axes is present by approximately 4 months of age if fusion and stereopsis have developed normally.[20] Fusion is the mechanism that keeps the eyes correctly aligned, and stereopsis is the reward. The critical period during which fusion and stereopsis may be developed, modified, or lost still has to be clearly established. However, stereopsis is present by 4 to 6 months of age.[1,5,8]

A bias for nasally directed eye movements, shown by testing optokinetic nystagmus, is present at birth. This disappears by 4 to 6 months of age in normal infants,[19] which is about the time that stereopsis develops and the visual system's ability to resolve contrast matures.[21,26] Optokinetic nystagmus remains asymmetrical in infants who have or who are likely to develop strabismus.[9] It also persists in patients whose congenital strabismus is not treated[28,30] and in adults who are stereo blind.[31]

Visual Maturity (Visual Adult)

Although good vision, stereopsis, and fusion are probably developed by 4 months of age, they do not become firmly established until around the age of 8 years. The younger the patient, the more vulnerable the various visual functions. Visual acuity deterioration and suppression are unlikely to occur in patients who develop a strabismus after the age of 5 years and are rare, although recorded, after the age of 8 years. For this reason, patients under the age of 8 years are usually referred to as being visually immature and those over the age of 8 as being visual adults. This division is used throughout this book.

From a practical standpoint, this means that any abnormality of the visual system that would interfere with the clear image falling on the fovea, or any misalignment of the eyes that would interfere with normal binocular vision, may cause permanent damage to the system if left untreated in a visually immature person. Once the visual system has matured, after the age of 8, vision is fixed for life and amblyopia does not occur unless there is organic damage to the visual system. Stereopsis and fusion are also firmly entrenched by the age of 8 years, but occasional deterioration of binocular function can occur after prolonged interruption in visual adults (see section on Central Fusion Disruption in Chapter 19).

Development of Normal Monocular Visual Acuity

In order for normal monocular visual acuity to develop, it is essential that the fovea receives a clearly focused image throughout the period of visual immaturity, that is, at least to the age of 8 years. Normal monocular visual acuity is then firmly established for the rest of the individual's life. If these conditions are not met, a visual defect called amblyopia may result.

Development of Normal Binocular Vision

The term *binocular vision* is potentially confusing, because it has been used differently in the literature by different disciplines. This term has been used to describe a wide range of functions. At the most basic level, it only implies that both eyes can see. However, the term has been used to imply some level of cooperation or coordination between the eyes, even the ultimate of bifoveal fusion and 40 seconds of arc of stereopsis. The term *normal binocular vision* usually implies the latter, and that is what it means in this context.

It is necessary for the eyes to be correctly aligned during visual immaturity for normal binocular vision to develop. Sometimes a child is born with "wandering" eyes and the eye alignment stabilizes within the first 3 months of life. It is necessary to have the alignment of the eyes arranged so that the clearly focused image of the object of regard falls onto the fovea of each eye to allow fusion and stereopsis to develop normally. Once these faculties have been developed and maintained to visual maturity, they will remain with the patient permanently. The occasional exception to this rule is central fusion disruption, which is discussed in Chapter 19.

Normal Binocular Fusion (Bifoveal)

This is one of our most highly developed senses and is contingent on the one-to-one relay from ganglion cells of corresponding points from each retina to a shared cortical cell in the brain. Because fusion is such a highly developed sense, it is also highly vulnerable and is readily disrupted in the visually immature years by any of the conditions that may cause amblyopia. It is essential that equal input from correspond-

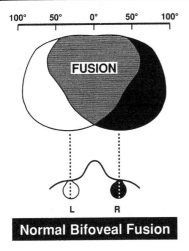

Figure 1–1. Normal binocular field of vision showing area of fusion and the monocular temporal crescents of visual field from each eye.

ing retinal points reaches the same cortical cell. If there is any significant difference in the input from each eye, it causes competition between the two. The clearer image prevails, and the other image is inhibited. The visual fields of the two eyes overlap in an area approximately 60° to either side of fixation to provide stereopsis and central and peripheral fusion. There is a monocular temporal crescent of each visual field that can only be seen by the ipsilateral eye, which provides more peripheral visual field (Fig. 1–1). Normal binocular vision is characterized by excellent stereoacuity of 60 seconds or better with the Titmus test.[4] Normal fusional amplitudes for near fixation are 8 prism diopters of divergence, 50 prism diopters of convergence, and 1 or 2 prism diopters of vertical amplitude when tested with prisms.

Retinal Correspondence, Fusion, and Stereopsis

There must be correspondence between the retinas of the two eyes before fusion can develop. If there is normal fusion, the patient has normal retinal correspondence.

The term *corresponding retinal points* has been used frequently in the past but it has largely been replaced by *corresponding retinal areas*. This is because retinal correspondence seems to be more flexible than just a point-to-point relationship.

Normal Retinal Correspondence

The foveas normally correspond and therefore have a common visual direction, as do areas that are displaced the same distance and in the same direction (e.g., to the right, left, up, or down) from the fovea in each eye. This means that anatomically corresponding points from each eye localize to the same point in space. This is accomplished by the crossing of optic nerve fibers in the optic chiasm. This brings fibers from the corresponding points from each eye to the same lateral geniculate body but to different layers there. In the cortex these fibers share a cell. Once normal retinal correspondence has been firmly established and has been maintained until visual adulthood, it is not possible to change it to anomalous correspondence. If both foveas fix an object in space, the visual axes will intersect there and a single image will be seen because the foveas are corresponding retinal areas. This is the basis of fusion.

Fusion

Fusion has been artificially subdivided into motor and sensory; from a practical point of view, however, both parts are needed to maintain normal binocular function. Sensory fusion is the result of the joining together of the images from corresponding points of each eye in the same cell in the striate cortex to form one image.[10]

Bifoveal fusion is called central fusion. There will be points to either side of the fixation object whose images also fall on corresponding retinal points peripheral to the foveas. This is the basis of peripheral fusion.

An imaginary line in space connecting all these points is known as the horopter. Images from objects on the horopter are normally seen singly because they are fused. On either side of the horopter is a narrow area known as Panum's fusional space or Panum's space of binocular single vision. The images of objects within this area, although they fall on noncorresponding retinal elements, are still seen singly. This is a basis for stereopsis. Motor fusion (fusional amplitude) is the brain's mechanism to keep the position of the eyes aligned so that both foveas project to the same point in space and sensory fusion can occur.

Motor Side of Fusion

The stability of sensory fusion depends on corresponding retinal areas being kept in proper alignment in different gaze directions and under stress. It therefore requires complex motor alignment of the eyes involving all the extraocular muscles and cranial nerves III, IV, and VI. Ordinary pursuit movements would seem to depend on the interrelation of cranial nerves III, IV, and VI in the midbrain. It has been shown that there are specific cells in the midbrain of the monkey, just rostral to the oculomotor nucleus, that respond specifically to convergence and others specifically to divergence.[12,16,17] This area of the midbrain therefore might represent the motor area of fusion and fusional amplitudes. Clinical evidence for convergence cells in this area of the midbrain is provided by the development of esotropia or convergence abnormalities from lesions demonstrated to be in that area.[2,7,13,23] Central fusion disruption (see Chapter 19) may result from a lesion in this part of the midbrain.

The Connection Between Sensory and Motor Fusion

The corticofugal projection from the striate cortex to the motor fusion area in the midbrain is still conjectural, and there is no general agreement among researchers on a pathway.

Visual Acuity

Visual acuity (the form pathway) and fusional movements (the motion pathway) are conveyed via different pathways from the retinal ganglion cells to the cortex.[18,25] It appears that the motion pathway provides a signal for pursuit eye movements[29] and possibly vergence.[11,15] This motion pathway emphasizes the parafovea and periphery, in contrast to the form (visual acuity) pathway, which emphasizes the central visual fields and foveal function.[14]

Prolonged visual deprivation in visual adults may cause loss of fusion but does not seem to cause visual acuity loss. Fusion may be governed by a period of cortical plasticity that is different from that covering visual acuity. It seems that the fusion pathway is distinctly different from the form pathway. The fusion pathway projects initially to different cells in the lateral geniculate body from the form pathway and then to different layers and zones of striate cortex before going to different areas of the extrastriate visual cortex. It is physiologically possible that fusion and visual acuity might have different critical periods of development.

Stereopsis

Stereopsis depends on input from slightly disparate retinal points from each eye, as happens in Panum's space. Different neurons representing coarse and fine stereo tuning have been located in the striate cortex of the monkey.[15,24] Information about fine stereo tuning from the foveal area appears to travel via the form (visual) pathway to specified zones within the striate cortex. However, coarse stereo tuning appears to travel via the motion pathway to other layers and zones of the striate cortex.

Images outside Panum's area, either closer than or farther away from the fixation image, give rise to physiologic diplopia because they do not fall on corresponding retinal areas. Physiologic diplopia also plays a role in stereopsis. Temporal displacement of the images causes crossed physiologic diplopia and therefore the sensation of relative nearness. Nasal displacement of the images causes uncrossed physiologic diplopia and therefore the sensation of being relatively more distant than the fixation object.

References

1. Archer, S.M., Helveston, E.M., Miller, K.K., Ellis, F.D.: Stereopsis in normal infants with congenital esotropia. Am J Ophthalmol 101:591–596, 1986.
2. Barraquer-Bordas, L., Illa, I., Escartin, A., Ruscelleda, J., Marti-Vilalta, J.L.: Thalamic hemorrhage. A study of 23 patients with diagnosis by computed tomography. Stroke 12:524–527, 1987.
3. Dobson, V., Teller, D.Y.: Visual acuity in human infants: A review and comparison of behavioral and electrophysiological studies. Vision Res 18:1469–1483, 1978.
4. Fisher, N.: The optic chiasm and the corpus callosum: Their relationship to binocular vision in humans. J Pediatr Ophthalmol Strabismus 23:126, 1986.
5. Fox, R., Aslin, R.N., Shea, S.C., Dumais, S.T.: Stereopsis in human infants. Science 207:323–324, 1980.
6. Fulton, A.B., Hansen, R.M., Manning, K.A.: Measuring visual acuity in infants. Surv Ophthalmol 25:325, 1981.
7. Gomez, C.R., Gomez, S.M., Selhorst, J.B.: Acute thalamic esotropia. Neurology 38:1759–1762, 1988.

8. Held, R., Birch, E., Gwiazda, J.: Stereoacuity of human infants. Proc Natl Acad Sci USA 77:5572–5574, 1980.
9. Hooper, A.: Opticokinetic strabismus and the age at onset of strabismus. Br Orthop J 47:44–47, 1990.
10. Hubel, D.M., Wiesel, T.N.: Binocular interaction in striate cortex of kittens reared with artificial squint. J Neurophysiol 28:1041, 1965.
11. Jampel, R.S.: Representation of the near-response on the cerebral cortex of the macaque. Am J Ophthalmol 48:573–582, 1959.
12. Judge, S.J., Cumming, B.G.: Neurons in the monkey midbrain with activity related to vergence eye movements and accommodation. J Neurophysiol 55:915–929, 1986.
13. Kawachara, N., Sato, K., Muraki, M., Tanaka, K., Kaneko, M., Uemura, K.: CT classification of small thalamic hemorrhages and their clinical implications. Neurology 36:165–172, 1986.
14. Livingstone, M.S., Hubel, D.H.: Psychophysical evidence for separate visual channels for the perception of form, color, movement and depth. J Neurosci 7:3416–3468, 1987.
15. Maunsell, J.H.R., Van Essen D.C.: Functional properties of neurons in middle temporal area of macaque monkey. J Neurophysiol 49:1148–1167, 1983
16. Mays, L.E.: Neural control of vergence eye movements. Convergence and divergence neurons in the midbrain. J Neurophysiol 51:1091–1107, 1984.
17. Mays, L.E., Porter, J.D., Gamlin, P.D., Tello, C.A.: Neural control of vergence eye movements: Neurons encoding vergence velocity. J Neurophysiol 56:1007–1021, 1986.
18. Mishkin, M., Ungerlieder, L.G., Mocko, K.A.: Object vision and spatial vision: Two cortical pathways. Trends Neurosci 6:414–417, 1983.
19. Naegele, JR, Held, R.: The postnatal development of monocular optokinetic nystagmus in infants. Vision Res 22:341–346, 1982.
20. Nixon, R.B., Helveston, E.M., Miller, K., Archer, S.M., Ellis, F.D.: Incidence of strabismus in neonates. Am J Ophthalmol 100:798, 1985.
21. Norcia, A.M., Tyler, C.W.: Spatial frequency sweep VEP: Visual acuity development during the first year of life. Vision Res 25:1399, 1985.
22. Norcia, A.M., Tyler, C.W., Allen, D.: Electrophysiological assessment of contrast sensitivity in human infants. Am J Optom Physiol Optics 63:12–15, 1986.
23. Pillai, P., Dhand, U.K.: Cyclic esotropia with central nervous system disease. J Pediatr Ophthalmol Strabismus. 24:239–241, 1987.
24. Poggio, G.F., Fisher, B.: Binocular interaction and depth sensitivity in striate cortical neurons of behaving rhesus monkey. J Neurophysiol 40:1392–1405, 1977.
25. Schiller, P.H.: The central visual system. Vision Res 26:1351, 1986.
26. Sokol, S.: Measurement of infant visual acuity from patterns reversal evoked potentials. Vision Res 18:33, 1978.
27. Teller, D.Y.: Visual acuity for vertical and diagonal gratings in human infants. Vision Res 14:1433–1439, 1974.
28. Tychsen, L.R., Lisberger, S.G.: Maldevelopment of visual motion processing in humans who had strabismus with onset in infancy. J Neurosci 6:2495, 1986.
29. Tychsen, L.R., Lisberger, S.G.: Visual motion processing for the initiation of smooth pursuit eye movements in humans. J Neurophysiol 56:953, 1986.
30. Tychsen, L.R., Nurtig, R., Scott, W.E.: Pursuit is impaired but the vestibulo-ocular reflex is normal in infantile esotropia. Arch Ophthalmol 103:536, 1985.
31. Van Hof-Van Duin, J., Mohn, G.: Stereopsis and optico kinetic nystagmus. In: Lennarstrand, G., ed. Functional Basis of Ocular Motility Disorders. New York: Pergamon, 1982:113–115.

2

What Happens if the Development of Vision, Fusion, and Stereopsis Is Interrupted?

As discussed in more detail in Chapter 1, different visual functions mature at different times. Visual acuity is approximately 6/30 at 6 months[2,17] and 6/6 at about 2 years of age.[3] The critical period for the development of fusion and stereopsis has yet to be defined. Although good vision, stereopsis, and fusion are probably developed by 4 months of age, they do not become firmly established until around the age of 8 years. The younger the patient, the more vulnerable the visual functions.

Different inputs to the cortex for each eye during visual immaturity may cause amblyopia or a strabismus or both. Any untreated abnormality of the immature visual system that prevents a clear image from falling on the fovea or any misalignment of the eyes that interferes with normal binocular vision may cause permanent damage, such as amblyopia. Fusion and stereopsis may not develop properly or may deteriorate and be irretrievable. Amblyopia and suppression are unlikely to occur in patients who develop a strabismus after the age of 5 years and are rare after the age of 8 years. Once the visual system is mature, generally considered to be after the age of 8, vision is fixed for life and amblyopia does not occur unless there is organic damage to the visual system. Stereopsis and fusion are also firmly entrenched by the age of 8 years, but occasional deterioration of binocular function can occur after prolonged interruption in visual adults[14] (see section on Central Fusion Disruption in Chapter 19).

Asymmetric Optokinetic Nystagmus

Infants under 3 months of age have been shown to have an asymmetry of optokinetic nystagmus (OKN). There is a bias toward temporal to nasal motion, and the response to nasal to temporal motion is reduced or absent. OKN remains asymmetrical in infants over the age of 3 months who have or are likely to develop strabismus under the age of 12 months.[5] This asymmetry between nasalward and temporalward motion persists in patients whose congenital strabismus is not treated or who do not develop fusion after treatment of their congenital strabismus.[18,19] It is also present in adults who are stereo blind.[20] If fusion and stereopsis develop normally, this asymmetry disappears.

Amblyopia

Amblyopia occurs in approximately 19% of untreated cases of congenital esotropia[1] and in over 50% of treated cases.[9] This is presumably because the patient develops a dominant eye if the esotropia is reduced to a small angle. Therefore, it is essential to explain to the parents that aligning the eyes of a child with congenital strabismus is just the beginning of many years of close observation to ensure that the child not only looks nice but also has good vision in both eyes. In our experience, 100% of patients who acquire esotropia under the age of 3 years develop strabismic amblyopia if not treated immediately after onset.

Suppression

Suppression is the mechanism used to eliminate an unwanted image caused by, for example, strabismus or anisometropia. Suppression develops in visually immature individuals as a response to the differing inputs from each eye to the cortex. Suppression is a barrier to the development of fusion. Its presence also can eradicate the fusion and stereopsis that have developed if it occurs during visual immaturity.

The whole area of the visual field of the deviating eye that overlaps the visual field of the fixing eye is suppressed. The remainder of the visual field of the deviating eye is not suppressed.[13] Thus, the deviating eye always contributes to the overall binocular field of vision in a strabismic patient. This binocular field is smaller (narrower) in esotropic patients and larger (wider) in exotropic patients (Fig. 2–1A,B,C).

In a strabismic patient with suppression, when the image of the fixation target crosses the midline of the retina from the nasal side to the temporal side or vice versa, it operates a "trigger" mechanism (the hemiretinal trigger mechanism), which determines whether diplopia or suppression occurs.[13] This mechanism has been wrongly interpreted as hemiretinal suppression.[6,13] A strabismic patient with suppression will experience either diplopia or suppression, depending on which side of the retina the image of the fixation target falls. Diplopia or suppression occurs wherever the visual fields of the two eyes overlap in patients with strabismus. The retinal midline divides the temporal retina and one side of the brain from the nasal retina and the other side of the brain. Suppression develops in the visually immature patient in order to avoid diplopia. The image of the fixation object always falls on the same side of the retina of the deviating eye and is suppressed. As long as the deviation is unchanged, suppression will persist. If the deviation is overcorrected by surgery or prisms, however, this is a new situation. Suppression has not been developed for this, so diplopia is triggered (Fig. 2–1D,E).[13] In the visually immature patient suppression will develop in response to the new eye position,

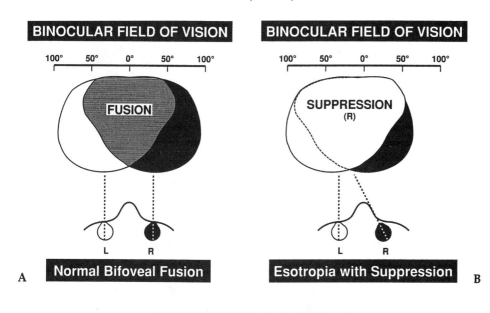

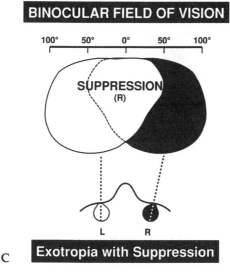

Figure 2–1. Fusion and suppression. (*A*) Normal fusion. (*B*) Binocular field of vision in esotropia with suppression is slightly smaller than normal. (*C*) Binocular field of vision in exotropia with suppression is larger than normal. (*Figure continued on next page.*)

but a visual adult is unable to suppress again and diplopia persists. It is the change in position of the retinal image from one half of the retina to the other half that triggers the change from suppression to diplopia and vice versa wherever the visual fields overlap. Whenever suppression or diplopia occurs, both halves of the retina are involved, not just the nasal or the temporal half, and suppression or diplopia occurs throughout the overlapping areas of the visual fields.[13]

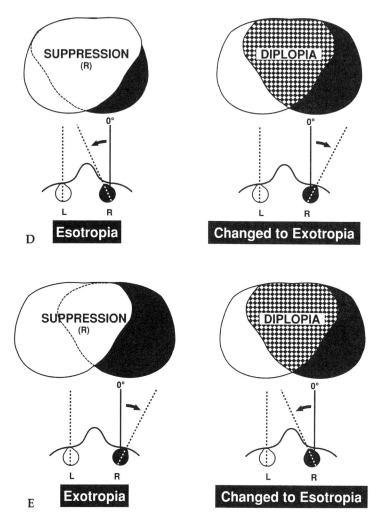

Figure 2–1 *(Continued).* (*D*) Right esotropia with suppression changed to right exotropia provokes diplopia in a visual adult. (*E*) Right exotropia with suppression changed to right esotropia provokes diplopia in a visual adult.

Innate Inability to Fuse

Even after early treatment and stable alignment of the eyes to within 10 prism diopters of being straight, normal bifoveal fusion and fine stereopsis do not develop in patients with congenital strabismus.[9] In approximately half the cases so aligned, even peripheral fusion and gross stereopsis fail to develop.[9] This may be because of a congenital sensory anomaly resulting from an innate inability to fuse, as suggested by Worth.[21]

Patients with a strabismus that develops after a period of perfect visual alignment may regain completely normal fusion if realignment of their eyes is undertaken soon after the onset of the strabismus.[10,11]

How the Patient Functions if Fusion and Stereopsis Do Not Develop

Patients without fusion, and the parents of children without fusion, should be told that it is wrong to think that the deviating eye is not being used. The binocular field of vision should be demonstrated to them (Fig. 2–1B,C). An adaptation of the confrontation test is helpful. The patient has both eyes open, and a target is brought in from the temporal side of the deviating eye until the patient sees it. The deviating eye should then be covered and the patient asked if the target is still visible. The target will have disappeared from the visual field, proving that it must have been seen only by the deviating eye. This is important information for patients and parents to have because it helps them to understand how someone can function well despite having a strabismus. It also helps alleviate an adult's fears of amblyopia occurring or recurring.

The advantages of a dominant eye should also be explained to patients. Adult patients without fusion may note a shift in the apparent position of objects when they alternate fixation and may be disturbed by this.[7] Therefore, every effort should be made to prevent the development of spontaneous alternation so as to avoid this problem. A deviation may be more unsightly fixing one eye versus the other. This is another reason for promoting the development of fixation (and therefore dominance) of the eye that gives the best cosmesis if the patient has no fusion.

It is important for parents and patients to understand that stereopsis is just one method of judging depth, and everyone uses additional uniocular clues for depth perception. People can function very well without stereopsis. Adult patients who suddenly lose their stereopsis will be very aware of their loss until they adapt to judging depth entirely on monocular clues. Patients who have never developed stereopsis seldom have a problem as a result of this.

Lack of fusion or stereopsis does not affect reading but may affect ball games, although it is difficult to assess this accurately for sports because other factors are involved. As an example, it is not unusual for someone with perfect stereopsis and no physical disabilities to be unskilled at tennis or baseball, yet there are several famous baseball players who were or are legally blind in one eye from childhood.

The Monofixation Syndrome

The monofixation syndrome is characterized by a "Flick," a small heterotropia, usually with a latent component.[8] This is the best result that is obtained in cases of congenital strabismus. There is suppression of the macula of the deviating eye only. This permits peripheral fusion to develop. The peripheral fusional amplitude varies from a few prism diopters to near normal. This is a stabilizing factor for eye alignment. Some patients also develop gross stereopsis. Investigation includes the cover-uncover test to detect the small manifest "Flick" strabismus. This is followed by the cross-cover test, which will reveal the accompanying larger latent component.

Stereopsis is never normal. Patients with a monofixation syndrome always have difficulty with the TNO or the Lang stereotests, that is, stereotests involving random dots, and frequently they cannot do these tests at all, although they can still appreciate gross stereopsis with the Titmus test. The Titmus test result is rarely better than 100 seconds of arc.

There is further discussion of this syndrome in Chapter 8 (Congenital Esotropia Syndrome), and the tests listed above are described in detail in Chapter 4 (Sensory Evaluation of Strabismus). It is a matter of some debate as to whether retinal correspondence is normal or abnormal in these cases. The small angle of strabismus makes it difficult to resolve this argument.

Abnormal Retinal Correspondence

Abnormal retinal correspondence (ARC) is an adaptation to the presence of a strabismus in early childhood. The foveas cease to be corresponding areas. Instead, the fovea of the fixing eye corresponds to an extrafoveal area in the deviating eye. In most cases little or no fusion is demonstrable. However, in some cases ARC is so highly developed that some fusion and even stereopsis are demonstrable. The incidence of ARC seems to have declined markedly, possibly because of the early referral and treatment of childhood strabismus. The presence of ARC is only of practical importance when surgery is planned to improve cosmesis. Patients may become aware of paradoxical diplopia (i.e., crossed diplopia despite esotropia on the cover test), but this is usually transient.

Failure to Develop Fusion or Suppression (Intractable Diplopia)

We reported on two patients treated for unilateral congenital cataract by cataract extraction and contact lens correction of the resulting aphakia. Good vision but no fusion was achieved. The patients were aware of diplopia. The phakic eye had been patched for 90% of the waking day from earliest infancy until the patients were 6 years old. This appears to have prevented sufficient interaction of the eyes for either fusion or suppression to develop.[16] Care therefore should be taken to allow sufficient binocular interaction for fusion or suppression to develop and to obtain optimum visual acuity.

Loss of Fusion in Visual Adults

We also have reported on a group of patients who lost their ability to fuse when they were over 10 years old. This central disruption of fusion was due to an insult to the brain.[12] The most common cause was trauma involving serious head injuries and resulting in unconsciousness for several days.[12,14] Acceleration forces generated within the skull produce a shear force that concentrates in the brain stem. In addition, there is a downward displacement of the brain stem with a blow to the head.[4] The most interesting cases of loss of fusion in visual adults have been those in which there did not appear to be any particular etiology. Patients suddenly became aware of diplopia that they were unable to eliminate except by closing one eye.[14] No fusion was demonstrable despite detailed orthoptic evaluation. Four patients had a presumed vascular lesion, and two had suffered a pyrexial flulike illness just preceding the onset of diplopia.[14]

Patients with a central loss of fusional amplitude have definite clinical characteristics typified by their ability to superimpose the images from each eye only momentarily, suggesting that the sensory side of fusion may be intact. There is no fusional amplitude despite good ductions and, in many cases, normal versional movements. These findings point to a lesion affecting the motor part of fusion, probably in the midbrain. If the images from each eye are artificially superimposed with the aid of a major amblyoscope, or with prisms in free space, there seems to be an avoidance of fusion. The patient notices a vertical bobbing movement of the image seen by the deviating eye whenever the images are made to approach each other. Sometimes the examiner can see a slight vertical bobbing movement of one of the patient's eyes. This phenomenon is only present when both eyes are open.[14] Prolonged sensory deprivation of one eye in visual adults may cause a similar central disruption of fusion, but it does not seem to cause visual acuity loss.[15]

Sensory Deprivation Resulting in the Loss of Fusion in Visual Adults (Central Fusion Disruption)

Adult patients who have had visual deprivation even for decades do not seem to have any loss of visual acuity once a clear image can be formed on the retina. Some patients lose their ability to fuse, however. Fusion may have a period of cortical plasticity that is different from that of visual acuity. We have described a series of patients who have had a unilateral traumatic cataract as visual adults. Visual deprivation has resulted either from the cataract being left in place or from uncorrected aphakia following removal of the cataract. In some patients, if the visual deprivation continued for longer than 2 1/2 years, fusion was totally lost, although the corrected visual acuity remained unaffected. The patients suffer from intractable diplopia with no suppression.[15] Another example of loss of fusion in a visual adult is a 49-year-old woman who had herpetic keratitis causing severely blurred vision (6/60 or worse) for 18 years before regaining 6/9 vision with a penetrating keratoplasty. She had constant diplopia with the characteristic vertical bobbing of the image from one eye when an attempt was made to superimpose the images. She had lost the ability to fuse or suppress. All these patients have objective and subjective findings similar to those of patients with a loss of fusion from organic insults to the brain. Central fusion disruption is described in more detail in Chapter 19 (on diplopia).

Social Implications of Strabismus

Living with a strabismus or having a child with strabismus affects all aspects of daily life. For the parents there is the expense of occlusion, glasses, and visits to the ophthalmologist's office. Even if they have some kind of insurance, the time and costs of transportation involved can be considerable. The endless questions and advice from family, neighbors, and even strangers in the supermarket, as well as the teasing that the child has to endure, all have a major impact on their lives. When surgery is needed, this is an additional cost and stress factor. Adults and older children are frequently asked "Who are you looking at?" "Why don't you look at me when you are speaking?" and so forth. This makes social occasions uncomfortable for them because they are worrying about their eyes. Applying for a driver's licence may involve additional visits to the ophthalmologist to have forms completed to show they are fit to drive because they do not have stereopsis. Similarly, a pilot's licence may be denied. These are just a few of the problems that patients encounter, particularly if they have a strabismus without potential fusion ability.

A strabismus may appear to most people to be a minor problem. However, adults who have grown up with a strabismus will describe it as a disability that has had a major impact on their social and working lives.

References

1. Calcutt, C.: The natural history of infantile esotropia. A study of the untreated condition in the visual adult. In: Tillson, G., ed. Advances in Amblyopia and Strabismus. Transactions of the 7th International Orthoptic Congress. Germany: 1991:3.
2. Dobson, V., Teller, D.Y.: Visual acuity in human infants: A review and comparison of behavioral and electrophysiological studies. Vision Res 18:1469–1483, 1978.
3. Fulton, A.B., Hansen, R.M., Manning, K.A.: Measuring visual acuity in infants. Surv Ophthalmol 25:325, 1981.
4. Haller, K.A., Miller-Meeks, M., Korlon, R.: Early magnetic resonance imaging in acute traumatic internuclear ophthalmoplegia. Ophthalmology. 97:1162-1165, 1990.
5. Hooper, A.: Opticokinetic strabismus and the age at onset of strabismus. Br Orthop J 47:44–47, 1990.
6. Jampolsky, A.: Characteristics of suppression in strabismus. Arch Ophthalmol 54:683–696, 1955.
7. Lyons, C.J., Oystreck, D.T.: Presbyopia and strabismus: Old patients, new symptoms. In: Pritchard, C., et al., eds. Orthoptics in Focus—Visions for the New Millennium. Transactions of the IXth International Orthoptic Congress, Stockholm, Sweden 1999. Nuremberg: Berufsverband der Orthoptistinnen Deutschland e.V., 1999:200–204.
8. Parks, M.M.: The monofixational syndrome. Trans Am Ophthalmol Soc 67:609, 1969.
9. Pratt-Johnson, J.A.: Fusion and suppression: Development and loss. J Pediatr Ophthalmol Strabismus 29:1–7, 1992.
10. Pratt-Johnson, J.A., Barlow, J.M.: Binocular function and acquired esotropia. Am Orthop J 23:52–59, 1973.
11. Pratt-Johnson, J.A., Barlow, J.M., Tillson, G.: Early surgery in intermittent exotropia. Am J Ophthalmol 84:689–694, 1977.
12. Pratt-Johnson, J.A., Tillson, G.: Acquired central disruption of fusional amplitude. Ophthalmology 86:2140, 1979.
13. Pratt-Johnson, J.A., Tillson, G.: Suppression in strabismus—An update. Br J Ophthalmol 68:174–178, 1984.
14. Pratt-Johnson, J.A., Tillson, G.: The loss of fusion in adults with intractable diplopia (central fusion disruption). Aust N Z J Ophthalmol 16:81–85, 1988.
15. Pratt-Johnson, J.A., Tillson, G.: Intractable diplopia after vision restoration in unilateral cataract. Am J Ophthalmol 107:23, 1989.
16. Pratt-Johnson, J.A., Tillson, G.: Unilateral congenital cataract: Binocular status after treatment. J Pediatr Ophthalmol Strabismus 26:72–74, 1989.
17. Teller, D.Y.: Visual acuity for vertical and diagonal gratings in human infants. Vision Res 14:1433–1439, 1974.

18. Tychsen, L., Lisberger, S.G.: Maldevelopment of visual motion processing in humans who had strabismus with onset in infancy. J Neurosci 6:2495, 1986.
19. Tychsen, L.R., Nurtig, R., Scott, W.E.: Pursuit is impaired but the vestibule ocular reflex is normal in infantile esotropia. Arch Ophthalmol 103:536, 1985.
20. Van Hof-Van Duin, J., Mohn, G.: Stereopsis and optico kinetic nystagmus. In: Lennarstrand, G., ed. Functional Basis of Ocular Motility Disorders. New York: Pergamon, 1982:113–115.
21. Worth, C.: Squint: Its causes, pathology and treatment. Philadelphia: Blakiston, 1903:55.

3

Looking for Strabismus: The First Visit

"You Cannot Get Anywhere without the Full Data"

Strabismus and amblyopia affect approximately 5% of the population.[3,4] Amblyopia is the leading cause of unilateral visual loss in childhood.[1] The conditions most often requiring surgery in ophthalmology are cataracts and strabismus. Amblyopia was the leading cause of monocular visual loss in the 20 to 70+ age group, surpassing diabetic retinopathy, glaucoma, macular degeneration, and cataract in the Visual Acuity Impairment Study sponsored by the National Eye Institute of the United States.[8] Amblyopia can be eliminated largely by appropriate treatment in childhood.

What You Need to Know from the History

1. Does the eye go in, out, up, or down? This is an important question. If the parents say the eye goes in and this cannot be confirmed, it is probably a pseudostrabismus caused by broad epicanthal folds. This is especially likely if the parents say that the adducted eye "goes in too far" when the child looks to the side. If the parents say one eye turns outward, this is usually a true strabismus, especially if the patient also closes one eye in bright light. In order to elicit the deviation, the patient may need to be tested looking in the far distance or observed in the waiting room. Sometimes the deviation may only become manifest after half an hour of occlusion of one eye. If parents mention that one eye goes up and this is not immediately apparent, there may be dissociated vertical divergence, Brown's syndrome, etc.

2. Is it always the same eye that deviates? Which eye is it? If one eye is always preferred for fixation, the other eye is likely to become amblyopic.

3. Is the deviation constantly present, or are the eyes sometimes straight? This question is asked to assess whether fusion potential is likely to be present or not. If the eyes are sometimes straight, some fusion may be present.

4. Is there a family history of strabismus or preschool glasses? If the answer is yes, one should be suspicious of the presence of strabismus even if the eyes appear to be straight in a preliminary examination. In addition, it is important to tell parents with a positive family history about the dangers of acquired esotropia (see Chapter 9).

5. Was the baby the product of a full-term normal delivery after a normal pregnancy? What did the baby weigh at birth? If the baby was premature, was oxygen used? These questions are asked because cataracts and esotropia are common in the rubella syndrome. Strabismus and high myopia may be associated with retinopathy of prematurity in a premature baby who has received oxygen.

6. Is there a head tilt or face turn that the patient assumes regularly? This might suggest a paretic strabismus or nystagmus. Other causes rarely seen by an ophthalmologist include torticollis from congenital fibrosis of one sternocleidomastoid muscle or unilateral deafness.

7. Is the child healthy? Are there any developmental problems? How does the child's development compare with the others in the family? Any condition that affects the tone of the muscles in general also may affect the eye muscles. Delayed general development may be associated with delayed development of visual function as well.

8. When did the parents first notice the strabismus, even momentarily? The answer to this question indicates the probable level of development the child's vision and fusion had reached prior to being disrupted.

9. Has any treatment been given for this such as patching, glasses, or surgery? What was the result of this treatment? The answers to these questions may determine the prognosis.

The Examination

The examination should include a sensory and motor evaluation. If normal vision is present in each eye, a full motor evaluation is indicated at the first visit. An approximate motor evaluation only is indicated if there is defective visual acuity in one or both eyes because the tests will all have to be repeated once the cause of the visual deficit has been determined and, if possible, corrected. An accurate and thorough assessment of the sensory and motor aspects of strabismus is more meaningful when any amblyopia has been treated and when the full optical correction is worn.

Examination of very young children often yields suboptimal results because some objective tests may be difficult to perform and subjective tests are not possible in most children under $2\frac{1}{2}$ years of age.

All tests mentioned in this chapter are discussed in detail in Chapters 4 and 5. Before performing any tests, however, it is important to look carefully for a head tilt or face turn or whether the eyes appear to be straight in any position of gaze at near or distance, because testing occasionally may disrupt fusion temporarily (see also Chapter 18).

The tests used in the examination should provide an answer to the following questions:

1. Is a pseudostrabismus present? Apparent esotropia due to broad epicanthal folds is the classic example of pseudostrabismus. The child may appear to be esotropic in side gaze but not when looking straight ahead. In the primary position, the red reflex of the fundus of each eye viewed at approximately 1 m through a direct ophthalmoscope are equally bright, indicating bifoveal fixation (Brückner test[7]; see also Chapter 4). All the tests for latent or manifest strabismus will be negative. Less commonly, the eyes may appear to be convergent (esotropic) or divergent (exotropic) due to a positive or negative angle kappa. With a positive angle kappa, the corneal light reflex appears to be on the nasal side of center when the patient fixates a light straight ahead, giving the appearance of an exotropia (see Fig. 5–1B). This diagnosis is supported by negative tests for latent and manifest strabismus.

2. Is a manifest or latent strabismus present? A brief nondissociating cover-uncover test for distance and near fixation is used to see if there is a manifest strabismus (heterotropia) or if the eyes are aligned. The occluder should be placed over one eye for only a few seconds before removal. Then, after a pause of about 20 seconds, it should be placed over the other eye. If there is no heterotropia, fusion is likely to be present. The red reflexes of the fundus of each eye when viewed at 1 m through a direct ophthalmoscope are unequal in brightness in the presence of a strabismus, the brighter reflex belonging to the deviating eye (Brückner test[7]).

Sensory Evaluation

See Chapter 4.

VISUAL ACUITY

Visual acuity should be assessed at both distance and near. If the visual acuity is subnormal in one or both eyes, a pinhole should be used to see if a refractive error accounts for the reduction in visual acuity. In infants or children unable to perform reliable subjective tests, the fixation pattern of each eye is observed to detect poor vision, particularly in one eye compared with the other.

THE TITMUS STEREOTEST

The Titmus stereotest is useful for screening children 3 years or older. If some stereopsis is present, one can presume that some fusion is present. However, the absence of stereopsis does not exclude fusion.

THE LANG STEREOTEST

The Lang stereotest can sometimes be done on children as young as 2 years of age. It is used as evidence for the presence of stereopsis and therefore fusion.

Motor Evaluation

See Chapter 5.

PRISM COVER TEST

The prism cover test should be done for distance fixation in the primary position, in side gaze, and in up and down gaze. The deviation should also be measured at near.

SIMULTANEOUS PRISM INTRODUCTION AND COVER-UNCOVER TEST

The simultaneous prism introduction and cover-uncover test should be done with all patients who have an esotropia. This is essential in the assessment of a monofixation esotropia.

SUBJECTIVE VERIFICATION OF THE PRISM COVER MEASUREMENTS

This may be obtained by deliberate overcorrection of the deviation in order to elicit diplopia (see report on hemiretinal trigger mechanism[5] and Chapter 2).

OCULAR MOVEMENTS

Both ductions and versions should be tested, ductions to show the extent of movement of each eye individually, and versions to show the alignment of both eyes in the various gaze directions. Convergence also should be checked.

Refraction and Fundus Examination

EVERY PATIENT BEING EXAMINED FOR STRABISMUS NEEDS A REFRACTION

Refraction at the first visit is usually performed after the motor and sensory screening tests. Cyclopentolate (Cyclogyl 1%) eye drops are used routinely for refraction in a strabismic patient under the age of 9 years. In patients with very dark irides or patients whose pupils fail to dilate properly with cyclopentolate 1%, cyclopentolate 2% should be used. The patient is examined approximately 30 minutes after the instillation of the drops. Refraction may be repeated using atropine 1% eye drops three times a day for 3 days (prior to the next visit) if more than +5.0 D refractive error is detected with cyclopentolate. Atropine is only used if it is essential to detect and correct all the hypermetropia present, as in a case of esotropia with a possible accommodative element particularly with a high accommodative convergence to accommodation (AC:A) ratio. In children over 8 years or age or in adults, a manifest refraction should be performed to exclude the presence of a significant unilateral or bilateral refractive error. A significant hypermetropic refractive error that could affect the angle of an esotropia can be found in the presence of normal unaided visual acuity. It is important to make sure that a hypermetropic correction has not been discontinued or the hypermetropia undercorrected in an effort to reduce a consecutive exotropia after strabismus surgery for an esotropia.

The media and fundi are examined, directing particular attention to the disc and fovea in the deviating eye to exclude any organic disease that could disrupt fusion, causing a secondary strabismus. Cataract, retinoblastoma, or an organic lesion at the fovea (e.g., toxoplasmosis) may cause strabismus by interfering with fixation.

THE CYCLOPLEGIC COVER TEST AT NEAR

This is performed with full cycloplegia and is the final part of the examination. This test is particularly important in an infant suspected of having strabismus whose examination has hitherto been normal. An interesting object (e.g., a small toy) should be held directly in front of the child while the child's head is straight. Once the child is fixing the toy, it is brought closer to the child's eyes. Although the cycloplegic agent prevents the child from accommodating, the effort to see will precipitate an esotropia if there is any tendency toward strabismus. This will not happen in a patient who has no strabismus tendency. It is therefore a useful test in those patients in whom the parents report that an esotropia is sometimes present but that has not been confirmed prior to the cycloplegia.

The Uncooperative Child

Even though a child may appear to be totally uncooperative—yelling, shrieking, kicking, and resisting all efforts to examine the eyes—it is frequently possible to obtain much useful information. Patients who have traveled a long way for the visit may be tired and fretful and yet unable to come again. In this scenerio, the following tips may help.

1.   Allow the child to return to the waiting room to play with toys and then observe the child's behaviour, head position, and eye alignment from a distance.

2.   Suggest that the parents give the child something to eat and drink and then observe the child during this time.

3.   Sometimes an older sibling may assist by doing the tests initially while the patient watches. The older sibling also may help administer the tests. The Lang stereotest is often helpful here.

4.   Hirschberg[2] and Brückner tests[7] (undilated pupils) are performed before any cycloplegic drops are instilled. The tests can be done when the child is standing, sitting on someone's lap, or sitting alone, provided the child's attention is momentarily focused on the light from the ophthalmoscope. It is an advantage, but not essential, to dim the room's illumination. Both eyes are simultaneously illuminated by the light from a direct ophthalmoscope, while the examiner focuses the ophthalmoscope from about 1 m away. The position of the corneal light reflex in each eye and the brightness of the fundal red reflex in each undilated pupil are compared. Results are: (1) The position of the light reflexes will be asymmetrical if a strabismus is present (Hirschberg's test[2]); and (2) the brightness of the red reflex in the undilated pupils will be different if strabismus is present, the brighter red reflex belonging to the eye with a manifest strabismus (Brückner test[7]) (see Fig. 4–5).

The above techniques, combined with the detailed history, should allow a gross evaluation of eye alignment.

5.   Cycloplegic evaluation: At this stage a cycloplegic evaluation is necessary, and the use of cycloplegic drops often destroys any hope of further cooperation. If an orthoptist, nurse, or parent can put in the cycloplegic drops while the ophthalmologist is busy elsewhere, the child may be less uncooperative with the ophthalmologist. The child might not associate the ophthalmologist with the drops. The child has time to recover from the upset of the drops before the next stage of the investigation. The rest of the examination is forced on the child if necessary. First the child is examined for strabismus at near with a squeaky toy or flashing light as a fixation target. This may precipitate a previously undetected strabismus. Then the child is refracted.

6. Cycloplegic refraction and fundus examination: This is best forced on the child by one parent sitting in the examination chair holding the child. The parent hugs the child, effectively restraining the arms and hands. The child's kicking feet are restrained by being gripped between the parent's legs. An assistant holds the patient's eyelids open while restraining the child's head against the parent's chest. Loose lenses are used for the enforced refraction. The fundus examination is usually confined to a quick glance at the fovea and disc, usually with an indirect ophthalmoscope with a powerful plus lens (28), which gives a large field with small magnification. Disc pathology such as hypoplasia can easily be missed by this type of examination but gross pathology that could cause strabismus by preventing fixation such as a retinoblastoma at the posterior pole or a central choroidal scar should be detectable.

This part of the examination often leaves patient, parents, and doctor exhausted, but usually the essential information has been obtained.

7. For children who live nearby, a different approach may be taken in this situation because, presumably, repeat visits can easily be arranged within a few days. This allows the patient to get used to the office and personnel. The cycloplegic refraction and fundus examination can be done at a subsequent visit by the parents instilling atropine 1% eye ointment three times to both eyes the day prior to the next visit.

Action at the End of the First Visit

Treatment of Amblyopia

If amblyopia is present, treatment should begin immediately and detailed instructions should be given at the end of the first visit according to the principles outlined in Chapter 7 (Amblyopia). The presence of amblyopia is determined by the detection of a visual acuity defect that does not have an optical or organic cause and does not improve with pinhole. In the case of a preverbal child, it is detected by the child's inability to fix properly with one eye.

The Prescription of Glasses if a Significant Refractive Error Is Present

The prescription of glasses depends on the amount of refractive error found, with cycloplegia, and the type of strabismus present. The full optical correction is given if a refractive error is present that could affect the treatment of the strabismus or the amblyopia.

What Is the Full Optical Correction?

Empirically, cyclopentolate or atropine abolishes the ciliary tone, which accounts for up to 1 diopter of plus refraction in hypermetropes. The principle is to prescribe the maximum plus the patient will accept without degrading the visual acuity. Generally this equals the full cyclopentolate or atropine refraction up to the age of 2 years because the patient's environment is close at hand and subjective tests are not possible. In older hypermetropic children, 0.50 diopter sphere (DS) should be subtracted when using cyclopentolate 1% and 1.0 DS when using cyclopentolate 2% or atropine. In some cases of accommodative strabismus there may be an indication to try to give the maximum plus because an extra 0.50 DS could make some difference to the strabismus.

Example: A 3-year-old with +2.0 DS under cyclopentolate 1% has an acquired esotropia of 20 prism diopters, no amblyopia, and there is a chance of fusion. Plus 2.0 DS should be given, and if the vision is blurry, cyclopentolate 1% should be used in the morning for a week. If the child is 4 years of age or older, it is important to always check subjectively that the maximum plus correction does not interfere with optimal visual acuity.

Guidelines Regarding the Prescription of Plus Lenses

CONGENITAL ESOTROPIA

Usually there is 50 prism diopters or more of esotropia. No glasses should be prescribed preoperatively if the hypermetropia is under +3.0 DS. However, glasses may be needed postoperatively.

If there is +3.0 DS or more of hypermetropia, glasses should be tried before operating. This may be a good reason to delay surgery. For example, if the child is 9 months old, the clinician should wait until the child is 18 months old to evaluate the effect of glasses before operating.

In the event of a postoperative recurrence of the esotropia or under correction of an esotropia, any plus refractive error present should be corrected by glasses. As an example, the deviation is less than 10 prism diopters postoperatively but 3 months or so later 20 prism diopters of esotropia recurs. Cycloplegic refraction reveals +1.0 hypermetropia. Glasses with +1.0 DS should be prescribed to try to reduce the angle to 10 prism diopters again.

ACQUIRED ESOTROPIA

If there is fusion potential, any refractive error over +1.0 DS should be corrected. If a manifest deviation persists with glasses and there is no amblyopia, surgery should not be delayed (refer to Chapter 9, Acquired Esotropia). This management differs from that of congenital esotropia.

HIGH AC/A RATIO

Any uncorrected (hypermetropic) refractive error will trigger convergence, therefore, even +0.50, should be fully corrected for distance. The prescription of bifocals also may be necessary (see Chapter 9, Acquired Esotropia).

HYPERMETROPIA WITH "STRAIGHT" EYES

Should glasses be prescribed if the eyes are straight and if the refraction shows +2.0 to +4.0 for each eye? If there is no anisometropia, if there is no strabismus (not even at near with cycloplegia), if there is no family history of strabismus or amblyopia, and if the patient can return for a follow up visit within 6 months, glasses need not be prescribed.

The parents should be informed about the possibility of accommodative esotropia and the need for urgent care should the strabismus occur (see Chapter 9, Acquired Esotropia). The child should be seen every 6 months until subjective evaluation is possible, usually by the age of 4 years, and the child is able to complain of diplopia if strabismus occurs.

If an error of more than +4.0 DS is detected in a patient without strabismus, glasses should be prescribed for visual comfort provided corrected vision is normal. Ideally, the hypermetropia should be undercorrected. Bilateral amblyopia has been reported in patients with a high plus error in both eyes that was not corrected during visual immaturity.[6,9]

SHOULD THE REFRACTIVE ERROR OF THE NONFIXING EYE OF A PATIENT
WITHOUT FUSION POTENTIAL BE CORRECTED?

The Visually Immature Patient. If the patient is amblyopic, it may be necessary to prescribe glasses to correct the refractive error of the deviating eye prior to treating the amblyopia, even if the dominant eye is emmetropic. Amblyopia responds better to occlusion if the refractive error is corrected, particularly if there is hypermetropia in excess of 4.00 DS or astigmatism.

The Visually Mature Patient. If there is no refractive error in the fixing eye there is no point in prescribing glasses for the nonfixing eye because the fovea of this eye will be suppressed when both eyes are open. The deviation of the nonfixing eye will be affected only by uncorrected errors in the dominant fixing eye. This is because accommodation occurs equally in each eye and only the amount of accommodation needed to give a clear image in the fixing eye will be exerted.

ASTIGMATISM SHOULD ALWAYS BE FULLY CORRECTED

Cross-cylinder verification is rarely reliable in patients under the age of 10 years. A keratometer is a very accurate method of assessing the amount and axis of astigmatism because astigmatism is commonly corneal.

A FULL CORRECTION OF MYOPIA IS IMPORTANT IN INTERMITTENT EXOTROPIA

This encourages accommodation, and therefore convergence, which might establish control of the exotropia.

Subsequent Visits

Once the full optical correction is in place and the amblyopia cured, the patient should return for a full sensory and motor assessment so that all the information can be gathered about the strabismus and the goal of treatment established.

Action if a Strabismus Is Present

If the patient has no significant amblyopia or refractive error, further, more detailed tests to evaluate the sensory and motor characteristics of the strabismus can be undertaken at the initial visit, preferably before instilling a cycloplegic agent, which may disrupt the tests. If amblyopia or a significant refractive error is present, the patient should return for further assessment when these have been treated. If a manifest or latent strabismus is then present, tests to evaluate in greater detail the sensory and motor characteristics of the strabismus may be indicated.

Prognosis and Treatment

The prognosis for the strabismus can be determined by studying the data provided by the history and the sensory and the motor evaluation performed when the patient is wearing the full optical correction of the refractive error and after the treatment of any amblyopia has been completed. The prognosis differs for the various types of strabismus and is discussed in detail in the appropriate chapter. In the congenital strabismus syndrome, the best prognosis is for a monofixation syndrome with peripheral fusion if the child is under the age of 2 years with good vision in each eye when first seen. In acquired esotropia, the prognosis for a complete cure with central fusion depends on the age at onset of the deviation and the duration of the constant strabismus prior to treatment. The older the child at the onset of the strabismus, the better the prognosis, and the shorter the duration, the better the prognosis. It is important to establish the goal in treatment as soon as possible.

Is the Goal to Obtain Fusion or Just to Improve the Appearance?

The history, as well as the sensory and motor assessments, must be closely analyzed to establish the logical goal to which all efforts of treatment must be directed. This important decision will influence the correction of refractive errors, treatment of amblyopia, type and time of surgery, and preoperative and postoperative management of the case.

Discussion with Parents

Once strabismus has been diagnosed parents wonder what has gone wrong.

Questions Frequently Asked by the Parents

"Are the muscles too weak?" "What has caused the strabismus?" The muscles usually look normal macroscopically and microscopically and are usually attached to the eye in the normal place. A positive family history of strabismus may indicate a genetic or hereditary influence. The same type of strabismus is not necessarily inherited; for example, the parent may have had a congenital esotropia and the child an intermittent exotropia or Duane's retraction syndrome. Nothing further is known.

"Will exercises help?" Usually not. Exercises can only help in special cases, for example, cooperative patients over about 8 years of age who already have some ability to use their eyes together.

"Will this affect my child's reading ability?" No. There is no greater incidence of children with reading problems among those who have strabismus than among those who do not (American Academy of Ophthalmology Policy Statement 1984 and Canadian Ophthalmological Society Policy Statement 1987).

"Will this be a problem for my child when playing sports?" No. If there is amblyopia or a lack of fusion and stereopsis because of the strabismus, it may influence the patient's ability in ball games. However, it is not a reason to give up because some do not seem to find it a hindrance.

Commitment and Compliance

The importance of compliance with the management of strabismus and amblyopia should be stressed to the parents with children under the age of 8 years. This management, particularly where occlusion is necessary, can be stressful and frustrating for all the family. However, inadequate treatment of amblyopia may result in a legally blind eye, which could have been prevented by occlusion therapy.

References

1. Ehrlich, M.I., Reinecke, R.D., Simons, K.: Preschool vision screening for amblyopia and strabismus. Programs, methods, guidelines 1983. Surv Ophthalmol 28:145–163, 1983.
2. Hirschberg, J.: Über die Messung des Schielgrades und die Dosierung der Schieloperation. Zentralbl Prakt Augenheilkd 8:325, 1885.
3. Nelson, L.B.: Paediatric Ophthalmology. Philadelphia: WB Saunders, 1984:110.
4. Parks, M.M.: Strabismus: An overview. In: Spaeth, G.L., ed. Modern Concepts of Eye Care for Children. New Jersey: Slack, 1986:51.
5. Pratt-Johnson, J.A., Tillson, G., Pop, A.: Suppression in strabismus and the hemiretinal trigger mechanism. Arch Ophthalmol 101:218, 1983.
6. Schoenleber, D.B., Crouch, E.R.: Bilateral hypermetropia and amblyopia. J Pediatr Ophthalmol Strabismus 24:75, 1987.
7. Tongue, A.C., Cibis, C.W.: Brückner test. Ophthalmology 88:1041–1044, 1981.
8. The Visual Acuity Impairment Study (VAIS), sponsored by the National Eye Institute. In: Flynn, J.T.: Amblyopia revisited: 17th Annual Frank Costenbader Lecture. J Pediatr Ophthalmol 28:183–201, 1991.
9. Werner, D.B., Scott, W.E.: Amblyopia case reports—Bilateral hypermetropic ametropic amblyopia. J Pediatr Ophthalmol 22:203–205, 1985.

4

Sensory Evaluation of Strabismus

"You Cannot Get Anywhere Without the Full Data"

This chapter discusses the many tests used to evaluate the sensory aspects of strabismus. Although for convenience sensory and motor evaluations are addressed in separate chapters, the consideration of both evaluations together is essential in establishing the prognosis and plan of management for all types of strabismus. The tests in general use are described in some detail. These tests are then just noted, as appropriate in the various chapters, without further description. The cover test can be used for both sensory and motor assessment, as can the major amblyoscope and Brückner test, but they are described in detail only in this chapter.

Observation of the Patient

Before any tests are attempted, the patient should be observed for the presence of any obvious strabismus, nystagmus, or unusual head tilt or face turn. A compensatory head position may be used to avoid diplopia (e.g., superior oblique palsy) or to improve visual acuity (motor nystagmus). It is advisable to screen for a manifest deviation by doing a quick cover test for near and distance, covering each eye in turn for just a few seconds so that the dissociation of the eyes is minimal. This helps in assessing the responses obtained on sensory testing. The occlusion of each eye during most visual acuity tests may temporarily disrupt fusion; therefore, it is suggested that, in the absence of a manifest deviation, stereopsis be assessed before visual acuity.

The Cover Test

The cover test for near and distance fixation is the most important part of any examination for strabismus or amblyopia. It conveys both sensory and motor information. It can be done with patients of all ages and requires only the minimum of cooperation from a patient. Without a cover test, there is no check on the patient's responses, and many tests need to be done in conjunction with a cover test in order to interpret the results. The cover test is often combined with prisms to measure the deviation.

The term *cover test* refers to the whole test. The cover test has been subdivided into parts, which are variously described as the cover-uncover, cross-cover, and alternate cover test, but these terms may be confusing because they are used differently in the literature.

In this book the following terms are used throughout:

1. Cover test: the test in general.

2. Cover-uncover test: This is characterized by having an interval between removing the cover from one eye and placing it over the other.

3. Cross-cover test: This is characterized by having no interval between removing the cover from one eye and placing it over the other eye.

The cover test is used to detect the presence of a manifest deviation (heterotropia) or a latent deviation (heterophoria) at the testing distance and in the required direction of gaze. The difference between a manifest deviation and a latent deviation is that the latent deviation is controlled by the patient's fusion ability. The only equipment needed for the cover test is a fixation target and an occluder such as an opaque card or paddle.

All cover tests should be done with the patient wearing the appropriate optical correction for any refractive error that may be present and then repeated without glasses, fixing a target straight ahead at distance and near. It also may be necessary to repeat the cover test with the patient fixing a target in different gaze positions if there is an incomitant deviation. The first and most important thing to be watching for with a cover test is a manifest deviation because its presence can adversely affect the patient's vision and fusion ability. A latent deviation (heterophoria) may cause ocular discomfort in many cases, however, it may be symptomless and not require treatment.

Fixation Targets

When doing a cover test, it is fundamentally essential to hold the patient's attention with a fixation target at the required distance. The choice of target is dictated by the patient's age and visual acuity. It is necessary to be specific, and it is not enough to say "find something to look at at the end of the room." Whenever possible, a target should be chosen that will not only keep the patient's interest but will also control the patient's accommodation. A letter consistent with the patient's visual acuity in the eye with the worst vision at near and distance is the best choice. Children need small detailed toys at near and either animated toys or pictures for distance fixation. Figure 4–1 shows the variety of toys that must be used to keep a child's attention during the cover test. Figures 4–6A,C,D show Worth Lights, which can also be used as a fixation target in addition to their primary use. Figure 4–6B shows an amusing picture that flashes on and off to attract fixation for distance. A child's attention span is short, necessitating frequent changes of the

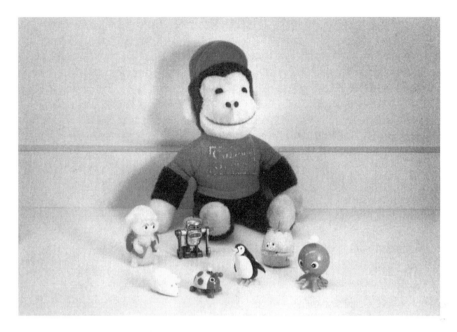

Figure 4–1. Fixation targets for a child.

target resulting in the aphorism, "One toy, one look; many toys, many looks." The cover test should be done first for distance fixation, then for near with patients over the age of about 4 years. Before that, it is better to establish a rapport by starting with a cover test for near fixation using "fun" fixation targets. With very shy children and with infants, a cover test for near fixation may be all that is possible. Distance fixation is the most difficult with preliterate children; having someone at the end of the room waving attractive toys is helpful in maintaining a child's attention. A light may be most effective with infants, especially if it is made to flash on and off. It is also useful when the influence of accommodation on the control of the deviation needs to be minimized.

Occluder

The use of an opaque card or paddle is preferable to ensure that an eye is properly occluded. Infants and young children often look at the occluder or are frightened by it; in that case, the examiner's hand with the fingers closely pressed together may be used instead. It is also important not to touch the child in this situation because many children are upset by having their head or face touched.

   Caution: Because the cover test appears to be such a simple test to do, the temptation is to try to take in too much information at the same time.

Cover-Uncover Test to Detect a Manifest Deviation (Heterotropia)

Once the patient is fixing the required target, one of the patient's eyes is occluded and the uncovered eye observed as the cover is placed over its fellow eye. If there is no movement of the uncovered eye to take up fixation, it was already fixing the target foveally. Any movement of the uncovered eye to take up fixation indicates a manifest deviation of that eye. The eye has had to move in order to take up fixation with its fovea. This shows that it was not aligned with the target. The occluder should be removed and the patient again instructed to fix the target. The test is repeated with the previously uncovered eye now being covered (Fig. 4–2A,B). It is important to remember to watch only the uncovered eye as the cover is being placed in front of the other eye. It is also important to have both the patient's eyes uncovered briefly before checking the second eye. If there is a manifest deviation, the usually fixing eye will always deviate when the patient is made to fix with the deviating eye and will be seen to move when the cover is removed (Hering's law). If neither eye has to move to take up fixation, then the patient has bifoveal fixation in the direction of gaze and at the distance the test was done. A latent deviation (heterophoria) should then be sought.

Cover-Uncover Test to Detect a Latent Deviation

If only a latent strabismus (heterophoria) is present, the eyes will be kept straight by fusion (Fig. 4–2C). The same test is repeated as described to detect a manifest deviation, except that attention is now directed to the eye that is covered. Once the patient is steadily fixing the required target with one eye occluded, the clinician should watch the eye behind the cover to see if it makes a movement to resume fixation as the cover is removed. It is also useful to note how quickly this recovery takes place because this shows how well the patient can control the latent deviation. The latent deviation will be revealed with either eye covered (Fig. 4–2D).

Cross-Cover Test (Alternate Cover Test)

In the cross-cover test the occluder is transferred from one eye to the other, this time without any interval. The examiner watches the eye that was behind the occluder as the occluder is being transferred to the other eye. The longer the occluder is left over one eye before transferring it without an interval to the other eye, the more disruptive it is to fusion, which helps reveal the full extent of any strabismus. Repeating the test is more dissociative to fusion than doing the test once and may then bring out a very well controlled latent deviation. This test shows both the latent deviation in the absence of any manifest strabismus, as well as the combined manifest and latent features of a strabismus if both features are present.

The Best Combination of the Cover Test

1. The cover-uncover test to detect a manifest strabismus is followed by the cross-cover test to detect any latent strabismus if none has been revealed by the cover-uncover test.

2. The prism cross-cover test is then used to measure the whole deviation (Fig. 4–2E).

Monofixation Syndrome and the Cover Test

There may be a combination of a small manifest deviation and an underlying larger latent deviation. This will be detected most easily by first looking for a

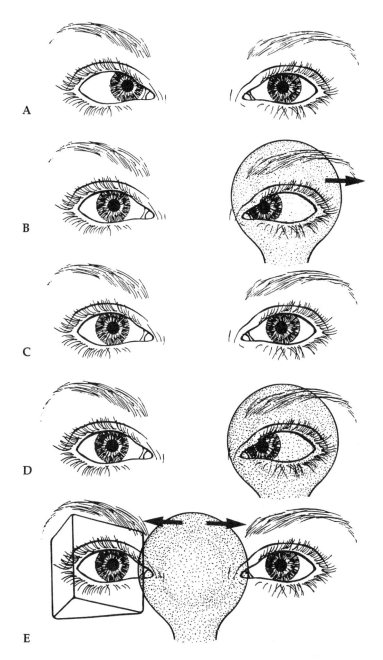

Figure 4–2. Cover-uncover test. (*A*) Right esotropia. (*B*) Cover-uncover test confirms a manifest right esotropia (see text). Arrow indicates movement of opaque occluder on and off fixing eye while observing the other eye for manifest strabismus (cover/uncover). (*C*) A different patient with a latent deviation. Eyes held straight by fusion. (*D*) Cover-uncover test detects the latent deviation (esophoria), the eye behind the occluder becoming es-otropic with the disruption of fusion. (*E*) Appropriate base out prism neutralizes the es-odeviation so there is no movement of either eye with alternate occlusion. Arrows indicate movement of opaque occluder from one eye to the other (cross-cover test).

manifest deviation and then for a latent deviation, as already described. The recovery will occur from the latent deviation to the small manifest deviation originally detected. This condition is usually managed like a latent deviation, but it is necessary to be aware of the easily missed manifest deviation because it will explain many of the sensory deficits found on more detailed testing and may avoid unnecessary surgery.

Major Amblyoscope: Synoptophore and Troposcope

Because the major amblyoscope can be used for both sensory and motor evaluation, it is discussed in detail here and then just listed under sensory and motor tests without additional comments. There are many versions of the major amblyoscope. The most widely used are the Clement Clarke synoptophore (Fig. 4–3) and the troposcope. The troposcope is no longer manufactured but is still used in many orthoptic clinics. These devices make use of Hirschberg's method combined with a cover test to measure the deviation. The test presents known targets to each eye.

The targets are pairs of slides that are placed in slide holders and viewed through an internally lighted optical system (Fig. 4–4). Each eye sees one of the pair of slides. The test uses slides that hold a child's interest. It is a great favorite of children and may be the best way of obtaining detailed measurements of a complex strabismus in a child. It can generally be used in children starting at 3 or 4 years of age. This is a particularly useful tool in the hands of an experienced orthoptist because, in addition to measuring the angle of deviation, it can be used to assess retinal correspondence and the potential for fusion and stereopsis. This

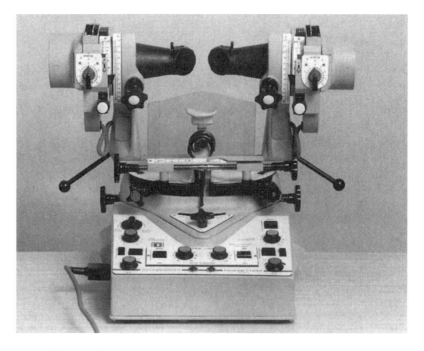

Figure 4–3.   Clement Clarke synoptophore.

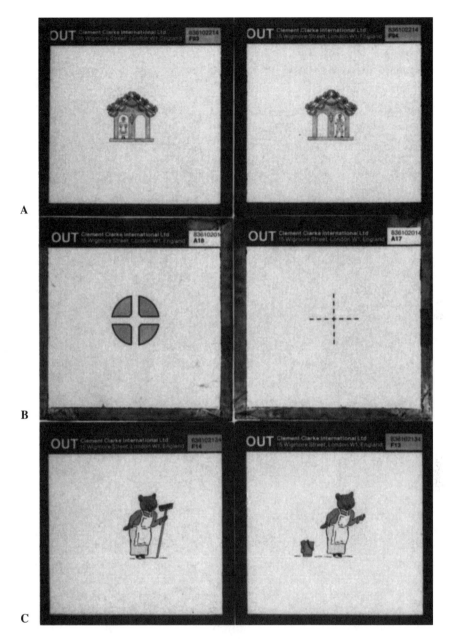

Figure 4–4. Slides for synoptophore (Clement Clarke). (*A*) Fusion slides with central control: man in one archway and woman in the other act as controls. (*B*) Simultaneous perception slides for measuring torsion. (*C*) Fusion slides with peripheral control: broom and bucket act as controls.

information is needed to give a prognosis for the functional outcome in patients. Worth divided binocular vision into three parts. Over the years this subdivision of binocular vision has become modified and called *grades of fusion*. However, this term is misleading and has contributed to the unfortunate neglect of this very useful piece of equipment. Grade I became defined as the ability to see superimposed two dissimilar slides. This is an abnormal situation in everyday life and should not be considered as fusion. The brain requires similar images from each eye in order to be able to fuse them. Grade II was defined as the ability to superimpose similar slides and to keep them superimposed through a range of convergence and divergence. This is the most important aspect of binocular function because it is what keeps the eyes aligned in everyday life and is real fusion. This is what is referred to throughout this book as fusion. Grade III refers to stereopsis. To avoid confusion, it is preferable to refer to fusion and to stereopsis without subdivisions by grades.

Measuring the Deviation with a Major Amblyoscope

The deviation may be measured objectively and subjectively. Simultaneous perception slides are used, such as the circle and the plus sign (Fig. 4–4B) or the dog and the dog house. The choice of slides is influenced by the patient's age and visual acuity. To measure the deviation objectively, the angle between the slide carriers is adjusted by the examiner until the corneal reflections appear symmetrical (Hirschberg's test). The angle of presentation of the slides can be read from scales giving the angle of the deviation. The patient is instructed to keep looking at the targets, and the illumination in front of one eye is switched off briefly while the other eye is observed for any movement to take up fixation (cover test) on the target that is still illuminated. The angle of the slide carriers is adjusted until there is no movement and the angle is read off the scales. To measure the angle of deviation subjectively, the patient adjusts the angle between the slide carriers until the images appear to be superimposed. The angle should then be checked objectively. If the objective and subjective angles are the same, this indicates normal retinal correspondence. If the angles are different, it indicates abnormal retinal correspondence and the need for further investigation of retinal correspondence. It is important however to rule out just a variable angle of deviation causing a difference between the two measurements.

The synoptophore versions of this test can be used to measure the deviation in the nine cardinal positions of gaze with either eye fixing with or without the presence of fusion and can measure any or all of the possible components of a deviation, that is, horizontal, vertical, and torsional. It can therefore also be used to assess the role of torsion as a barrier to the patient regaining fusion and thus aid in the planning of surgery to correct the deviation. This is an advantage over the prism cover test. The testing conditions are controlled and therefore repeatable. The theoretical testing distance is infinity, but in many cases there is some so-called machine convergence, which tends to give a relatively more esotropic measurement of the horizontal deviation.

Angle Kappa and the Major Amblyoscope

Angle kappa can be measured with the major amblyoscope and a special slide with zero as the center of the slide and targets to either side of zero at 1° intervals. The corneal reflection in the eye being checked is observed as the patient looks at each target in turn on the appropriate side of zero until the corneal reflection appears central. The angle kappa may be measured in a similar fashion using prisms and a flash light. Angle kappa may influence any measurements based on corneal reflections.

Assessing Fusion with the Major Amblyoscope

Slides designed to help assess fusion are similar in design in all respects except for a control that can be seen only by one eye. This is essential to be able to distinguish between fusion, when both eyes are used, and suppression when only one eye is used. Depending on whether the patient sees only one or both controls simultaneously, suppression or fusion is revealed (Fig. 4–4A,C). The presence of both controls when the patient has superimposed the slides shows fusion.

Example: A house with two arched doorways appears on both slides of a pair but on one slide there is a man in one archway and on the other slide there is a woman in an archway (the man and the woman are the controls). When the slides are correctly fused, the patient sees a house with a man in one archway and a woman in the other. The angle between the slide carriers can then be increased or reduced until the patient is no longer able to see one image with both controls. This gives a measurement of the patient's fusional amplitude. The choice of slides is influenced again by the patient's age and visual acuity. Slides are available that can assess foveal or peripheral fusion. The major amblyoscope is a particularly useful tool in the hands of an experienced orthoptist because it can be used to assess the potential for fusion and stereopsis in down gaze as well as straight ahead. It can also isolate which components of a deviation need to be corrected by surgery before a patient can regain fusion in everyday seeing conditions. For example, a patient may have a combination of a vertical strabismus and an exodeviation. Correction of only the vertical deviation may be sufficient for stable fusion. In another example, a patient with a marked excyclotorsion following a bilateral superior oblique palsy may be able to maintain comfortable fusion with correction of the vertical or horizontal elements alone. In some cases, correction of the excyclotorsion in addition is critical for stable fusion, especially on down gaze. Prisms cannot measure or neutralize excyclotorsion, making the major amblyoscope essential for this diagnosis. The major amblyoscope also can help make the differential diagnosis between central fusion disruption and other causes of diplopia in a patient. This information is needed to give a prognosis for the functional outcome of strabismus therapy, especially when surgery is being planned.

The patient's responses may be checked objectively by the examiner observing the corneal reflections. They should appear symmetrical (Hirschberg). The patient is instructed to keep looking at the targets, and the illumination in front of one eye is switched off briefly while the other eye is observed for any movement to take up fixation (cover test) on the target that is still illuminated. There should be none.

Assessing Stereopsis with the Major Amblyoscope

It is a test for potential stereopsis, that is, evidence that if the patient's eyes were correctly aligned, the patient would appreciate stereopsis. It can therefore be used to detect the potential for stereopsis in patients whose angle of deviation is so large that it prevents assessment with any of the other tests mentioned in this chapter. These other tests cannot be used unless the deviation is neutralized by prisms, which is often impractical. Specially designed slides for use in an amblyoscope can be presented at an angle that is the same as that of the strabismus. The images therefore fall on the retinas of each eye as they would if the eyes were correctly aligned. The most often used slides do not have a stereoacuity provided by the manufacturer. Random dot slides for use with the synoptophore were designed by Braddick and give a stereoacuity from 720 to 90 seconds of arc. As with all random dot stereotests, it may take a while for the patient to detect the effect, and approximately a minute should be allowed before deciding that the patient cannot appreciate stereopsis with that particular slide.

The major amblyoscope also can be used to measure fusional amplitudes and stereoacuity in patients without a strabismus. The angle between the tubes of the amblyoscope would be 0°.

Assessing Retinal Correspondence with the Major Amblyoscope

The synoptophore version of the major amblyoscope also may be used to assess retinal correspondence by inducing an afterimage in each eye. It has special slides (Clement Clarke S3 and S4) and a switch that allows the normal illumination to be increased enough to give an afterimage. The slides are black except for a central clear bar with a small red fixation target at the center. One bar is vertical (slide S3) and the other horizontal (slide S4). The test is performed in the same way as the Bielschowsky afterimage test as described later in this chapter, and the responses are interpreted similarly.

The Brückner Test

The Brückner test is administered with the patient's pupils undilated (Fig. 4–5). The red reflexes are observed through a direct ophthalmoscope focused for the test distance with the bright light shone simultaneously into both the patient's eyes from about 1 m away. The brightness of the red reflex in each eye is compared. If the illumination of the red reflex is brighter in one eye than the other, strabismus is likely to be present in the eye with the brightest reflex (Fig. 4–5B). A young child is best seated on the parent's lap and encouraged to look at the light. This test is particularly useful in children who will not tolerate a cover test and hate having one eye covered. It also can be performed when the child is looking in different gaze positions. This makes it particularly useful if trying to assess why an uncooperative child has an unusual head position. Is it because the eyes are better aligned in one particular direction of gaze? Any attempt to hold the head straight so that the eye gaze position can be assessed will upset the child and prevent any useful conclusions.

Visual Acuity

Ideally, visual acuity should be tested for near and distance both uniocularly and binocularly with a Snellen's test type and the patient wearing the appropriate correction of any refractive error.

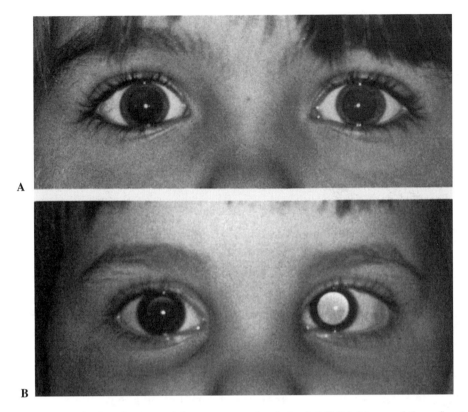

Figure 4–5. The Brückner test (photoscreener simulation). (*A*) Brightness of the reflex in each eye is equal because eyes are straight. (*B*) Left esotropia: Reflex is brighter in left eye. (Photos courtesy Dr. Ross Kennedy.)

Tests of Visual Acuity

TESTS BASED ON SNELLEN'S PRINCIPLES

If the patient knows the alphabet, the ordinary Snellen chart should be used; otherwise, a matching test such as the HVOT test can be used. The HVOT test can be used with children as young as 2 ½ years of age and certainly at 3 years in most cases. If this test is not available, the Snellen illiterate E test can be used, but this is more difficult for children under 5 years of age because of laterality problems. Many children find the stylized drawings used to assess visual acuity on most picture charts difficult to identify even when they are large enough for them to see. They have to be coached first, and by the time they are ready to do the test, they are also capable of doing the HVOT test, which is more closely aligned with Snellen letter charts.

Recording Visual Acuity

There are different methods of recording the visual acuity (Table 4–1). It is useful to be able to understand any of them and to convert from one to another in the context of global ophthalmology.

Table 4–1. Examples of Some of the Ways that Visual Acuity Can Be Recorded

Meters	Feet	Decimal	Percentage	Minutes of arc
6/120	20/400	0.05	3	20.0
6/60	20/200	0.10	20	10.0
6/45	20/150	0.133	31	7.5
6/36	20/120	0.17	41	6.0
6/30	20/100	0.2	49	5.0
6/24	20/80	0.25	58	4.0
6/18	20/60	0.33	70	3.0
6/15	20/50	0.4	76	2.5
6/12	20/40	0.5	84	2.0
6/9	20/30	0.67	91	1.5
6/7.5	20/25	0.8	96	1.25
6/6	20/20	1.0	100	1.00
6/4.5	20/15	1.33	104	0.75
6/3	20/10	2.0	109	0.5

Visual acuity should be assessed at 33 cm. It is important to do this before instilling cyclopentolate. Near vision measurement is essential data in assessing patients with nystagmus, cataract, asthenopic symptoms at near, or with strabismus with an accommodative element.

TELLER ACUITY CARDS

An estimation of visual acuity may be obtained by using the Teller acuity cards, which have vertical gratings on them.[1,3] These cards are particularly useful in comparing the vision in one eye with the fellow eye and can be used in infants and in all patients who cannot cooperate with other tests of visual acuity. Teller visual acuity and Snellen acuity do not always correlate, an under- or overestimation occurring in certain conditions.

THE FIXATION ABILITY OF EACH EYE

Fixation is a useful reliable way of determining the presence or absence of amblyopia, in the presence of strabismus. Spontaneous alternate fixation is consistent with equal vision, holding fixation through a blink approximately 6/12 vision and holding fixation but not through a blink about 6/21. If there is no strabismus but amblyopia is suspected, a strabismus can be artificially created by holding a 10-prism diopter prism vertically in front of one eye and the fixation pattern of each eye studied as described above. Fixation may become "wandering" or even steadily eccentric in cases of dense amblyopia (see Fig. 7–1). A visuscope or an ophthalmoscope incorporating a fixation graticule should be used to check for either of these conditions (see also Chapter 7, Amblyopia).

Stereopsis

Tests for stereopsis are useful screening tests for fusion. If stereopsis is present, fusion of some degree is always present. The converse does not hold true because peripheral fusion with amplitudes may be present without stereopsis.

Tests for Stereopsis

Most tests for stereopsis are performed for near fixation; whenever possible, however, stereopsis should be tested for distance fixation as well. Tests may be possible for only one distance because of the type of strabismus present, but demonstrated stereopsis at one distance indicates the possibility of establishing stereopsis at the other distance with appropriate treatment. Responses should be recorded as a score in seconds of arc and a note made of the test used.

Stereopsis Tests for Use at Near

TITMUS STEREOTEST

The Titmus stereotest is probably the most widely used of the tests for stereopsis. It is a vectograph and uses Polaroid dissociation and glasses. The design involves representations of a house fly, animals, and circles. The test measures stereopsis from 3000 seconds (house fly) to 40 seconds of arc (circles) if held at 16 inches or at 40 cm from the patient.

Caution: There is often a comprehension problem with children so that the initial response may be worse than might be anticipated on the basis of other tests; however, most 4-year-olds without strabismus and amblyopia will demonstrate 40 seconds of arc stereopsis with a little encouragement. If the response is consistently below this, the patient may have a monofixation syndrome, and further tests of binocular function are needed. This test is widely used in screening tests, and children soon realize what response is being sought and may fake it. This is particularly true with larger disparities, where monocular clues can help the patient who has no stereopsis guess the correct response. If the test is occasionally presented first upside down when the targets appear recessed instead of coming up out of the picture as the patient is expecting, the reliability of the patient's responses can be checked. A response of 100 seconds or worse suggests peripheral fusion and a monofixation syndrome at best.

TNO RANDOM DOT STEREOTEST

This test is an anaglyph, which put simply means that the dissociation is by color instead of Polaroid filters. The patient wears complimentary red and green glasses to see the images, which are made of computer-generated random dots, and to be able to appreciate the stereopsis. The first three plates are simple test plates; the largest disparity is 1900 seconds of arc. The other plates have disparity ranges from 480 seconds to 15 seconds of arc. There are no monocular clues, so this is an advantage over the Titmus test, but random dot stereotests seem to be more difficult for patients of all ages, not just children. The reason for this difference is not clear. Random dot tests can probably be compared only with other random dots, even though all stereotests are quantified in the same way (seconds of arc of disparity). Patients with any defect of binocular function generally cannot do this test.

LANG STEREOTESTS

There are two versions of this random dot test. Each test consists of a card that is approximately the size of the average post card. The random dots are incorporated in a panagraph and dissociation of the eyes is by cylindrical lenses

laminated onto the surface of the card. This test has the great advantage of not requiring the patient to wear glasses so it can be used with children as young as 1
year, who often do not tolerate anything touching their faces. Disparity ranges
from 1200 seconds to 550 or 200 seconds of arc depending on the version of the
test. Again, there are no monocular clues and the test seems more difficult for patients than a vectograph like the Titmus test. Adults sometimes take longer than
children to recognize the objects on the card. Patients with any defect of binocular
function cannot do this test.

OTHER STEREOTESTS FOR NEAR

There are other stereo tests mainly for near, many of which use the random dot
principle, but very little information is available that compares the results obtained with the various tests. The choice of test is therefore one of availability, personal experience, and preference. The tests described above are the ones in most
common use.

Stereopsis Tests for Use at Distance

There are few clinical tests available for assessing stereopsis for distance. They are
usually not as practical as the tests for near, because they use either a projector or
are incorporated in other equipment. They are also less portable.

1.   American Optical (A/O) vectograph slides are used with the same projector
that is used for Snellen's visual acuity tests. One slide has four rows of five circles; '
one circle on each line appears closer to the patient than the other circles when
viewed through Polaroid glasses. Another slide has a group of shapes that appear
to be at different distances from the patient. Disparity ranges from 480 to 30 seconds of arc, depending on the test. This test can be used with children as young
as 4 years provided they are given a card to hold with either a row of five circles
or the appropriate shapes drawn on it. The child can then indicate which circle or
shape appears to "stick out the most." It is also helpful to project just one row of
circles at a time when testing children.

2.   The Mentor B-Vat system of assessing visual function also can incorporate a
test of distance stereopsis. Special goggles connected to the unit allow the patient's
stereopsis to be tested with circles similar to the Titmus stereotest or by random
dot tests. Patients are impressed by the use of modern computer-driven technology to test their eyes. The equipment is very expensive initially but has the
advantage of incorporating many other tests of visual function in one piece of
equipment, making it easy and efficient to switch from one test to another.
Stereoacuity of 15 seconds can be detected with this equipment.

   It is very difficult to compare the various tests used for assessing stereopsis. Differences in the disparities used and the methods of dissociation are common. Random dot stereograms seem to be assessing different aspects of stereopsis from
nonrandom dot tests and are more challenging for the patients. As an approximate guideline, the following values may be of help.
   A patient who achieves 100 seconds or better with the Titmus test can be expected to achieve 180 seconds or better with the A/O vectograph, 120 seconds or

better with the TNO, and 550 seconds with the Lang stereotest. Suggestions than stereoacuity improves with age should be doubted; it is more likely that there is improvement in comprehension and ability to communicate responses.[4]

Stereopsis as an Indicator of Fusion

Although stereopsis and fusion are not the same, the presence of stereopsis can be used as a screening device to confirm the presence of fusion and therefore binocular single vision. Most of the tests for stereopsis that are in common clinical use confirm the actual presence of stereopsis at the time and distance the test is being used. The patient therefore has binocular single vision, with either a monofixation syndrome and only peripheral fusion, or with bifoveal fixation and with both central and peripheral fusion in normal seeing conditions. Stereopsis is usually recorded as the minimum angle of disparity, in seconds of arc, that the patient can detect on a particular test. The smaller the disparity that can be detected, the better the stereopsis. A major amblyoscope can be used to detect the potential for stereopsis in patients whose strabismus is too large for stereopsis in normal seeing conditions, only the Braddick random dot slides are produced with information about their disparity in seconds of arc.

Tests for Fusion

Worth Four-Dot Test (Worth Four-Light Test)

This test is used to confirm that a patient is actually fusing at the testing distance. It also may be used to determine the patient's dominant eye. The original design, which is still the most widely used, consists of four circular panes of glass arranged in a diamond pattern in one side of a box that has its own internal illumination. The lower pane of glass is white, the upper one red, and the two side ones are green (Fig. 4–6A). The test should be administered with the patient seated 6 m away from the lights. The patient wears red and green glasses or goggles which are complementary to the lights. It is customary to place the red glass in front of the right eye but it may be placed in front of either eye. This is a very dissociative test, so a patient who can maintain fusion under these circumstances usually can maintain it well in more natural circumstances.[2]

Possible responses include:

1. Bifoveal or peripheral fusion: four lights in the correct formation. The color of the lower light may be pink or green, depending on the dominant eye. When the patient is closer to the lights than the correct distance for the size of the test (thus displacing the images outside the fovea), then peripheral fusion rather than bifoveal fusion may be present when the patient sees four lights.

2. Diplopia: five lights. If the original design is used, then the patient will report two red and three green lights. The diplopia may be crossed (heteronymous) or uncrossed (homonymous) depending on the type of horizontal deviation present. The lights will be displaced vertically if a vertical deviation is present.

3. Suppression: two or three lights. This indicates suppression of one eye. There may be alternation between two and three lights, indicating alternating suppression.

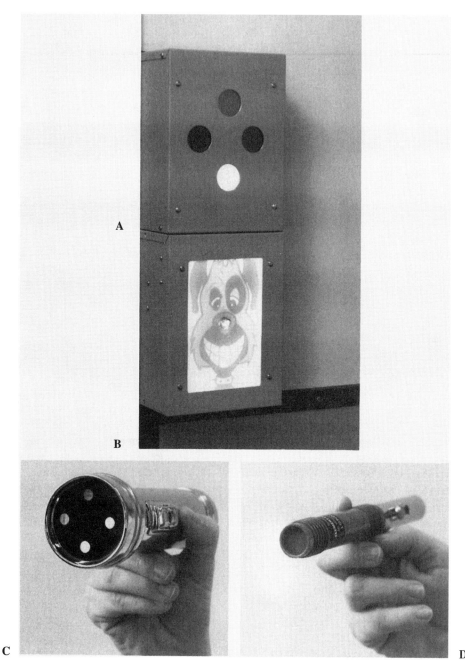

Figure 4–6. Worth four-dot test. (*A*) Worth four-dot test for viewing at 6 m. (*B*) Smiling dog face with light on the nose useful for fixation at 6 m in young child. (*C*) Worth four-dot large flashlight test. (*D*) Worth four-dot penlight test for use at 33 cm.

Caution: (1) Some patients who can maintain binocular single vision under more natural conditions may give a diplopia response because of the dissociation caused by the red/green glasses; and (2) some patients whose visual axes are not aligned and who suppress normally may give a diplopia response because of the disruption to their suppression caused by the test, especially if the red glass is placed over the deviating eye.[2]

Test responses should be recorded as fusion, diplopia, or suppression because there are many variations in the design of this test (Fig. 4–6A,C,D). These are differences in size of the dots and the testing distance, and in the arrangement and shape of the lights. Sometimes there are two red lights, one green light, and one white light. There is also a version using Polaroid dissociation that might be less dissociative than the red/green version. It is therefore important to take these variations into consideration when performing the test and interpreting the results. The patient can only be said to be fusing bifoveally if four lights are seen at the correct distance designed to place the images in the foveal area. If the patient is tested at a closer distance, then a response of four lights may indicate peripheral rather than central fusion, because the images are peripheral to the foveal area. If suppression is then recorded at the correct distance designed to place the images in the foveal area, this would further indicate peripheral fusion. There are hand-held versions of the test, usually in the form of a flashlight, which may be used for near and intermediate test distances. The correct distance for the test should be provided by the manufacturer but can be calculated by determining the angle subtended at the eye by the lights.

Fusional Amplitudes Measured with Prisms in Free Space

Fusional amplitudes may be measured with a prism bar or rotatory prism using a target in free space. The end point is diplopia. It is more accurate if one can identify when both eyes are participating by assessing fusional amplitudes using the Worth four-dot test and red/green glasses. Even in 1-year-old children, a rotary prism may be used objectively to assess fusion by watching for convergence movements and the break point when one eye diverges, showing that the fusional amplitude is exceeded. This is best done while the child fixes a toy which will keep his or her attention.

An older patient fixes a small isolated target at the required distance while prisms of increasing strength first base out and then later base in are used to assess the patient's convergence and divergence fusional amplitudes. When the fusional amplitude is exceeded, the patient will experience diplopia. If the patient has a manifest deviation, it should be corrected by prisms and then the amplitudes assessed with additional prisms as already described. In these circumstances it is often easier to use a major amblyoscope.

Fusion Assessment with Major Amblyoscope, Synoptophore, or Troposcope

From the age of 3 years, evaluation of fusion using a synoptophore or troposcope may be possible. This has been described earlier in the chapter.

Tests of Retinal Correspondence

In normal retinal correspondence the fovea in each eye localizes an image as straight ahead and in the same place as the fovea of the other eye. However, in abnormal retinal correspondence, an area of the retina, other than the fovea in the deviating eye, develops correspondence with the fovea of the fixing eye. This phenomenon occurs in some cases of childhood-onset strabismus (for a more detailed description of retinal correspondence, see Chapter 2).

There are two tests commonly used to assess retinal correspondence, and the principles of these tests are markedly different. The afterimage test assesses fovea-to-fovea correspondence involving individual stimulation of the foveas, which are normally corresponding retinal points. It therefore is independent of the alignment of the eyes when both eyes are open. Bagolini glasses present images to both eyes simultaneously so that in the presence of a strabismus the fovea of the fixing eye and a more peripheral area of the retina of the deviating eye are stimulated, thereby assessing fovea-to-extrafoveal correspondence.

Afterimage Test

Bielschowsky modified this test, which was originally described by Tschermak, as a means of determining retinal correspondence. This test provides bifoveal but not simultaneous stimulation. It is a test of foveal localization and correspondence. At one time, the afterimage was produced by a cylindrical bulb with a glowing filament. The synoptophore or a modified camera flash unit are the methods most often used for producing an afterimage these days. The reflecting surface of a battery-powered flash unit for a camera may be masked with tape except for a narrow line across the middle. Across the center of this line should be a piece of a different-colored tape that serves as the fixation target. The test is best administered in a darkened room with the flash unit held about 1m from the patient's eyes. A horizontal line afterimage is induced in one eye and then a vertical line in the other. Each eye must be completely occluded in turn while the fellow eye receives its afterimage. It is important to always give a vertical afterimage to the deviating or nondominant eye because suppression is usually less dense vertically than horizontally. It is also important to give this vertical afterimage second, because there is less time for suppression to take place. When both afterimages have been presented, the patient is asked to describe, or draw, the resulting afterimage. It is easier for the patient to see an afterimage with both eyes closed or by staring at a blank wall. The afterimage seen by each eye should be in the shape of a line with a break in the middle. The break represents the fixation target and therefore the fovea if central fixation is present. The synoptophore has special slides (Clement Clarke S3 and S4) and a switch that allows the normal illumination to be increased enough to give an afterimage similar to that with the flash.

Results

When the results are recorded, a simple line drawing with a notation of which eye received which image and what the response indicates should be included in the patient's chart.

NORMAL RETINAL CORRESPONDENCE

The test stimulates both foveas. Because the foveas are corresponding points in patients with normal retinal correspondence, the afterimages will be seen superimposed. The patient will describe, or draw, a symmetrical cross with a hole in the center where the horizontal and vertical lines intersect (Fig. 4–7A). The hole represents the foveas that were not stimulated by the light because they were fixing the central masked area of the line targets. Because this is a test of foveal projection in which the foveas are stimulated individually, the relative position of the eyes when both are uncovered does not influence the outcome. This response will be given by patients whose eyes are correctly aligned under normal circumstances, because by definition their retinal correspondence will be normal, as well as by patients with a strabismus who have retained normal retinal correspondence. The cover test differentiates between the two cases.

ABNORMAL RETINAL CORRESPONDENCE

If the foveas are no longer corresponding points, the patient will see an asymmetrical cross or the images may not touch at all. The images will be crossed in esotropia because the fovea behaves like a temporal retina and projects nasally (Fig. 4–7B). An area of nasal retina in the deviating eye has become the corresponding point with the fovea of the fixing eye in this case. In exotropia the afterimages are uncrossed (Fig. 4–7C). This can be confusing to the examiner because this projection of the afterimages is opposite to the usual projection of diplopic images.

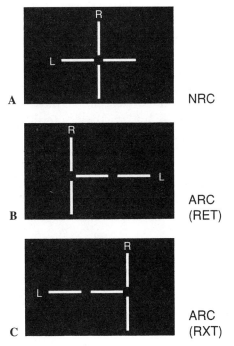

A — NRC

B — ARC (RET)

C — ARC (RXT)   **Figure 4–7.** (*A–C*) Afterimage test.

SUPPRESSION

Only one afterimage will be perceived by the patient. This is an unusual response because the nature of the test precludes the need for suppression.

Bagolini Striated Glasses or Lenses

The terms *glasses* and *lenses* are used interchangeably in the literature when referring to this test. This test assesses fovea-to-extrafoveal correspondence in cases of strabismus by providing images that fall on the fovea of the fixing eye and a nonfoveal area of the deviating eye. These areas do not normally correspond. Plano lenses with fine striations are placed in front of the patient's eyes. The striations are arranged diagonally at right angles to each other (Fig. 4–8A). The patient fixes a small light 6 m or 33 cm away. Because the lenses have small striations, a white line is seen crossing through the light, just as it does with a Maddox rod. However, the line is thinner and the patient's eyes can be observed through the Bagolini lenses. In addition, the patient can be aware of peripheral objects surrounding the fixation light, which also minimize dissociation. There is therefore minimal dissociation of the eyes, and the testing conditions are close to normal. It is useful to ask patients to draw what they see. If the lenses are left in place while they do this, the patients can check the accuracy of their responses and a cover test can be done to aid in interpreting the response.

Results

NORMAL RETINAL CORRESPONDENCE

If there is no manifest deviation, the patient will describe a symmetrical cross (shaped like the letter X or a St. Andrew's cross) with a light at the intersection of the lines (Fig. 4–8A). It is important to check with the cover-uncover test that there is no manifest deviation at that time. If there is a strabismus and the patient is not suppressing during the test, the patient will see two lights (diplopia), each with a line through it if the retinal correspondence is normal. The lines may intersect above or below the lights, depending on the deviation. The intersection of the lines will be above the lights (uncrossed) in the case of esotropia (Fig. 4–8C) and below (crossed) in exotropia (Fig. 4–8D). The separation of the lines may be less than that expected from the deviation, suggesting the possibility of unharmonious abnormal retinal correspondence, but this is difficult to check accurately because it requires the addition of prisms and great concentration from the patient. There may just be a variable angle giving this impression.

ABNORMAL RETINAL CORRESPONDENCE

If the response is a symmetrical cross (shaped like the letter X or a St. Andrew's cross) with a light at the intersection of the lines, then the retinal correspondence is abnormal if there is a strabismus (Fig. 4–8A). The presence of a manifest strabismus can be detected with the cover-uncover test even when the Bagolini lenses are in place.

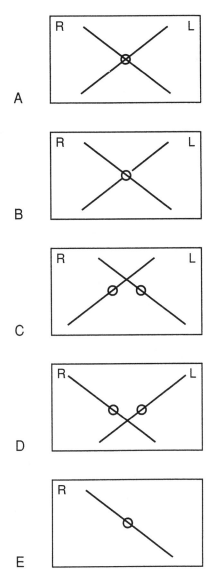

Figure 4–8. Bagolini striated glasses test. (*A*) Orthophoria with normal retinal correspondence (NRC) or strabismus with abnormal retinal correspondence. (*B*) Left monofixation syndrome. (*C*) Estotropia with diplopia and NRC. (*D*) Exotropia with diplopia and NRC. (*E*) Left suppression.

SUPPRESSION

The patient will see one light with a line through it (Fig. 4–8E shows suppression of the left eye).

MONOFIXATION SYNDROME

The patient will describe a cross that is symmetrical except for a small gap on the line seen by the eye with the small angle strabismus. This demonstrates foveal suppression in that eye (Fig. 4–8B shows a left monofixation syndrome). Sometimes the patient does not report the gap unless asked specifically about it.

Caution: Cover-uncover and cross-cover tests must be used to check the patient's responses to determine whether or not a manifest deviation is present; otherwise, the results may be misinterpreted.

The Bagolini glasses also may be used to detect and measure cyclotorsion in a manner similar to that used with the double Maddox rod and described in Chapter 5 (Motor Evaluation of Strabismus).

Four-Diopter Prism Test

This test has been used to confirm the presence of a monofixation syndrome, which has been suggested by the results of sensory evaluation using tests already described in this chapter. The patient fixes a small penlight with both eyes open. A four-diopter prism is held base out and introduced from the temporal side in front of the eye suspected of having foveal suppression. A positive test result, indicative of foveal suppression, shows no movement of the fellow eye. If there is bifoveal fusion and no suppression, the fellow eye makes a small corrective movement. Results of the four-diopter prism test are not infallible, and other tests should be used to confirm the presence of foveal suppression.

Near Point of Convergence

The near point of convergence is tested with an object that is both interesting to the patient and has fine detail. The object is moved toward the patient in the midline from about 50 cm away. When the near point of convergence has been reached and fusion lost, one eye will diverge. The patient is asked to indicate when the object appears to be double. Patients do not always appreciate diplopia when their convergence breaks at the near point. They suppress one image instead. This is an indication of a long-standing convergence problem, particularly if associated with a near point that is more remote than 8 to 10 cm. Sometimes a child who has a history of intermittent esotropia will not relax convergence binocularly when the fixation target is removed; one eye may remain esotropic, revealing the deviation that had not been obvious previously with other tests.

Near Point of Accommodation

Accommodation is tested in each eye individually and binocularly. It is most easily tested by a near point rule such as the RAF Near Point Rule. The patient should be wearing the appropriate optical correction for distance. One of the patient's eyes should be covered. The reading target that the patient can see clearly at the end of the rule should be moved toward the fixing eye until the patient first notices that the print is blurred. This distance from the eye is measured and recorded as the near point of accommodation. The size print used should be noted. The test is repeated for the other eye and then with both eyes open. The near point recedes with increasing age.

Special Tests

Contrast Sensitivity

This may be recorded by using special linear visual acuity charts hung on the wall or displayed on a television monitor. Alternatively, contrast sensitivity using sinusoidal gratings may be tested. The clinical significance of these measurements in the treatment of strabismus and amblyopia is still not clear; data are still being accumulated and studied. Recording contrast sensitivity has been shown to be useful in charting the progress in cases of optic neuritis.

Visually Evoked Potential

The accuracy of sweep visually evoked potential (VEP) acuity is dependent on the steady fixation and attention of the patient. Generally, however, this is still regarded as a research tool. VEP may be useful in confirming the diagnosis of a severe visual deficit such as that accompanying optic atrophy.

Electroretinogram

Retinal abnormalities, such as retinitis pigmentosa, congenital stationary night blindness, or Leber's congenital amaurosis, may be associated with poor vision or strabismus. The diagnosis of these conditions, especially in the early stages, may be detected by the use of the electroretinogram.

Photographic Screening for Strabismus and Refractive Errors

Several different screening techniques are being investigated for the detection of strabismus and refractive errors. It is hoped that a reliable, and simple to use, screening method will be developed to detect amblyogenic factors in infants.

References

1. Dobson, V., Teller, D.: Visual acuity in human infants: A review and comparison of behavioral and electrophysiological studies. Vision Res 18:1469–1483, 1978.
2. Oystreck, D.T., Parsons, C.: Can "Worth" be found in the 4 dot test? In: Pritchard, C., et al., eds. Orthoptics in Focus-Visions for the New Millennium. Transactions of the IXth International Orthoptic Congress, Stockholm, Sweden. Nuremberg: Berufsverband der Orthoptistinnen Deutschland e.V., 1999:273.
3. Teller, D.Y.: Visual acuity for vertical and diagonal gratings in human infants. Vision Res 14:1433–1439, 1974.
4. Tillson, G.: Two new clinical tests for stereopsis. Am Orthop J 35:126–134, 1985.

5

Motor Evaluation of Strabismus

This chapter describes in some detail the tests generally used to evaluate the motor aspects of strabismus. The tests are then only cited, as appropriate, throughout the book without further description.

Although the motor and sensory evaluations of strabismus are addressed in separate chapters for convenience, both are necessary to establish the prognosis and plan of management of all types of strabismus. They are an essential part of the investigation of every patient.

In the presence of normal vision and a normal manifest refraction, a full motor evaluation is indicated at the first visit. If amblyopia or an uncorrected refractive error is present or a cycloplegic agent has been used, an approximate motor evaluation only is indicated because the tests will all have to be repeated. An accurate and thorough assessment of the motor aspects of strabismus are more meaningful when any amblyopia has been treated and when the full optical correction is worn. In very young children some of the information ideally required may be difficult to obtain.

Tests Used in Motor and Sensory Evaluation

The cover test, major amblyoscope, and Brückner tests may be used for both motor and sensory evaluation. For simplicity they have been described in detailed only in Chapter 4 (Sensory Evaluation of Strabismus).

Tests to Measure the Deviation

All measurements should be obtained for near and distance fixation whenever possible. The patient should be wearing the appropriate correction of any refractive error when measurements of the deviation are taken.

Hirschberg's Test (Corneal Reflections Test)

This test is usually performed for near fixation. A small spotlight is held directly in front of the patient approximately one third of a meter from the patient's eyes.

It is important that the examiner is directly behind the light. The position of the light's reflection on each cornea is checked. If the eyes are correctly aligned, the corneal reflections appear symmetrical and usually central in each cornea (Fig. 5–1A). However, slight displacement from the center nasally (positive angle kappa) or temporally (negative angle kappa) may occur, giving the impression of a strabismus when in fact the eyes are correctly aligned as shown by a cover test (Fig. 5–1B). One millimeter of displacement is taken to indicate 7° of strabismus. As a guideline, it is generally taken that displacement of the corneal reflection to the pupillary margin is 15° (Fig. 5–1C), midway between the pupillary margin and the limbus is 30° (Fig. 5–1D), and at the limbus is 45° of deviation (Fig. 5–1E).

Caution: The measurement is for near fixation, so accommodative factors may influence the measurement even though a light is being used for fixation. It is difficult to do the test for distance fixation and still position oneself to correctly observe the corneal reflections without blocking the patient's view. The angle kappa, if significant, may mask or exaggerate a deviation (Fig. 5–1B). This is of concern only if the patient is visually immature, in which case missing a small deviation also might mean missing amblyopia, or if there is a pseudostrabismus and the patient or parents are concerned about cosmesis. This test has been in use for over 100 years and still may be the only possible way of estimating the angle of deviation in a variety of patients, for example, infants, the severely disabled, and patients who have less than 6/120 vision in one eye.

Krimsky's Test (Prism Reflex Test, Prism Reflection Test)

This test is performed in the same way as Hirshberg's test, except that prisms are used to move the corneal reflection in the deviating eye to a position similar to that of the corneal reflection in the fixing eye. The prism should be held in front of the deviating eye with the apex pointing in the direction that the corneal reflection has to move, that is, in the same direction as the eye is deviated. As an example, in an esotropic eye the corneal reflection is displaced temporally and needs to be moved nasally, in order to become more central (Fig. 5–2A). Therefore, the prism is placed in front of the esotropic eye with its apex pointing toward the patient's nose (this is also the direction that the eye is pointing) (Fig. 5–2B). The base of the prism is pointing temporally. The size of the prism is adjusted until the corneal reflections appear symmetrically placed in the two eyes. The prism needed to achieve this is always recorded according to strength and the direction of its base, in this example base out.

A modification of this test is necessary if the deviating eye is densely amblyopic or blind (Fig. 5–3A). The examiner should sit in front of the deviating eye. Prisms of increasing strength are placed in front of the fixing eye until the corneal reflection in the deviating eye becomes central (Fig. 5–3B).

Caution: The same problems as discussed in the caution for the Hirschberg's test also apply here.

Prism and Cover Test

This test is probably the most widely used method of measuring an angle of deviation. It can be used for measuring the manifest, latent, or combined manifest and latent deviation at any distance, with either eye fixing, in any direction of gaze. In addition, the effect of accommodation on the deviation can be assessed by

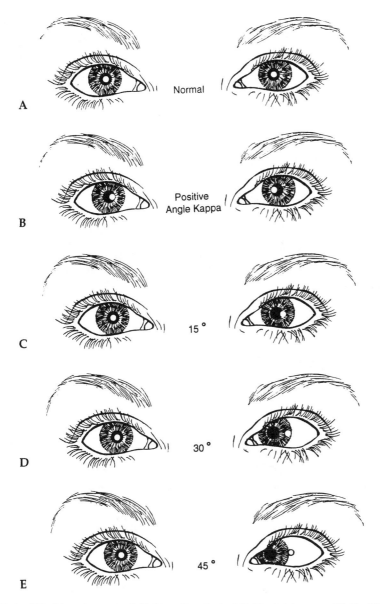

Figure 5–1. Hirshberg's corneal light reflex test. (*A*) Straight eyes. (*B*) Positive angle kappa. (*C*) 15° left esotropia. (*D*) 30° left esotropia. (*E*) 45° left esotropia.

varying the fixation target. It can be used to measure horizontal and vertical deviations but not to measure torsional deviations.

SIMULTANEOUS PRISM INTRODUCTION AND COVER TEST
(PRISM COVER-UNCOVER TEST)

This test measures the manifest strabismus only. To measure the deviation with the minimum of dissociation, the prism should be placed before the deviating eye

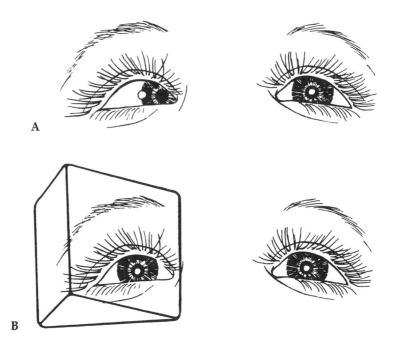

Figure 5–2. Krimsky's prism and corneal light reflex test. (*A*) Right esotropia. (*B*) Esotropia neutralized by appropriate base out prism placed over deviating eye.

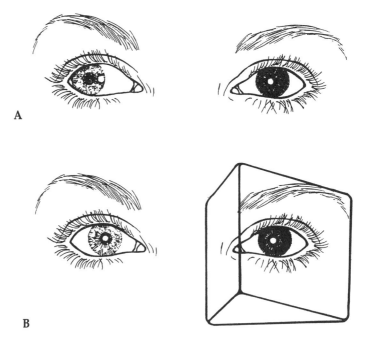

Figure 5–3. Krimsky's test if one eye is blind. (*A*) Blind right exotropic eye. (*B*) Appropriate base in prism over normal left eye measures deviation of blind right eye.

at the same time that the fixing eye is covered (Fig. 5–4A,B). It is essential to do this part of the prism and cover test before doing the prism and cross-cover test in the monofixation syndrome.

PRISM AND CROSS-COVER TEST

This test measures the manifest and, if present, latent components of the strabismus as well as the total deviation present. If no manifest strabismus is present, it measures any latent deviation. The patient is instructed to fix the chosen target, and a prism is placed in front of the deviating eye, the fixing eye is covered, and the eye behind the prism is watched to see if it makes any movement to take up fixation. The strength of the prism is adjusted and the test repeated until no movement is detected (see Fig. 4–2E). As always, the apex of the correcting prism points in the same direction that the deviating eye is pointing.

A target that encourages accommodation should be used to obtain the maximum deviation. Once the measurement has started, the eyes should be totally dissociated, that is, they should not be both uncovered at the same time until the deviation has been neutralized.

If a strabismus is present, the following measurements of the deviation (using a prism cover test) are required:

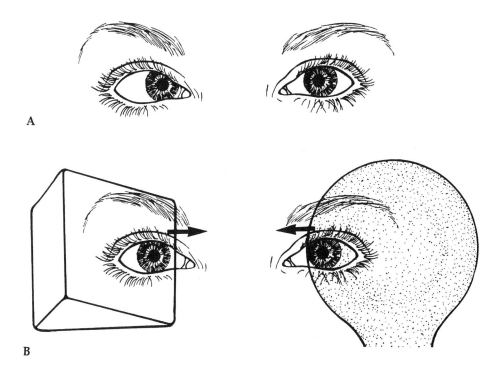

Figure 5–4. Simultaneous prism introduction and cover test. (*A*) Right esotropia. (*B*) Base out prism slipped over the right eye at the same time that the occluder is slipped over the left eye.

1. Using an accommodative target at 6 m, that is, the smallest Snellen letter that the patient can see with the poorer eye and the head straight (primary position), with the chin tilted up approximately 25° and with the chin down 25°. If the child does not know the alphabet yet, any interesting small toy or object should be used as the target. The measurements are also recorded in side gaze using a target at 6 m by turning the patient's head to the left so that the left eye can just see the fixation target past the nose in right gaze and vice versa.

2. Using a nonaccommodative target at 6 m, e.g., a light.

3. Using a small accommodative target that can be seen by the poorer eye at 1/3 meter straight ahead.

4. In the primary position with fixation at infinity, that is, beyond 20 feet, getting the patient to look out of the window at some interesting object in the distance. This is particularly important in intermittent exotropia because this may bring out the maximum deviation in patients with divergence excess.

HOW TO PLACE PRISMS WHEN MEASURING A DEVIATION

The prisms must be held upright in front of the eye and not tilted. When measuring a horizontal deviation, the base of the prism should be parallel to the vertical midline through the nose, and when measuring a vertical deviation the base should be parallel with the orbital floor or lower lid. This applies whatever the patient's head position (Fig. 5–5).

It is usually recommended that prisms not be stacked in front of one eye if the deviation is large because this causes inaccurate measurements mathematically and optically. However, from a clinical point of view, it probably makes little difference in planning treatment when deviations are that large. Prisms should be placed in front of the deviating eye whenever practicable.

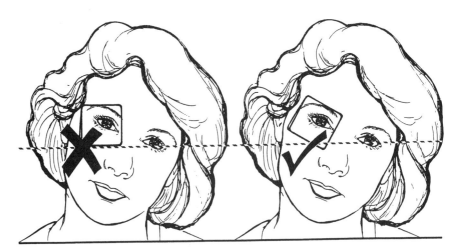

Figure 5–5. The base of the prism is held parallel to lower lid for measuring a vertical deviation with a head tilt.

INDUCING DIPLOPIA BY OVERCORRECTING PRISMS AND
MAKING USE OF THE HEMIRETINAL TRIGGER MECHANISM TO HELP
MEASURE THE DEVIATION

Patients who have horizontal strabismus with suppression will experience diplopia if their strabismus is overcorrected, that is, reversed by surgery (see also Chapter 2). This is a common finding when using adjustable sutures in adults. For instance, if an esotropia is made exotropic or vice versa, the instant the transition occurs from one to the other, the patient will appreciate diplopia. This overcorrection can be simulated by progressive prism neutralization of the horizontal strabismus angle until an overcorrection is produced and the image from the fixation object crosses the midline of the retina, triggering diplopia. This is a reliable and sensitive test and should be done on all adults and children old enough to report accurately. This can be used as a check on the angle of strabismus in any gaze direction, at distance or near fixation, to confirm the measurements. This should be part of the routine examination in all patients with strabismus who can reliably respond to subjective testing.

HOW TO MEASURE A DEVIATION WITH PRISMS IF THE PATIENT
HAS A LARGE "BOUNCING" END POINT OR NYSTAGMUS

Some patients have a large "bouncing" end point in which the eye appears to wobble horizontally at the point close to neutralization. Similarly, it is difficult to measure the end point in a patient with nystagmus, particularly if the nystagmus is of large amplitude. In such a situation the most reliable way of recording the amount of manifest strabismus present is by exploiting the hemiretinal trigger mechanism. This is done by using a prism bar and increasing the strength of the prism to neutralize the deviation until the patient first appreciates diplopia. The prism, which first gives rise to diplopia, is taken as the measurement of the strabismus.

PRISM MEASUREMENTS OF THE DEVIATION IF ONE EYE IS BLIND

The cover test is not possible in these cases. Prisms are placed over the fixing eye with the full optical correction in place until the blind eye appears to be straight (Fig. 5–3).

RECORDING THE RESULTS OF THE PRISM AND COVER TEST

If a horizontal deviation is found, measurements should be recorded in diagrammatical form for up and down gaze and side gaze to right and left (Table 5–1). If a vertical deviation is found, these measurements also should be recorded for head tilt to left and right and other gaze positions as indicated (Table 5–2).

If there is both a horizontal and a vertical deviation, the prism neutralization measurements of both elements are done together, but it is easier to see the change in each gaze direction by recording the results of the horizontal deviation in one diagram and the vertical in another (Table 5–2).

The Maddox Rod

Prisms combined with a Maddox rod may be used to measure the deviation at any distance or in any direction of gaze, although the test is generally used for distance

Table 5–1.   A Simple Method of Recording a Horizontal Strabismus in Up/Down and Side Gaze: Left Esotropia (LET)

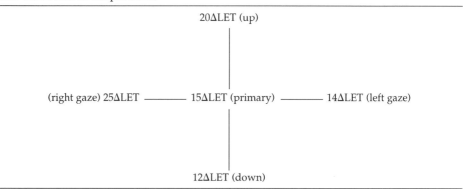

fixation. The patient fixes a small light and the Maddox rod is placed in front of the other eye (the deviating eye). The grooves of the Maddox rod are placed horizontally to measure a horizontal deviation (the patient sees a vertical line) and vertically to measure a vertical deviation (the patient sees a horizontal line). The line will appear to pass through the light if there is no deviation. If there is a deviation, the strength of the prism needed to superimpose the line on the light is the measure of the deviation. Prisms should normally be placed in front of the Maddox rod and the patient encouraged to maintain fixation on the small light throughout the test. Although usually described as a test for measuring heterophoria, this test does not differentiate between heterophorias and heterotropias but merely measures any deviation that may be present.

The Maddox Wing

The Maddox Wing was designed to measure heterophorias at near. Like the Maddox rod, the Maddox wing is usually described as a test for measuring heterophoria, but neither test differentiates between heterophorias and heterotropias.

Table 5–2.   A Simple Method of Recording a Left Esotropia (LET) and Hypertropia (LHT) in the Same Patient (Fixing Right Eye)

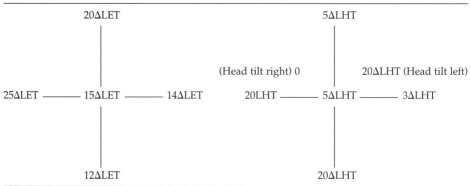

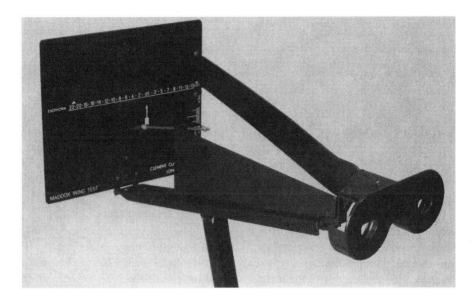

Figure 5–6.   The Maddox wing (Clement Clarke).

They merely measure any deviation that may be present. Using the Maddox wing, the eyes are dissociated by septa so that the right eye sees the arrows and the left eye the scales. There are three scales: horizontal, vertical, and torsional. The numbers to which the arrows appear to be pointing are the measurement of the deviation (Fig. 5–6).

Double Maddox Rod Test

This test is used to detect and measure torsion. A Maddox rod is placed in front of each eye in a trial frame. Each Maddox rod should be a different color if possible. The grooves are placed vertically to produce a pair of horizontal lines when the patient looks at a spotlight. If the lines appear parallel, there is no torsion. If either or both lines appear tilted, there is torsion and the patient should be asked to adjust the position of the rods until the lines appear parallel. The amount of axis change (i.e., torsion) can then be read off the scale on the trial frame. If a line appears tilted toward the patient's nose, there is excyclotorsion. It is essential to ensure that the trial frame is correctly placed on the patient's nose and the head is upright throughout. Bagolini glasses may be used in a manner similar to that described for the double Maddox rod. It is often easier to measure torsion with a major amblyoscope.

Tests to Assess Ocular Movements

Ductions: Does Each Eye Move Normally?

The ductions of each eye should be checked to determine if there is any weakness of a muscle or a restrictive syndrome. One of the patient's eyes is covered and the movements of the uncovered eye are observed as the patient fixes on a moving, interesting small target. Ductions may be recorded in various ways.

PRISMS

A vertical and horizontal measurement using full prism neutralization may be used. The vertical and horizontal measurements should be recorded separately in each direction of gaze.

LIGHT REFLEX DISPLACEMENT IN DEGREES

This is done using the same principles and calculations as those used in the Hirschberg test described in the beginning of this chapter. The amount that the eye moves away from the primary position is estimated in degrees, that is, abduction 20° meaning that abduction to 20° past the straight ahead midline position is the maximum possible for this particular patient.

FIELD OF UNIOCULAR FIXATION RECORDED ON A PERIMETER

Recording the field of uniocular fixation provides a diagrammatic and quantitative measurement of the limits of an eye's movement with the head held still. A perimeter is used. The patient maintains fixation on the target as it is moved from the center to the periphery in the required directions of gaze until it begins to blur. If the patient is unable to move the eye to fix on a central target, the target is moved to the place where the patient can fix it and then the range of movement is recorded. A Goldmann, or similar, perimeter with a small target just above threshold can be used but it is difficult to observe the patient's eye as it moves from the straight ahead position. It is preferable to use an arc perimeter and a target with a small letter or word printed on it. This makes it easier for the patient to notice the blur point, and, equally importantly, allows the examiner to closely observe the patient's eye, thus providing an objective check to a subjective test.

Versions: Do the Eyes Move in Unison?

Versions are tested by observing the patient's eyes as they follow a small interesting object as it moves into each of the diagnostic gaze positions. This test compares the primary action of the ipsilateral muscle involved and the primary action of its contralateral yoke muscle. Any underaction or overaction of extraocular muscles relative to each other is noted.

RECORDING VERSIONS

If the muscle balance is normal, there will be no overaction or underaction (weakness) observed. If, however, the action of one muscle appears to be restricted in one eye, the yoke muscle in the other eye will overact according to Hering's Law. Versions are best recorded by dividing overaction into four categories (+1 to +4) and underaction into four categories (−1 to −4) in the primary field of action of all muscles.

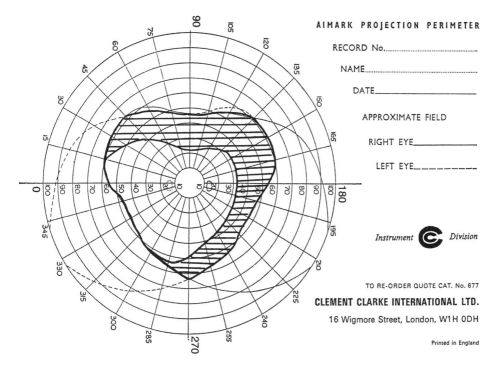

Figure 5–7. Field of binocular single vision (unshaded area); shaded area indicates diplopia.

FIELD OF BINOCULAR SINGLE VISION (FIELD OF BINOCULAR FIXATION)

Recording the field of binocular fixation provides a diagrammatic and quantitative measurement of the area over which a patient can maintain this with the head held still (Fig. 5–7). A perimeter is used. The patient maintains fixation on the target as it is moved from the center to the periphery in the required directions of gaze until diplopia is appreciated or the target moves into an area where it can only be seen by one eye. If there is diplopia straight ahead, the target is moved to an area where the patient can fix binocularly and then moved from there and this area is outlined. This test is best recorded on a single arc perimeter because this allows the examiner to closely observe the patient's eyes and even do a brief cover test to detect when binocular fixation is lost, thus providing an objective check to a subjective test. This is especially important in patients who tend to suppress when binocular fixation is lost. A Goldmann, or similar, perimeter may be used, but both of the patient's eyes cannot be observed even when they are in the straight ahead position. It is impossible to observe when binocular fixation is lost using this type of perimeter.

BINOCULAR FIELD OF SINGLE VISION

This is another confusing term and is often used to described the total field of vision over which the patient sees singly with both eyes open and head still whether or not there is binocular fixation. It is recorded on a perimeter with the target again moved from the center to the periphery until it disappears from sight; therefore, the type of perimeter is not so important.

FIELD OF DIPLOPIA

Although most clinicians prefer to record the area of single vision, some prefer to record the field in which the patient sees double. The test is again usually done with a perimeter, although various screens have been devised for the same function.

Tests for Paresis

COMPARING THE DEVIATION WITH EITHER EYE FIXING
(PRIMARY AND SECONDARY DEVIATIONS)

If a paretic element is suspected, the tests in Chapter 13 should be completed, with particular emphasis on repeating the prism cover test with the patient fixing the right eye and then fixing the left eye. This may give different values for the strabismus if a paretic or mechanical element is involved. The deviation fixing with the affected eye (secondary deviation) will be greater than that fixing with the unaffected eye (primary deviation) in this case.

TANGENT SCREENS

These tests use either red/green (Hess, Lancaster) or mirror (Lees) dissociation of the eyes. The projection of the nonfixing fovea is recorded on a chart. The accuracy of the test depends on the presence of normal retinal correspondence. The test is recorded with each eye fixing in turn.

Hess Screen (Hess Tangent Screen). This screen is used to chart the relative position of each eye in the nine diagnostic positions of gaze (Fig. 5–8). The resulting Hess chart aids in detecting an under- or overaction of an extraocular muscle. There are various adaptations of the original screen, but the underlying principle remains the same, as does the resulting chart and its interpretation. The Hess screen is done at 50 cm distance. The patient wears complimentary red and green goggles to dissociate the eyes. The original screen was of black cloth like a Bjerrum screen with the tangent screen outlined in red. An inner square and an outer square were formed by special marks at the places where the lines intersected at 15° and 30° from the center. The patient originally used a pointer with a green tip. Variations of this test include the introduction of a red-tipped pointer for the examiner to indicate to the patient the next spot to be recorded, and the replacement of the pointers with red and green lights from special flashlights, which produce line images on a metal screen. An electronically operated board with small red lights that can be illuminated as needed also has been developed, in this case the patient still holds a flashlight, which produces a streak of green light to be placed on the red target light. The patient has to try to place the green light on each of these points in turn. The place indicated by the patient is recorded on a chart printed with similar markings and with the name of the extraocular muscle whose action is greatest in

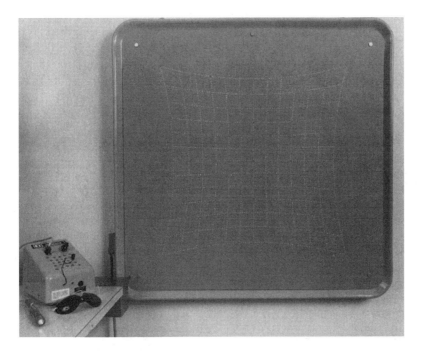

Figure 5–8.   The electronic Hess screen test (Clement Clarke).

each of the diagnostic positions of gaze (Fig. 5–9). Variations of this chart are still used today.

Recording and interpreting the Hess chart test is done first with the red glass over the right eye and then repeated with the goggles reversed so that the red glass is over the left eye. The eye that has the red glass in front of it is the fixing eye, and the movements being checked are those of the other eye. The recorded points are joined to form an inner and an outer square. The eye that has the smallest squares is the eye with the paretic element. The greatest shrinkage away from a particular gaze direction will be in the field of action of the affected muscle. This is particularly easy to see if the outer square is checked.

LEES SCREEN

This is an adaptation of the Hess screen (Fig. 5–10). It consists of two tangent screens whose markings can only be seen when illuminated from behind. The screens are placed at 90° to each other with a double-sided mirror angled at 45° between them. The screens may be illuminated individually or simultaneously. One screen is illuminated and the patient is seated so that one eye can see the illuminated screen in the mirror and the other eye sees the blank screen. The fixing eye is the eye that is looking into the mirror. The examiner indicates a spot on the illuminated screen with one pointer, and the patient places a ring on the end of another pointer over where the examiner's pointer appears to be on the blank screen. The result is recorded in the usual way on a Hess chart with each eye fixing in turn (Fig. 5–9).

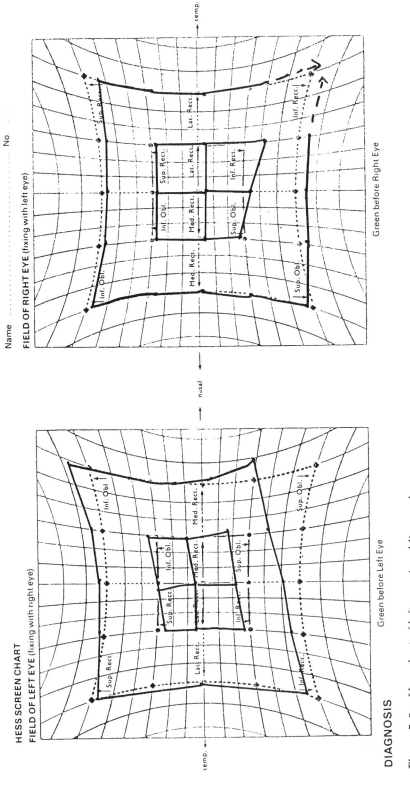

Figure 5–9.   Hess chart of left superior oblique palsy.

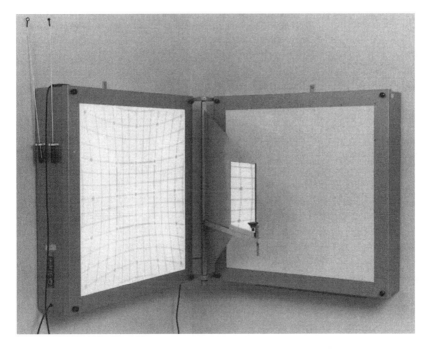

Figure 5–10. Lees screen uses a mirror to dissociate the eyes.

LANCASTER RED/GREEN TEST

This test is similar to the Hess screen test. However, it is recorded at a distance of 2 m. The special flashlights used project red and green slits on the screen, and the patient is asked to superimpose the two (one seen by each eye). The projected streak is long enough for the effects of torsion to be graphically noted, in which case one linear slit will be projected tilted when the patient attempts superimposition of the streaks.

SACCADIC VELOCITIES

Clinically the relative speed of saccadic movements in each eye can be compared as the patient looks from one specified target to another in the field of action of the suspected paretic muscle.

Saccadic velocities also may be recorded graphically and quantitatively with equipment using skin electrodes and based on electrooculography. Using this method, better results seem to be obtained recording horizontal rather than vertical movements. More sophisticated methods are being developed for clinical use as well as research, and the test may then become more widely used. The normal values vary according to the equipment and method used, so it is always important to establish normal values for the test.

ACTIVE FORCE GENERATION TEST

See Chapter 13.

PASSIVE DUCTION TEST /FORCED DUCTION TEST

See Chapter 13.

MEASUREMENT OF COMPENSATORY FACE TURN

An estimate of the amount of compensatory face turn adopted by the patient can be obtained by seeing how much the corneal light reflex is displaced when a light is directed from the same side to which the patient's face is turned. This is based on Hirschberg's principle, as described earlier in this chapter.

THE BRÜCKNER TEST

See descriptions earlier in Chapters 3 and 4.

CROSS-COVER TEST AT NEAR WITH FULL CYCLOPLEGIA

Once the child's pupils have been dilated, an interesting accommodation inducing object should be held 1 m away and then brought very close to the child's face. The object should then be moved back and held 20 cm from the child's eyes while a cross-cover test is performed. This test almost invariably exposes any strabismic tendency, particularly esotropia. If the eyes remain straight under this stress, it is unlikely that any strabismus tendency is present. This test should be done routinely on all cases in which the history relates to apparent crossed eyes or apparently intermittently crossed eyes. If this test is normal, that is, does not provoke a strabismus, it is unlikely that any strabismic tendency is present.

6

Esophoria, Exophoria, and Convergence Insufficiency

Esophoria

Definition

Esophoria is a convergent strabismus (esodeviation) kept latent by the presence of bifoveal fusion.

General Characteristics

A latent convergent strabismus becomes manifest when (1) fusion is disrupted or (2) when the ocular muscles, which keep the eyes straight, become tired or undermined by drugs, alcohol, or disease. Diplopia is experienced immediately when esodeviation becomes manifest.

Esophoria is prevented from becoming manifest, that is, from becoming an esotropia, by divergence fusional amplitudes that keep the eyes straight. Normally, these divergence fusional amplitudes are rarely greater than 10 prism diopters. Therefore, if there is an esophoria of 10 prism diopters, a patient may experience intermittent diplopia when the muscles get tired or their strength is undermined by drugs such as alcohol or sedatives. Alcohol seems to undermine esophorias more than most sedatives, and the patient may experience diplopia after drinking only one glass of wine at dinner, making it necessary to patch one eye before driving home. A patient who has not had many symptoms may become increasingly aware of tired sore eyes and double vision with increasing age.

Diagnostic Tests

Patients with esophoria, like all patients with strabismus, must have a refraction and wear their full optical correction before evaluation.

SENSORY TESTS

Diplopia Test. The eyes should be dissociated with an occluder as in a cross-cover test, and the patient must be asked not to blink when the cover is removed. The patient will experience diplopia while the esodeviation is manifest. The speed of recovery to single vision is an indication of the patient's ability to control the esophoria; the faster the recovery, the better the control.

Worth Four-Dot Test. An uncrossed diplopia response or a fusion response should be expected.

Stereopsis. The following normal responses can be expected: Titmus test, 40 seconds of arc; Lang test, 200 seconds of arc; TNO test, 60 seconds of arc or better.

Fusional Amplitude. By definition, all patients with a heterophoria have fusion. They should nevertheless have their fusional amplitudes assessed. This should be done preferably by an orthoptist using a major amblyoscope or prisms in free space. Some patients do not have a large enough fusional amplitude to allow them to keep their eyes straight without symptoms.

MOTOR TESTS

Cover-Uncover Test. This test will reveal no manifest deviation of the eyes.

Cross-Cover Test. This test will reveal a latent esodeviation.

Prism Cover Test. The deviation must be measured with prisms and the cross-cover test in all positions of gaze for distance and for near in the reading position. The measurements are usually the same in all directions of gaze except at near fixation, when the deviation is frequently less.

Treatment

PRISMS

Prisms may be effective in eliminating the symptoms and are more acceptable to the patient if the patient is already wearing glasses. However, because the prisms required are base out, the side of the glasses will look thicker and will be relatively heavy. A base-out prism in each spectacle lens of approximately five prism diopters is the practical limit. A larger amount of prism in the Fresnel form could be used as a temporary measure, but stronger Fresnel prisms tend to blur the vision unacceptably and the lines of the prism may be noted.

SURGERY

If the distance deviation is greater than that at near, a bilateral lateral rectus resection is preferred, the amount of surgery being calculated to fully correct or slightly overcorrect the distance measurement with the full optical correction in place. If the deviation is the same at distance and near, a recession of the medial rectus and a resection of the lateral rectus of the same eye is chosen. The particular amount of surgery will depend on the measurements (see Chapter 16). If the patient is old enough for the adjustable suture technique, the aim should be to overcorrect the deviation in the immediate postoperative period, leaving an exophoria of 5 to 10 prism diopters in the distance with the full optical correction in place. The reason for this is that some patients may develop a recurrence of the esophoria. If they do not, their convergence fusional amplitudes are rarely disturbed by the small exophoria.

Exophoria

Definition

Exophoria is a divergent strabismus (exodeviation) kept latent by the presence of bifoveal fusion.

General Characteristics

Like esophorias, the exodeviation becomes manifest when (1) bifoveal fusion is disrupted or (2) the ocular muscles, which keep the eyes straight, become tired or are undermined by drugs, alcohol, or disease. The fusion-free position of the eyes is divergent, and diplopia is always present when the deviation is manifest.

The patient's convergence fusional amplitude controls the exophoria, and often the amplitude exceeds 50 prism diopters. Some patients with exophoria manage satisfactorily with deviations as large as 30 prism diopters when they are young. In most patients the deviation measures the same at infinity, at 20 feet, and at near, and their symptoms relate purely to the effort needed to maintain alignment of their eyes. Some patients experience double vision when they are tired or sick, and some complain of sore and uncomfortable eyes because of the extra muscular effort required to keep the eyes aligned. As they grow older, patients usually find they have more symptoms and may require treatment.

Exophoria is distinguished from intermittent exotropia by the absence of suppression and the presence of diplopia when an exodeviation occurs. Patients with exophoria are warned by diplopia that one eye is wandering outward, so they are able to correct it and it is rarely noticed by others. On the other hand, patients with intermittent exotropia are not warned by diplopia because of immediate suppression as soon as an eye wanders outward. Exophoria usually measures less than 20 prism diopters, whereas in intermittent exotropia the deviation is frequently more than 20 prism diopters. This greater amount has resulted in the visually immature child being unable to keep the exodeviation latent, so the child develops suppression and then a typical intermittent exotropia.

Diagnostic Tests

These patients, like all patients with strabismus, must have a refraction and wear their full optical correction before evaluation.

SENSORY

Diplopia Test. The eyes should be dissociated with a cross-cover test, the patient must be asked not to blink when the cover is removed, and the patient will experience diplopia while the exodeviation is manifest.

Worth Four-Dot Test. A crossed diplopia response or fusion response should be obtained.

Stereopsis. The responses with the various tests for stereopsis should be normal: Titmus test, 40 seconds of arc; Lang test, 200 seconds of arc; TNO test, 60 seconds of arc or better.

Fusional Amplitudes. Fusional amplitudes can be measured by using a rotary prism or prism bar in free space as well as a haploscope such as a synoptophore or troposcope.

MOTOR

Cover-Uncover Test. There will be no manifest deviation.

Cross-Cover Test. The deviation must be measured with the cross-cover test in all positions of gaze, both distance and near.

Treatment

PRISM TREATMENT

Because an exodeviation that is symptomatic is usually in excess of 15 prism diopters, it is unlikely that prisms will play a significant role in its management. The large prisms, even if plastic, will make the glasses too heavy. However, sometimes prisms may be tried, particularly if the patient is already wearing glasses. The prisms would be base in, the thick part therefore being adjacent to the nose, which is cosmetically acceptable.

SURGERY

The aim should be to fully correct but not overcorrect the deviation because the patient's divergence fusional amplitudes are often six prism diopters or less. Whenever possible, an adjustable suture technique should be used. Surgery should be planned according to the general guidelines in Chapter 16.

Convergence Insufficiency

This condition should not be confused with intermittent exotropia or exophoria of the convergence insufficiency (weakness) type. It is a separate clinical entity. The similarity of the terms is very confusing. Unfortunately, this confusion of terms is not unusual in strabismology.

General Characteristics

Some patients have difficulty in converging their eyes or maintaining convergence to the near point required for reading. Any muscle movement in the body that is voluntary is strongly influenced by the patient's will. Hence, convergence insufficiency may be functional in some patients. Patients with true convergence insufficiency may get asthenopic symptoms when performing visual tasks at the reading distance. Before a diagnosis of convergence insufficiency is made, it is important to rule out any paretic element by testing ocular movements and by measuring the eye alignment in all directions of gaze.

There may be orthophoria or a small exophoria or esophoria (of two to four prism diopters) for distance, and there is usually exophoria at near. This condition is not really a type of exophoria, although it may coexist with any heterophoria. Patients with a true convergence insufficiency rarely have a convergence near point that is more remote than 20 to 25 cm.

Defects of accommodation may cause an apparent convergence insufficiency. Therefore, all patients should have their accommodation checked with the appropriate optical correction for distance in place. It is important to differentiate between a true convergence insufficiency and paresis of convergence or accommodative problems (see Chapter 13). Accommodative problems may include presbyopia, accommodative insufficiency for the age of the patient, or even accommodative paresis. Because the near synkinesis involves accommodation and convergence, a defect of accommodation could cause a secondary defect of convergence.

Tests

NEAR POINT OF CONVERGENCE, GRADUAL CONVERGENCE TO AN APPROACHING OBJECT

To test the near point of convergence, a detailed and interesting test object is shown to the patient and brought gradually closer in a straight line between the eyes. This is simplified by the use of a near point rule such as the RAF near point rule. The end point of this test can be noted objectively when one of the patient's eyes is seen to diverge or, subjectively, by the patient reporting when the fixation object appears double (see Chapter 4).

JUMP CONVERGENCE

It is often possible to show that the patient can converge at least momentarily by holding an interesting small target at the end of the patient's nose and asking the patient to identify it.

NEAR POINT OF ACCOMMODATION

In this test a detailed target such as small print is used to assess uniocular and binocular near points of accommodation. This is facilitated by the use of a near point rule. The patient is asked to indicate when the letters first appear to be blurred. The result of this test must be interpreted with regard to the age of the patient (presbyopia), and the test must be administered with the patient wearing the distance correction of any refractive error. The patient with an abnormal near point of accommodation, in addition to convergence insufficiency, rarely responds to orthoptic exercises.

Treatment of Convergence Insufficiency

ORTHOPTIC EXERCISES

Orthoptic treatment is the treatment of choice in most patients with convergence insufficiency and yields excellent results. Orthoptic treatment can usually improve convergence as well as the control of convergence so that the near point of convergence is well within the reading range. True convergence insufficiency may cause such severe symptoms that the patient is unable to perform any form of close work for more than a few minutes at a time. The prognosis is good if the patient cooperates with orthoptic treatment. Treatment consists of six half hour visits (preferably at weekly intervals) to an orthoptist, with homework between visits. The work that the patient does at home is a vital part of the treatment, even though it only requires 10 to 15 minutes of the patient's time daily. There are two main reasons why orthoptic exercises may not work: (1) failure to see the patient at weekly or biweekly intervals to check progress and give new homework exercises, or (2) failure of the patient to do the homework between visits.

It is often difficult for patients to accept that their symptoms can be relieved in such a short period by such a simple solution. Symptoms, particularly head and eye aches, often increase during the first 2 or 3 weeks of treatment, and patients should be warned of this in advance. Nevertheless, it is tempting for patients to stop their homework exercises, so they need the encouragement and reinforcement of frequent visits.

BASIC CONVERGENCE EXERCISES

Gradual Convergence. The patient's attention must be maintained by using an interesting test object that encourages maximum participation. If the patient is familiar with the alphabet, a reduced Snellen's test type is a useful target because the patient can be asked to try to read the chart as it is moved closer. It is important that the patient can maintain, as well as obtain, a near point of 6 cm. When practicing convergence exercises, the patient needs to be taught to always try to fuse the diplopic images when convergence fails and not immediately move the target away in order to get single vision again. If fusion cannot be regained, the fixation target can be moved back slightly until fusion is regained, then the target can be moved toward the patient once more. This exercise is sometimes referred to as pencil pushups, but the term does not really convey the slow controlled way in which it should be performed. Patients often exercise their arm muscles only instead of their convergence. They do not take the time to regain fusion before pushing the target away from them when convergence fails. Simple instructions and explanation are needed for even the most intelligent patients to stress the aim of trying to establish a near point of about 6 cm.

Jump Convergence. The patient should be taught to change fixation from a near to a distance fixation target and vice versa with ease. The near target should be anywhere within arm's length of the patient, even placed at the tip of the patient's nose. Single vision of the fixation target at any distance should be rapidly obtained and held for approximately 10 seconds before attention is transferred to the other target.

Voluntary Convergence. Once the patient has a sustainable near point of 6 cm on both gradual and jump convergence, voluntary convergence should be taught. The patient should be able to maintain convergence once the fixation target is removed, that is, the patient is instructed to imagine that the fixation target is still in the same spot even though it has been removed. Thus, the patient is converging "on nothing." Eventually the patient should be able to "go cross-eyed" without the aid of a fixation target.

Exercises with prisms and with a major amblyoscope can be given by the orthoptist. Except for exercises involving the use of a major amblyoscope, the patient can work at the same exercises at home as they do in the clinic. Clinic time should be spent checking progress and instructing the patient in the next stage of treatment. Ten minutes a day practicing is required between visits to the orthoptist.

At the end of treatment the patient should:

1.   Be symptom free.

2.   Recognize diplopia when convergence fails.

3.   Be able to obtain and maintain for several seconds convergence to a target being slowly brought in from approximately 50 cm and then held at the tip of the nose.

4.   Have a prism vergence amplitude of 40 prism diopters base out and 4 to 6 prism diopters base in for distance fixation.

5.   Have a convergence fusional amplitude of 80 prism diopters and divergence of 6 prism diopters/8 prism diopters on a major amblyoscope.

6.   Be able to converge voluntarily (i.e., be able to converge without a fixation target).

These standards are in excess of what most untrained adults can do, but they establish a reserve of fusional amplitude for times of stress.

SURGERY

Surgery is only indicated if there is a combination of an exophoria and convergence weakness. Surgery should be designed to obliterate the deviation in the distance and alleviate the convergence weakness at near. In this situation, the surgeon should resect both medial rectus muscles. The amount of surgery is calculated to fully correct the distance deviation (for calculation see Chapter 16).

Convergence Weakness that Does Not Respond to Orthoptics

Infrequently, convergence weakness is associated not only with a near point of convergence more remote than 10 cm, but also with an associated weakness or absence of accommodation and a paresis of convergence. This possibility should be considered if orthoptic exercises are not helpful in a cooperative patient with convergence weakness.

Treatment of Patients with Abnormal Near Point of Accommodation and Convergence (Convergence Paresis)

Reading glasses incorporating both plus lenses and appropriate base-in prisms for the distance required are the only way to alleviate this problem. The only other option for the patient is to close one eye for reading and other close work. Surgery is only indicated if there is an exophoria for distance and is specifically planned to eliminate the exophoria for distance. Surgery will not relieve the problem at near (see Chapter 13).

Convergence Paralysis

Congenital convergence paralysis is occasionally seen and must not be confused with convergence weakness (Chapter 13). Convergence paralysis may be mistakenly diagnosed as convergence weakness presenting with no deviation in the distance and an exotropia of 25 prism diopters at 33 cm. A congenital absence of convergence may not be associated with asthenopic symptoms because these patients show a total and complete inability to converge the eyes, voluntarily or involuntarily, in the presence of full adduction of each eye. Patients have usually learned to suppress when looking at objects at the reading distance. No surgical treatment is possible for this problem. Plus reading glasses with base-in prisms provide limited help in those patients who have diplopia. A paralysis of convergence also may be acquired (see Chapter 13).

7

Amblyopia

The management of amblyopia is one of the most time-consuming chores in pediatric ophthalmology, but if successful, it is also one of the most rewarding. The management of amblyopia is one of the ways that an orthoptist can help in a busy ophthalmologic practice.

The successful management of amblyopia is the foundation stone of successful strabismus management. There are many definitions and classifications of amblyopia. However, the management is essentially the same for all types of amblyopia.

Management can be divided into two parts: (1) Provide the affected eye with as clear a foveal image as possible, as early as possible; and (2) occlude the better eye.

Amblyopia is a barrier to binocular function, and occlusion is still the best proven method of removing that barrier. In early life a threat to the development of monocular vision is also a threat to the development of normal fusion and stereopsis.

Abnormal binocular interaction is usually responsible for amblyopia. Amblyopia is usually associated with strabismus or anisometropia early in life. There is conflicting or unequal input from the two eyes to the visual cortex. This results in active suppression and amblyopia of the nondominant eye. This form of amblyopia is unilateral.

Amblyopia also may be the result of stimulus deprivation caused by a cataract or complete ptosis. Occasionally, bilateral large hypermetropic errors and especially marked astigmatic errors may cause amblyopia in both eyes, resulting in defective visual acuity after correction of the refractive error in both eyes. In these cases the retina looks normal. However, lesions of the retina or visual pathway may occasionally cause organic amblyopia There is evidence to suggest that the mechanism of the various types of amblyopia differs fundamentally. Fortunately, however, the management is similar.

Causes and Types of Amblyopia

The deviated, defocused, or deprived eye has significantly reduced visual acuity. A difference in the images from each eye leads to abnormal cortical interaction, inhibition of an image, and subsequently amblyopia.

Deviated Eye

STRABISMIC AMBLYOPIA

1.   The amblyopia is unilateral.

2.   It will develop in 100% of patients with a constant untreated acquired esotropia under the age of 3 years and result in a marked decrease of visual acuity in the deviated eye within a few weeks. Treatment of this type of amblyopia following acquired esotropia therefore becomes a daytime emergency.

3.   A milder form of amblyopia with a less severe decrease in visual acuity may be seen in congenital esotropia. It occurs in 19.7% of congenital cases if the esotropia is untreated and increases to more than 50% if the esotropia is reduced to within 10 prism diopters.[4,5,11]

4.   Strabismic amblyopia does not occur in intermittent exotropia (provided that there is no monofixation syndrome) because there is fusion at one distance.

5.   Any amblyopia associated with intermittent exotropia is either anisometropic or from some other cause.

Defocused Eye

AMETROPIC OR REFRACTIVE AMBLYOPIA

1.   This is caused by an uncorrected refractive error in which there is a blurred image at all distances.

2.   The amblyopia may be bilateral or unilateral.

3.   Bilateral amblyopia may occur when a high hypermetropic (over +4.00) or astigmatic refractive error or both is not corrected during visual immaturity.

4.   There may not be a strabismus or nystagmus present. If it is unilateral, this type of amblyopia is more commonly termed *anisometropic amblyopia*.

5.   If the blur caused by the refractive error is severe at all distances, amblyopia may develop even if the patient has only one eye.

ANISOMETROPIC AMBLYOPIA

1.   The amblyopia is unilateral.

2.   It may be associated with strabismus in about 30% of cases.

3.   Even if there is a difference of several diopters in the refractive errors of the two eyes, aniseikonia is not a problem and should not be used as a reason to delay treatment.[15] In cases of unilateral aphakia where the child will not wear a contact lens, glasses should be prescribed and occlusion performed to treat any amblyopia. Indeed, there is evidence that children can tolerate aniseikonia more readily than some adults.[17]

AMBLYOPIA FROM NYSTAGMUS

Amblyopia may result from nystagmus itself. Frequently, however, other causes coexist and differentiation may be difficult.

MERIDIONAL AMBLYOPIA

Uncorrected astigmatism may cause unilateral or bilateral amblyopia, especially in the habitually blurred meridian.

Deprived Eye

STIMULUS DEPRIVATION OR FORM VISION DEPRIVATION AMBLYOPIA

1.   This form of amblyopia may be unilateral or bilateral.

2.   Form vision deprivation or stimulus deprivation is caused by lack of adequate foveal stimulation and is especially devastating if the deprivation occurs during the first few months of life.

3.   Amblyopia may occur as a result of a complete ptosis or media opacity (either corneal or lenticular). Congenital cataracts or cataracts acquired within the first few years of life, corneal scars (either congenital or acquired), and vitreous hemorrhage occurring during visual immaturity all may lead to amblyopia.

4.   If the amblyopia is unilateral, it will probably be associated with a strabismus.

5.   It also may be associated with anisometropia if, for example, a unilateral cataract is removed and the aphakia is not corrected by the appropriate glasses or contact lens.

DEPRIVATION AMBLYOPIA CAUSED BY TREATMENT OF A
NONSTRABISMIC OCULAR PATHOLOGIC CONDITION

Deprivation amblyopia also may occur as a result of occluding a patient's eye all day for as little as a week during the early stages of visual development. It is important to bear this in mind when treating a corneal ulcer or a lid condition in a child under the age of 1 year. No patches of any sort should be used. However, if amblyopia is being treated in the first year of life, it is safe to occlude provided occlusion is not used for more than 80% of the waking day. This is discussed in more detail later in the chapter. Hemangiomas of the eyelids that are prominent at birth largely disappear in most cases without treatment by the age of 6 or 7 years. However, if a complete ptosis is present, extreme amblyopia reducing the visual acuity to hand movements only will result if measures are not taken to clear the visual axis within the first few weeks of life. It is also important to refract the child because astigmatism frequently is present. This astigmatism is caused by pressure of the hemangioma on the globe and if untreated can give rise to anisometropic amblyopia. Hemiangoma may therefore be responsible for deprivation amblyopia or anisometropic amblyopia or both.

These are the most commonly encountered types of amblyopia, but organic amblyopia also may occur and may have one of the other types of amblyopia superimposed on it, strabismic amblyopia being the most likely.

Organic Amblyopia

1.   Organic amblyopia results from a pathologic lesion affecting the fovea and surrounding retinal area such as toxoplasmic chorioretinitis, a retinoblastoma, or a traumatic retinal lesion that, of course, can cause a visual acuity defect at any age.

2.   Organic amblyopia also may be associated with an abnormality of the visual pathway.

3.   Although organic amblyopia can occur in any age group it may have functional amblyopia superimposed on it if it occurs during visual immaturity.

4.   The only way to differentiate between the two components is to try occlusion of the better eye and see how the child responds, although the prognosis must be very guarded.

COMMON FACTORS IN ALL CASES REGARDLESS OF THE ETIOLOGY

1.   Early detection and early treatment are essential for a successful outcome.

2.   Onset of amblyopia is generally in the first 6 to 8 years of life (although it may recur in older children following earlier successful treatment).

Investigation

Some of the tests cited in the investigation of amblyopia have already been discussed in greater detail in Chapter 4. However, they are also discussed briefly here.

Assessment of Visual Acuity

Visual acuity can usually be tested subjectively in children around the age of 3 years, particularly if some matching game based on Snellen's principles, such as the HVOT test, is used. Tests that can be used at 3 m seem to be easier for children in this age group to do. The illiterate E test or any test based on indicating the orientation of the optotype is difficult for children as young as 3 years because they often have more of a problem indicating direction than with discriminating detail. As early as possible, near vision as well as distance vision also should be assessed. [For a more detailed discussion of methods of assessing visual acuity at all ages and ability levels, see Chapter 4 (Sensory Evaluation of Strabismus).]

The Crowding Phenomenon (Separation Difficulties)

It is important to recognize this phenomenon clinically because the use of single or widely spaced optotypes when testing visual acuity may underestimate the problem of amblyopia. Better vision may be obtained with single or widely spaced optotypes than with Snellen rows of optotypes. This is sometimes an indication of the minimum level of linear acuity likely to be achieved by occlusion.

Pinhole

This is a rapid way of determining whether or not the patient has an uncorrected refractive error, particularly if reduced visual acuity has just been detected, amblyopia seems to have recurred, or it has not responded to treatment. The pinhole helps to confirm the presence of amblyopia if visual acuity is not improved with its use.

Assessing Visual Acuity in Infants and Other Patients Unable to Cooperate with Subjective Tests

The problem of assessing visual acuity in infants and other patients unable to co-operate with subjective tests is discussed in more detail in Chapter 4. The available tests assess the relative visual acuity in the two eyes.

FIXATION PATTERN AND AMBLYOPIA IN STRABISMUS

The most commonly used test is the ability of the patient to maintain fixation with either eye.[24] It is important to have an interesting fixation target to attract the patient's attention when doing this. Because a child's attention span is usually brief, many small toys and fixation objects should be available—"One toy, one look; many toys, many looks" (see Chapter 4). Fixation is studied when both of the child's eyes are open and looking at the target. The presence of free alternation indicates equal visual acuity. If the patient does not alternate fixation freely, the nonfixing eye is suspected of being amblyopic. However, if it can be shown that fixation can be maintained well with the eye suspected of being amblyopic, then amblyopia is probably less dense than if fixation is not well maintained. If fixation is steady and maintained when fixing with the strabismic eye, particularly if fixation is still maintained with that eye after a blink, the vision is likely to be equal and normal in each eye. If the suspect eye does not maintain fixation after a blink, the vision is probably about 6/21. The more difficult it is for the patient to maintain fixation with one eye compared with the other, the greater the probable difference between the visual acuity of the eyes.[24] In cases of profound amblyopia, eccentric fixation may occur. This can sometimes be detected by observing the position of the corneal reflex in the amblyopic eye when the patient attempts to fix with it as well as the speed with which fixation is taken up by that eye.

FIXATION PATTERN AND AMBLYOPIA IF THE EYES ARE STRAIGHT

If no manifest strabismus is present but amblyopia is suspected to be present in one eye, the fixation pattern is studied as in the preceding paragraph after artificially creating a vertical strabismus with a 10-prism diopter vertical prism. This test may be useful in detecting anisometropic amblyopia or diagnosing significant amblyopia after successful surgery for congenital esotropia when the eyes appear to be straight postoperatively.

BRÜCKNER TEST

This test is discussed in Chapter 4. It is useful in detecting strabismus and hence potentially detecting amblyopia.

TELLER ACUITY CARDS

These are being used increasingly in clinical situations to assess vision in patients who are preverbal and cannot do subjective tests.[8] Their use, advantages, and disadvantages are discussed in Chapter 4.

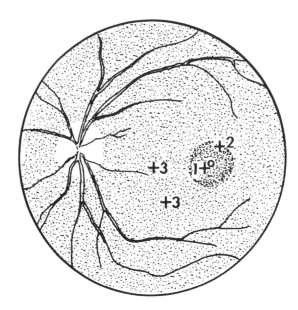

Figure 7–1. Checking fixation with a fixation ophthalmoscope. Target (+) projected onto the fundus while the patient is fixing the target with one eye open. 1: Normal foveal fixation; 2: paramacular eccentric fixation; 3: wandering (evasive) peripheral eccentric fixation.

Eccentric Fixation Assessment with a Fixation Ophthalmoscope

Patients with long-standing and dense amblyopia may lose the ability to fix centrally (i.e., with the fovea of the amblyopic eye) and instead fix with some other retinal area (i.e., fix eccentrically). This is best detected by the use of a visuscope or the fixation graticule that is incorporated in most ophthalmoscopes. One of the patient's eyes is occluded and the patient is asked to look at the fixation target that has been projected on to the patient's retina. The area used for fixation is noted (Fig. 7–1). As mentioned previously, it also may be possible to detect eccentric fixation by observing the corneal reflex when the patient attempts to fix with the amblyopic eye. In extreme cases, fixation becomes not only eccentric but also wandering. Nowadays most patients are seen and treated earlier, which prevents this phenomenon from occurring. In the tragic circumstances in which the patient with eccentric fixation of one eye loses the sight of the other eye to disease or most commonly in many developing nations from trauma, pleoptic treatment to try to reestablish foveal fixation and improve visual acuity should be tried even if the patient is an adult.[21]

Neutral Density Filters

A neutral density filter has been used to differentiate between organic and strabismic amblyopia.[16] Visual acuity in cases of organic amblyopia is reduced by diminishing the illumination with a neutral density filter, whereas the visual acuity in an eye with strabismic amblyopia remains relatively unchanged. This test was not considered to be useful in cases of anisometropic amblyopia because there is a depression of sensitivity throughout the visual field and not mainly at the macula, as in cases of strabismic amblyopia. However, a report has suggested using a neutral density filter to differentiate between strabismic and anisometropic amblyopia instead of between strabismic and organic amblyopia.[9]

Visual Fields

Monocular visual fields are usually recorded as normal in strabismic amblyopia. Although there is obviously a relative defect in the fovea, it is difficult to demonstrate it on a tangent screen or Goldmann perimeter. This clearly differentiates strabismic amblyopia from organic amblyopia, in which a scotoma involving the fovea area can be plotted.

Contrast Sensitivity

Strabismic and anisometropic amblyopes have poorer contrast sensitivity in the affected eye than in their normal eyes. The various methods of testing this are described in Chapter 4.

Electrodiagnostic Tests

These tests may be of help in detecting the presence of organic amblyopia in cases where there has been little or no response to treatment.

Prognosis

The earlier amblyopia is detected, the less dense it will be and the shorter the period of constant occlusion that will be needed to treat it. Close monitoring of the vision will be necessary until the child is a visual adult to try to maintain vision at the best possible level. Occlusion in one form or another is usually needed for prolonged periods of months or years as the child matures.

Treatment

The most effective way of treating amblyopia is still early detection, correction of any significant refractive error, and constant occlusion of the dominant eye. Occlusion has been used successfully for over 250 years. Knowledge of the mechanisms involved in amblyopia has increased tremendously. Pleoptics and other methods such as the CAM vision stimulator were developed as alternative methods of treatment, but they do not avoid the need for occlusion. Occlusion is still the most effective and economical treatment.[6,7,10,21] Pleoptics are best reserved for a visual adult whose dominant eye has been lost to trauma or disease and whose remaining eye has strabismic amblyopia with eccentric fixation. In this situation, pleoptics may be of help in reestablishing central fixation and thus encouraging improvement in visual acuity. In all other cases, occlusion remains the treatment of choice.

If the amblyopia is intractable, it is important to advise the wearing of protective glasses or goggles to safeguard the vision of the sound eye as much as possible.

Types of Occlusion

1.   Constant occlusion of the dominant eye is the best method in the treatment of amblyopia regardless of the fixation pattern of the amblyopic eye.

2.   Part-time occlusion and penalization are alternatives but are not as effective as constant occlusion. They should be reserved for patients where constant occlusion is not tolerated or practical, or where only maintenance occlusion is needed.

Age Limits for Occlusion

Occlusion can be used in children under 1 year of age if the child can be seen at least once a week.

The upper age limit is difficult to set and has to be determined for each individual. It is always worth trying occlusion in children with strabismic amblyopia who are under the age of 8 years. The older the patient, the slower the recovery of vision. This makes it difficult for children with dense amblyopia to be treated once they are in school. It is surprising how much progress can be made and how cooperative many children are in a very difficult situation. The most common reasons that children do not tolerate the occluder are the thoughtless comments and questions from family, friends and "concerned" strangers. Occlusion is not usually continued or restarted in strabismic patients beyond the age of 8 or 10 years. This is because of the poor prognosis as well as the social aspects and the practical problems associated with education. It is generally accepted that the best visual acuity obtained by visual maturity (8 years) is recoverable even if amblyopia recurs. This is the concept of the "spare tire." If the patient should ever need to rely just on this eye, it is likely that its visual acuity will improve to its previous best level provided that there is central fixation.

Anisometropes have a particularly good prognosis if they wear their glasses, even if treatment is commenced after the age of 8 years.

Occlusion

Method

Adhesive patches on the skin, over the eye (such as Opticlude) are the most effective way of occluding an eye. Parents may be instructed how to make their own occluders using hypoallergenic adhesive tape and gauze, or even transparent tape such as cellophane tape and paper tissues. Precautions must be taken to prevent peeking around the edges of the patch and to ensure that the patched eye is totally occluded in all gaze positions. It is important to instruct the parents to buy the adult size, if they use Opticlude or a similar oval-shaped adhesive patch, because the infant or children's size does not comfortably fit anyone over a few months of age. Many parents have found that their child only objected to the occluding patch when they accidentally bought the smaller size. Parents also should be instructed to make the adhesive patch very wet before removing it, because it then peels off more easily, without tearing the skin. It is unusual for children to be allergic to this particular occluder; the problem is much more likely to result from the skin being torn if the patch is not made very wet before it is removed. Parents should be particularly careful around the area of the lateral canthus, because this is where any sore areas are most likely to occur. Often the child dislikes the removal of the patch more than the actual wearing of the patch. Vaseline or cold cream rubbed into the skin where the patch is likely to stick makes it less adhesive and may make it easier to remove. Alternatively, cellophane tape may be used on the skin and the occluder stuck to it.

It should be remembered that the younger the child, the greater the risk of inducing occlusion amblyopia in the formerly dominant eye.

Reversal of Amblyopia (Occlusion Amblyopia)

This is a rare occurrence in which the eye being occluded becomes amblyopic and the vision in the previously amblyopic eye approaches or reaches normal. Occlusion amblyopia is a form of stimulus deprivation amblyopia. This special type of stimulus deprivation amblyopia may result from prolonged occlusion of one eye. This can be avoided in many cases by frequent monitoring of the vision in each eye (approximately every week). It is especially important to monitor the effect of occlusion in very young children. As a guideline, if they are under 2 years of age, they should be seen within 2 weeks; if they are 3 years of age, they should be seen within 3 weeks. However, some children "switch" after a much shorter period of occlusion of one eye. If a child arrives with one eye occluded, it is advisable to allow 15 minutes or so, after the occluder has been removed, before testing visual acuity to let the eye become accustomed to the light. Often fixation is again taken up by the initially dominant eye, with demonstrable good vision in that eye. If there is true occlusion amblyopia, switching to occlusion of the originally amblyopic eye for 2 or 3 days followed by observation of the fixation pattern is needed. The preferred eye should be occluded until alternation is achieved or vision is equal. The interval between checks should be determined by the progress of the child and, if necessary, telephone consultation with the parents. Fortunately, the end result is equal vision in most cases. Unfortunately, in a few cases one eye remains amblyopic, although it may not be the eye that was so originally. The other eye retains normal vision, so there has been no overall loss of vision from treatment when both eyes are considered.

Occlusion Programs

It is important to set up an occlusion program for each patient. This program depends on the age of the child, the density of the amblyopia, the cooperation of the parents, and the ease with which the child can be brought to the office for regular progress checks. These are such variables that it is difficult to set firm guidelines on how long a child should be occluded, but some general principles should be followed and modified slightly as needed to fit a particular set of circumstances.

PATIENTS WHO CAN BE SEEN REGULARLY

1.   Children under 4 months of age should not have an eye occluded for more than 50% of the waking day.

2.   Children under about 18 months of age should have the dominant eye occluded for 80% of the waking day and should be seen again in a week. This usually allows a short period each day when the child is awake without the patch, so the dominant eye is able to receive some stimulation every day. Alternatively, occlusion of the dominant eye for 3 days is followed by occlusion of the deviating eye for 1 day, the routine repeated, and the child seen again in a week.

3.   Once the child is over 2 years old, it is not necessary to let the child sleep without the patch, but it is a good idea for them to do so on the nights that the patch needs replacing. Even though children of 4 or older can probably go 3 or 4 weeks without being seen, it is better to see them in 2 weeks initially to check progress, reinforce instructions, and address any problems that might have occurred. Once occlusion is progressing well, the interval between visits can be adjusted appropriately. The parents may aid in the follow-up if they are provided with a distance vision chart and instructions on its use.

PATIENTS WHO CANNOT BE SEEN REGULARLY

The following program should avoid inducing occlusion amblyopia and is particularly useful when the parents are unable to bring the child to the office for frequent checks. Of course, it also can be used for children who can be seen regularly.

1.   For patients under the age of 3 years in whom visual acuity cannot be tested, part-time occlusion of the dominant eye should be prescribed for up to half of each day or all day on alternate days until the next visit.

2.   For patients 3 years of age or older, part-time occlusion as suggested above should be prescribed. However, visual acuity can usually be tested in these patients using the illiterate E test or other matching test. The parents can be provided with a photocopy of an E chart and shown how to use it to monitor their child's vision until their next visit. Occlusion should continue until vision is equal and is maintained over a period of several months or they are insturcted to stop by the ophthalmologist or orthoptist. Progress will be slower than with full-time occlusion in both these age groups, but this method can be used for patients who cannot return for several months.

This program is only a guide, the rules are not hard and fast. Provided that in the early stages of occlusion therapy the child is seen at frequent intervals, it is usually safe to later extend the periods of occlusion of the dominant eye beyond those suggested. One of the main reasons for failure to establish a good stable result in strabismus therapy is the failure to occlude adequately in the early stages of treatment.

STRABISMIC PATIENTS IN WHOM IT IS HOPED TO RESTORE
NORMAL BINOCULAR FUNCTION

It is better to change the occluder to the other eye from time to time in a child with strabismus who is having full-time occlusion than to leave the child entirely without occlusion for a day. This is particularly important when it is hoped to restore normal binocular function, that is, in children with a fairly recent onset of strabismus, because they have the potential for normal fusion. If the child is allowed to have both eyes uncovered at the same time, there is conflicting binocular input to the brain, which leads to active suppression of the deviating eye. As a result, some of the visual gain already achieved by occlusion is lost. In addition, this active suppression of the deviating eye is a barrier to the restoration of fusion.

If there is a possibility that normal binocular function can be restored and the eyes are not straight with glasses, then one eye or the other should be occluded until the visual acuity is equal and the child is being taken to the operating room for surgery (see Chapter 9). If there is no potential for fusion, then the aim of occlusion therapy is purely to improve visual acuity and it is not so important to prevent the child from having both eyes unoccluded at the same time.

FREQUENCY OF VISION CHECKS

1. Patients should be checked at regular intervals, every 1 or 2 weeks initially, with the younger the child the more frequent the checks. The interval between checks can be gradually extended to 3 or 4 weeks, depending on the child's age and progress. Even in children over the age of 4 or 5 years, the checks should be kept at about this interval whenever possible. It reinforces the instructions and encourages the child and parents.

2. The suggestion of occluding for 1 week per year of life refers only to the possible interval between vision checks and not to the total length of time a child should be occluded in any one year. However, an interval between progress checks of 4 weeks at most is preferable. There is a great variation in response to occlusion in children.

3. Treatment must be individualized and fixation preference determined at each visit.

Management of Problems Associated with Occlusion

The worst experience in patching is during the first few days before the amblyopia begins to improve. It is better to start occlusion of children who go to school or day care during the weekend so that they can adapt to wearing the occluder in familiar surroundings with the help and encouragement of their parents.

It is important to tell the parents how not to occlude. For example, a child may be able to use his or her occluded eye for near vision by tilting the head back and looking under the lower edge of the occluder. Pirate patches or patches that clip onto the spectacle lens are not recommended for full-time daily use because it is easy for the child to cheat by looking around them or even removing them. These forms of occlusion may have some use when worn for short supervised periods daily to maintain any improvement previously achieved by adhesive occluders over the eye.

Once an occlusion regimen is established, most children are cooperative and accept the daily wearing of an occluder. When vision improves, there is less of a problem.

One of the biggest problems is the curiosity of other children and of adults or even complete strangers. "Show and Tell" at school often provides an opportunity to address this curiosity in other children, but adults present a more difficult problem.

Most children show a gradual improvement in vision, achieving equal visual acuity after about 3 months of constant occlusion. It is not always possible to check a child's progress as frequently as one would like if that child lives in a remote area. However, changing the occluder to the amblyopic eye for an occasional day, as previously suggested, should be sufficient to gradually establish equal visual acuity without risking occlusion amblyopia.

If the child knows the alphabet, the parents can be given a chart to take home so that they can check the vision and occlude as necessary. The occluder should be worn all day until the vision is equal, and then the length of time it is worn each day can be reduced.

Failure of the visual acuity to improve should first be addressed by gradually increasing the length of time that the fixing eye is occluded, that is, not alternating the occlusion as frequently as before. Frequent vision checks should continue. If there is no progress, constant occlusion of the fixing eye should be continued until there has been a period of at least 3 months without progress before being abandoned.

If the child is old enough, detailed close work should be encouraged in addition to occlusion in an effort to achieve the maximum possible visual acuity.

Once equal vision has been obtained, or there has been no progress for 3 months, the length of time that the occluder is worn can be gradually reduced, trying to find the minimum amount of occlusion needed to maintain the optimum corrected visual acuity.

Occlusion to Maintain Recovered Vision: Suggestions for Success

Children may be kept on a maintenance regimen, that is, the minimum amount of daily occlusion that enables them to maintain the best level of visual acuity in the amblyopic eye. Maintenance basis occlusion should be continued at least until the child is 5 or 6, and preferably until 8 years of age, in an effort to stabilize the visual acuity and prevent a recurrence of the amblyopia.

It is most important during the latter stages of amblyopia therapy to maintain a routine; that way the parents are less likely to forget and the child is less likely to object to continuing with the patch. The occluder should be put on as soon as the child gets up in the morning-on with the clothes, on with the patch-but the occluder can be taken off slightly earlier in the evenings (e.g., 1 or 2 hours before bedtime). If the visual acuity is maintained for about a month, then a further reduction in the length of time the patch is worn each day is permitted.

Parents and children find it much easier to use the patch for short periods daily than for longer periods once or twice a week. Once the daily routine of occlusion is broken, it is very difficult to ensure that the patching will be kept up. Fortunately, young children do not have much concept of time, so the parents should be advised to put the patch on each day even if, for some reason, they can only leave it on for a brief period instead of the usual length of time.

When the occlusion is worn for only short periods each day, other forms of occlusion may be used instead of Opticlude, which is very expensive. For example, if a piece of opaque cloth held in place by cellophane tape is used, a different color patch can be used for each day of the week. MacTac on the spectacle lens is easily applied and removed, and it is reusable. If the patch can be made fun as well, it helps.

When a child is being occluded for short intervals, activities such as tracing, jig-saw puzzles, Legos, and reading are helpful during this time, as are Nintendo and other video games. The latter are very effective if the child is only allowed to play them while wearing an occluder.

Compliance is more difficult to obtain with a second bout of occlusion than with the first. The child is usually much older, more concerned with appearance, and fed up with the seemingly never-ending occlusion. A few hours of occlusion two or three times a week is harder to accept than a shorter period each day, such as an hour a day. A few helpful suggestions are provided here. Occlusion can be done first thing in the morning, then the rest of the day is free for enjoyment. The child is usually at home, thus avoiding comments and questions from others (children and adults). Maintenance basis part-time occlusion can be given a more "grown up" status by instituting close work activities called "homework" (like older brothers and sisters have). The child should be encouraged to draw pictures to be displayed on the clinic or office wall. Stickers, drawings, or designs done by sib-lings or parents on the patch make it fun and different each day, or patches made of soft cloth in different colors to match an outfit often encourages compliments instead of questions from other people. Favorite TV shows or games or Nintendo may be used as incentives to wear the occluder. A star on a calendar for each time the patch is worn can lead to a small reward after a certain number of stars. The timer on the kitchen stove or an alarm clock can be set for the required time so that the child knows when it is time to take off the patch. With younger children, it is better to do even 15 minutes than miss a day if it is not convenient to do the full session of occlusion; it is important to keep up a routine. With older children, once their concept of time improves, it is still better to do even 15 minutes of occlusion provided it is combined with detailed close work than miss a session. Any progress is slower with older children, so that even a few minutes a day may at least consolidate what has already been achieved. This reinforces the need to con-tinue maintenance basis patching until the child is past 8 years of age, reduce the risk of recurrence. There is no way of knowing who will have a recurrence of am-blyopia and who will not. It is easier to increase the length of time a patch is worn rather than start again after a period without patching.

Sometimes something as simple as the orthoptist or ophthalmologist speaking to the child on the phone encourages compliance with occlusion.

When to Stop Occlusion

If visual acuity becomes equal in the two eyes or if no progress has been made af-ter 3 months of good compliance with constant occlusion, then occlusion can be gradually stopped. Vision should be checked regularly to try to keep it at the best level obtained. Maintenance occlusion as discussed earlier in the chapter should be continued as long as possible during visual immaturity.

Some parents are keen to continue with almost full-time occlusion even when advised that further progress may not be achieved. For example, patient H.A.'s vi-sion did not improve beyond 6/60 after several months of occlusion at the age of 3 years. Parents continued with occlusion over the next 2 years, and his vision im-proved to 6/15 (6/6 persisted in the dominant eye). Vision has been maintained for 1 year so far without occlusion.

It is generally accepted that when the child becomes visually mature the best visual acuity obtained at that age is recoverable even if amblyopia recurs. This is the concept of the "spare tire." If the patient should ever need to rely just on this eye, it is likely that its visual acuity will improve to its previous best level. Occlusion is not usually continued or restarted in patients beyond the age of 10 years because of the practical problems associated with education and the social aspects.

Patients with Nystagmus

These patients should have their amblyopia treated in the same way as any other patient with amblyopia despite the fact that occluding one eye makes the nystagmus worse. Atropine has been suggested as an alternative to an occluder on the skin, but it is usually much less effective.

Special Remarks about Congenital Esotropia

Not all children who have strabismus and a strong fixation preference in the primary position develop amblyopia in the less preferred eye. This is especially true of the congenital esotropes (see also Chapter 8). If they can be shown to cross-fixate (i.e., use the right eye on gaze left and the left eye on gaze right), then they are probably not amblyopic and do not require occlusion preoperatively. However, a problem arises postoperatively when their strabismus has been changed to one of small angle esotropia with a dominant eye. Many of these children go on to develop amblyopia because they no longer alternate and no longer cross-fixate. Patients with congenital esotropia may obtain peripheral fusion and monofixation where a dominant eye is an advantage (see Chapter 8). The ideal is to have the visual acuity 6/6 in the dominant eye and 6/9 in the other eye.

It was disappointing to discover in a 1983 study that 50% of congenital esotropes who had had early surgery and whose angle of deviation was reduced to under 10 prism diopters were amblyopic when they were old enough to have their visual acuity tested.[19] Fortunately, in most cases this responded well to occlusion. As a result of the study, the preferred eye is now occluded part time postoperatively until visual acuity can be assessed. It is important to avoid causing the patient to alternate freely, which can cause symptoms in adult life (see Chapter 15, Strabismus in the Adult). Occlusion is used for 1 or 2 hours daily until an accurate assessment of visual acuity is obtained. It is possible to get a reliable estimate of visual acuity in many 2 ½-year-old and most 3-year-old children by using the HVOT test. Our clinical impression is that this policy reduces the incidence of amblyopia in these cases.

Refractive Amblyopia

It may take several years of wearing full time the appropriate correction of a high refractive error before vision develops to the 6/6 level even if the eyes are straight without nystagmus. Some children never achieve 6/6 if correction is delayed until school age.

Special Remarks about Anisometropic Amblyopia

Anisometropic amblyopia often responds just to the wearing of the appropriate correction of the refractive error, if it is worn full time. This is especially so if there is some astigmatism. However, if there is still some amblyopia 2 months after the glasses have been worn full time, occlusion should be used in conjunction with the glasses.

The Unilaterally Aphakic Infant

Unilateral aphakia before 2 months of age carries with it the ultimate challenge of the treatment of anisometropic amblyopia, if both good vision and fusion with stereopsis are to be obtained. The optical correction is invariably provided by a contact lens, because there are many problems associated with the use of intraocular lenses in patients under the age of 1 year. Originally, we advised occluding the good eye for about 80% of the waking day until Snellen visual acuity could be obtained. Occlusion was then adjusted according to the vision, until it was stopped when the patient was over the age of 8 years. We reported four children who retained 6/12 vision or better after occlusion had been discontinued. However, none of these patients showed evidence of fusion, and two were unable to suppress, giving rise to constant diplopia.[20] There are several reports of fusion and stereopsis resulting from a less vigorous occlusion regimen.[1,2,3,13,23] Most researchers seem to favor occluding for no more than 50% of the time and even reducing this further in the first 6 months, allowing 1 hour's occlusion per month of age to a maximum of 6 hours per day. These treatment schedules allow more time for binocular interaction, with rewarding results even with bifoveal fusion.[13] If a strabismus develops in the course of treatment, the ultimate prognosis for fusion is poor.

Esotropia Precipitated by Occlusion

This may happen occasionally in patients with anisometropic amblyopia. Usually leaving the child for a short period (even 30 minutes) without occlusion allows control of the esodeviation to be regained. If occlusion is still needed for amblyopia, leaving the child without occlusion for approximately 2 hours at the end of each day will usually be enough to maintain fusion.

Penalization

There appears to be little indication for this method of amblyopia therapy. Early and prolonged occlusion therapy is simpler and very effective in most cases. Penalization involves reducing the level of visual acuity of the dominant eye to below that of the amblyopic eye. This is achieved by atropinizing the dominant eye or by under- or overcorrecting the refractive error in the dominant eye. Graduated filters, cellophane tape, or one or more coats of clear nail varnish on one spectacle lens also can be used. In either case, this produces a blurred image in the dominant eye. However, care must be taken with anything put on the spectacle lens because it might not be removable without destroying the surface of the lens. It is important to remember that penalization is only effective at one distance, and then only if very carefully worked out on an individual basis for each patient. For example, atropinizing the dominant eye in an emmetropic patient only blurs the vision in that eye at near. If the child is densely amblyopic, even this blurred image at near may be better than the image from the amblyopic eye. The child will therefore continue to fix with the dominant eye at all distances despite the atropinization. It is important to regularly check which eye is being used for fixation at both distance and near when any form of penalization is being used. If the child is hypermetropic, removing the glasses in addition to atropinizing the dominant eye could reduce its near vision to below that of the amblyopic eye. The child would then be forced to use the amblyopic eye at near.

Caution: Unless penalization reduces the visual acuity of the dominant eye below that of the amblyopic eye, it is a useless form of treatment because the patient will continue to fix with the dominant eye. The American Optical Vectograph test uses Polaroid dissociation of the eyes so that the letter seen by each eye alone can be identified. In this way, the penalizing effect on the fixing eye can be checked to ensure that the patient has transferred fixation.

Will the Vision Stay Up?

It has been shown that 70% to 80% of patients achieve 6/9 or better after occlusion and 90% 6/12 or better. Figures vary considerably, mainly because patients were chosen by many different criteria for inclusion in the various studies published. This also makes it difficult to give any definitive answer as to how well this improvement is maintained once occlusion is stopped. Gregersen et al. have perhaps the longest follow-up reported.[12] In 1964 they recalled patients who had been without occlusion for at least 10 years. They found that 25% had maintained their entire visual gain and 58% had maintained half their visual gain. However, 50% of all patients in the study had maintained 6/12 or better in their amblyopic eye when reviewed 10 years after occlusion was stopped. In studies with a shorter follow-up period (2-3 years), the proportion of patients who maintained 6/12 or better in their amblyopic eye was 40% to 50%, which is similar to Gregersen's findings.[14,20] The restored visual acuity is more likely to remain the sooner treatment is started after the onset. If significant amblyopia has been present for years, the acuity may improve, with intensive patching only to recur when patching is reduced. All of these reports emphasize the need for close monitoring of visual acuity and repeated bouts of occlusion if amblyopia recurs. This can be achieved easily by giving the parents a vision chart with which to check the visual acuity at home. The parents can then use occlusion as necessary.

When Occlusion Is Stopped

Once the child is a visual adult and occlusion has been stopped, it is important to discuss with the child and the parents the prognosis for maintaining the level of vision obtained and alleviate any concerns they have.

In summary, constant total occlusion of the dominant eye is still the best method of overcoming amblyopia. It is especially effective when combined with detailed close work. Constant total occlusion can and should be used as soon as amblyopia is detected, even in children under 1 year of age. Careful monitoring of fixation and visual acuity throughout occlusion therapy is important no matter what the age of the patient. Once a routine has been established, most children will cooperate well with occlusion.

References

1 Birch, E., Stager, D.: Prevalence of good visual acuity following surgery for congenital unilateral cataract. Arch Ophthalmol 106:40–43, 1988.

2. Birch, E.E., Swanson, W.H., Stager, D.R., Woody, M.E.: Outcome after very early treatment of dense unilateral congenital cataract. Invest Ophthalmol Vis Sci 34:3687–3699, 1993.

3. Brown, S.M., Archer, S., Del Monte, M.A.: Stereopsis and binocular vision after surgery for infantile unilateral cataract. J AAPOS 3:109–113, 1999.

4. Calcutt, C.: The natural history of infantile esotropia. A study of the untreated condition in the visual adult. In: Tillson, G., ed. Advances in Amblyopia and Strabismus. Transactions of the 7th International Orthoptic Congress, Germany, 1991:3.

5. Calcutt, C., Murray, A.D.: Untreated essential infantile esotropia: Factors affecting the development of amblyopia. Eye 12(part 2):167–172, 1998.

6. Carruthers, J.D.A., Pratt-Johnson, J.A., Tillson, G.: A pilot study of children with amblyopia treated by the gratings method. Br J Ophthalmol 64:342–344 1980.

7. Downey, R.: New ideas gleaned in foreign clinics for the treatment of amblyopia especially that due to eccentric fixation. Br Orthoptic J 14:47, 1957.

8. Ellis, G.S., Harman, E.E., Love, A., May, J.G., Morgan, K.S.: Teller acuity cards versus clinical judgment in the diagnosis of amblyopia with strabismus. Ophthalmology 95:788-790, 1988.

9. France, L.W.: Luminance and the neutral density filter in the classification of amblyopia. Am Orthoptic J 47:109–117, 1997.

10. Gale, H.: Pleoptics. Br Orthoptic J 14:43, 1957.

11. Good, W.V., da Sa, L.C.F., Lyons, C.J., Hoyt, C.S.: Monocular visual outcome in untreated early onset esotropia. Br J Ophthalmol 77:492–494, 1993.

12. Gregersen, E., Rindziunski, E.: "Conventional" occlusion in the treatment of squint amblyopia: A ten year follow-up. Acta Ophthalmol 43:462–474, 1965.

13. Gregg, F.M.., Parks, M.M.: Stereopsis after congenital monocular cataract extraction. Am J Ophthalmol 114:314–317, 1992.

14. Little, J.G., Oglivie, M.: Amblyopia results with conventional therapy. Trans Can Ophthalmol Soc 26:240–248, 1963.

15. Lubkin, V., Linksz, A.: A ten year study of binocular fusion with spectacles in monocular aphakia. Am J Ophthalmol 84:700, 1977.

16. von Noorden, G.K.: Visual acuity in normal and amblyopic patients under reduced illumination. 1. Behavior of visual acuity with and without neutral density filter. Arch Ophthalmol 61:533, 1959.

17. Phillips, C.I.: Anisometropic amblyopia, axial length in strabismus and some observations on spectacle correction. Br Orthoptic J 23:57–61, 1966.

18. Pratt-Johnson, J.A., Tillson, G.: Unilateral congenital cataract: Binocular status after treatment. J Pediatr Ophthalmol Strabisimus 26:72–75, 1989.

19. Pratt-Johnson, J.A., Tillson, G.: Sensory results following treatment of infantile esotropia. Can J Ophthalmol 18:175–177, 1983.

20. Sparrow, J.C., Flynn, J.T.: Amblyopia: A long term follow-up. J Pediatr Ophthalmol Strabismus 14:333–336, 1977.

21. Tillson, G.: Pleoptic treatment of adult patients using simple equipment. Br Orthoptic J 24:116–119, 1967.

22. Tytla, M.E., Lewis, T.L., Maurer, D., Brent, H.P.: Stereopsis after congenital cataract. Invest Ophthalmol Vis Sci 34:1767–1773, 1993.

23. Wright, K.W., Matsumoto, E., Edelman, P.M.: Binocular fusion and stereopsis associated with surgery for unilateral congenital cataracts. Arch Ophthalmol 110:1607–1609, 1992.

24. Zipf, R.F.: Binocular fixation pattern. Arch Ophthalmol 94:401–405, 1976.

8

Congenital (or Infantile)
Esotropia Syndrome

At present, the terms *congenital esotropia syndrome* and *infantile esotropia syndrome* are used somewhat interchangeably. In this book, the syndrome will be referred to as congenital esotropia.

There has understandably been some confusion in the terminology. This strabismus syndrome is not present at birth but usually develops at about 2 to 3 months of age.[5,16] Because the esotropia is not present at birth, many authorities like to refer to this syndrome as the infantile esotropia strabismus syndrome. It never develops later than 6 months of age. However, it is likely that the defect that results in the esotropia at 2 to 3 months of age is present at birth[17]; therefore, this condition may be referred to correctly as congenital esotropia. An apparently reliable history from the parents may indicate that the condition started at 1 year or 18 months of age. What has probably happened is that the patient has had a small, cosmetically unnoticeable strabismus from the age of 3 months. In response to accommodating more and using the eyes for more detailed vision, at about 18 months of age the esotropia has increased, bringing it to the attention of the parents.

General Features

Congenital esotropia is not just crossed eyes in infancy but is a collection of signs and symptoms and is hence referred to as a syndrome.

The congenital esotropia syndrome consists of the following elements:

1. Large angle esotropia.

2. Deficient abduction.

3. It also may include any or all of the following: (1) cross-fixation; (2) dissociated vertical divergent strabismus (DVD); (3) inferior oblique overaction with V pattern; (4) nystagmus; (5) nystagmus blockage; (6) asymmetrical optokinetic nystagmus (OKN); and, rarely, (7) refractive errors in excess of 2.00 diopter sphere (DS).[17]

The angle of strabismus is usually in excess of 35 prism diopters. Both eyes may be turned in, especially if the nystagmus block feature is present (Fig. 8–1).

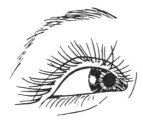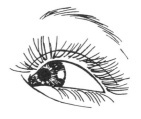

Figure 8–1.   Infant with congenital esotropia with both eyes turned in.

Many of the patients cross-fixate and alternate. These patients, if not treated surgically or some other way, will generally mature with 6/6 vision in each eye, alternating suppression and no fusion. Patients may be amblyopic if they do not alternate, but the amblyopia is rarely equivalent to that seen in acquired esotropia. It is usually in the 6/9 to 6/18 range, and it usually responds well to occlusion. In a study of adult patients who had the congenital esotropia syndrome and had never had any treatment, 19.7% had amblyopia of two lines or more.[1,2] There is more danger of significant amblyopia being provoked when the eyes are approximately aligned by glasses or surgery when the patient is under 2 years of age. In a study of such patients, over 50% had amblyopia.[21] The reason may be that the closer alignment causes more cortical cell interaction of the eyes, resulting in amblyopia.

Deficient Abduction in Congenital Esotropia: Does the Infant Have a Sixth Nerve Palsy?

Reduced abduction is a typical feature of the congenital esotropia syndrome. Many of these patients cross-fixate and, for this reason, never use abduction; instead, they just change fixation. It is therefore understandable why abduction is almost always reduced. It is sufficient if the patient can be shown to abduct each eye just past the midline. Sometimes fundus examination with the indirect ophthalmoscope through dilated pupils forces the child to look away from the light during the examination, showing abduction past the midline position. If occlusion of alternate eyes is performed, good abduction of each eye past the midline will be demonstrated within a few days.

It is rare for an infant to be born with a bilateral sixth nerve palsy. A unilateral sixth nerve palsy may occasionally be acquired during birth trauma or from other causes, but it invariably recovers before 6 months of age. Deficient abduction is a characteristic feature of cross-fixating congenital esotropia. If the other features of the syndrome are present and even if it has not been possible to demonstrate abduction of either eye past the midline, the correct diagnosis is still almost certain to be the congenital strabismus syndrome. After conventional strabismus surgery, these patients abduct their eyes fully.

Dissociated Vertical Divergent Strabismus

This condition is also referred to as alternating hypertropia or alternating sursumduction. Dissociated vertical divergent strabismus (DVD) occurs in at least half the patients with the congenital esotropia syndrome.[9,14,17,19] DVD is characterized by an eye floating up and extorting under cover. When the cover is removed, the eye comes down and rotates inward, returning to the same position as before dissociation. DVD may not become obvious until the age of 18 months or older. Most cases are bilateral, although the DVD may be less marked in one eye than in the other. Characteristically, with the cross-cover test, whichever eye is occluded in bilateral DVD will float up and come back down to its original position when the occluder is removed. If a unilateral DVD is present, there is no hypotropia of the other eye if the patient is made to fix with the eye with the obvious DVD. It does not cause a V pattern. In contrast there is a V pattern associated with overaction of the inferior oblique muscles. These features help to distinguish DVD from a vertical strabismus due to mechanical or paretic influences.

The etiology of DVD has been conjectural. Guyton et al.[7] concluded on the basis of observations and experiments that occlusion of one eye or even concentrating on fixing with one eye produces unbalanced input to the vestibular system, provoking cyclovertical latent nystagmus. This cyclovertical nystagmus tends to intort the fixing eye and depress it, which in turn causes the occluded eye to float up and extort. Simultaneously, upward versions occurring for the maintenance of fixation also contributed to the elevation of the eye behind the cover. This appears to be an example of Hering's Law of equal innervation, whereas previously it was thought that DVD did not obey this law. The nystagmus is frequently so small that it is not detectable unless sought using magnification. We have observed that the frequently occurring head tilt in DVD is also caused by micronystagmus, which is often undetected unless special methods are used to detect it. These methods may be helpful to detect the type of nystagmus reported by Guyton et al. (see later section on Tests Used When a Head Tilt or Face Turn Is Present).

Inferior Oblique Overaction

This condition is frequently misdiagnosed in the congenital esotropia syndrome. It may be difficult to distinguish whether a vertical deviation is due to inferior oblique overaction or DVD. It is also common to find both these conditions in the same patient. To avoid unnecessary or ineffective surgery, inferior oblique overaction should only be diagnosed in the presence of a V pattern characterized by a decrease of the esotropia in up gaze by at least 10 prism diopters. In some cases bilateral superior oblique underaction also may be seen. To differentiate between DVD and paretic strabismus, the patient should fix a test object with the eye with the hypertropic deviation in the field of action of its inferior oblique. The other eye should then be occluded. DVD is present if the eye floats up, under the cover, coming down to fix when the cover is fixed to the previously fixing eye. In contrast, if the patient has inferior oblique overaction, the nonfixing eye will be hypotropic and will come up to fix when the fixing eye is covered.

Example: The patient is made to look in the direction of the field of action of the left inferior oblique, that is, up to the right, and to fix an object in this position with the left eye (Fig. 8–2A,B). The behavior of the right eye behind the occluder is watched. If it floats up and then comes down to fix when the occluder is transferred to the left eye, it is probably caused by DVD (Fig. 8–2B). If the right eye goes down behind the occluder and comes up to the fix, the diagnosis favors

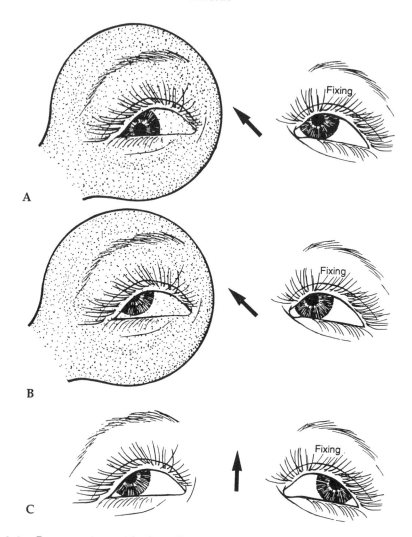

Figure 8–2. Postoperative residual small esotropia with vertical component. (*A*) Inferior oblique overaction. With left eye fixing up and to the right in direction of arrow, right eye is down behind the occluder. (*B*) DVD. With left eye fixing up and to the right in direction of arrow, right eye floats up behind the occluder. (*C*) V pattern associated with bilateral inferior oblique overaction resulting in exotropia in up gaze.

overaction of the inferior oblique muscle (Fig. 8–2A). However, the results of this test alone are only supportive evidence, and a V pattern also must be present for the diagnosis of significant overaction of the inferior obliques, which may require surgical correction (Fig. 8–2C). It is sometimes possible to demonstrate superior oblique underaction in those patients who obviously have inferior oblique overaction and a V pattern.

In some patients with bilateral inferior oblique overaction and a V pattern, the overaction is more marked on one side. If treatment is contemplated for this, a myectomy of both inferior obliques is recommended because the less affected inferior oblique will usually overact more markedly following a myectomy of only the inferior oblique muscle that was overacting the most.

Unilateral Superior Oblique Paresis and Congenital Esotropia

Occasionally, a congenital unilateral superior oblique palsy coexists with congenital esotropia. This may be accompanied by overaction of the direct antagonist inferior oblique. This strictly unilateral oblique dysfunction is associated with hypertropia of the affected eye when fixing with the unaffected eye and a hypotropia of the unaffected eye when fixing with the eye with the paretic superior oblique muscle. An increase of the hypertropia is typically seen on head tilt to the same side (positive Bielschowsky head tilt test) and gaze to the opposite side due to the antagonist inferior oblique overaction.

Does Primary Overaction of the Inferior Obliques Exist?

No principle in muscle physiology can explain primary overaction of any muscle. Overaction of a muscle takes place in response to a weakness of the direct antagonist. For instance, if there is a weakness of the superior oblique, then overaction of the ipsilateral inferior oblique may occur. However, largely due to the fact that many patients with congenital esotropia syndrome have what appears to be an overaction of both the inferior oblique muscles, without any obvious underaction of the superior obliques it has been referred to as primary overaction of the inferior oblique. Versions are gross tests, and paresis of the superior obliques may be difficult to demonstrate, especially in infants. It is hence more important to rely on the V pattern resulting from bilateral oblique dysfunction for the diagnosis. In the absence of a V pattern or of weakness of the superior oblique muscles, an alternating hypertropia should be regarded as being caused by DVD.

Evidence for this idea is provided by many of our patients who, as young children, have had recessions of both medial recti and myectomies of both the inferior oblique muscles for what was a congenital esotropia syndrome with presumed bilateral primary overaction of the inferior obliques. These same patients 20 years later have an exotropia with a significant A pattern. These patients are usually in the group of congenital esotropes who do not obtain peripheral fusion. The A pattern is associated with a very definite clinical overaction of both superior oblique muscles. This supports the suggestion that these cases did not have true inferior oblique overaction but had DVD when the inferior oblique myectomies were performed, resulting in the later overaction of the superior oblique muscles.

Guyton and Weingarten[8] proposed a plausible hypothesis to explain the phenomenon of "primary" oblique overaction as being secondary to sensory torsion. This torsion is associated with rotation of the planes of action of the horizontal and vertical rectus muscles about the visual axes, which could produce either an overaction or an underaction of the inferior obliques, depending on the direction of the rotation.[8]

Nystagmus

Approximately half the cases with congenital esotropia have micronystagmus.[17] It is particularly noticeable when one eye is occluded (latent feature), particularly when the nonpreferred eye is forced to fix by occlusion of the preferred eye. The reduction of light in one eye by an occluder or neutral density filter appears to increase the nystagmus in the other eye. Nystagmus, in these cases, is usually of small amplitude but has the features of motor nystagmus found in the absence of any strabismus (see also Chapter 20). Because it is usually of small amplitude, it is referred to as micronystagmus. It is common for the patient to find a null point in which better visual acuity may be obtained. This is the most frequent explanation of a head tilt or turn in patients with the congenital esotropia syndrome.

Convergence Block Nystagmus

Convergence is often used to dampen nystagmus. It has been postulated as one of the etiologic influences for the marked bilateral esotropia often found in congenital esotropia. Both eyes are frequently esotropic at the same time, simulating bilateral sixth nerve palsy. The esotropia may be present even if one eye is occluded; consequently, the infant adopts a face turn so that one esotropic eye can see straight ahead. The nystagmus may be of small amplitude but can often be seen when the infant is made to straighten or abduct the eye. The association of congenital esotropia with nystagmus and a head turn is sometimes referred to as Ciancia's syndrome.[3] Asymmetric OKN is present because there is no fusion.[11,22,23]

Refractive Errors

Many patients do not have a refractive error of more than two prism diopters when first seen. Glasses are seldom indicated before surgery, but more than half the patients will require glasses at some stage of their treatment.[19]

Natural History of Untreated Congenital Esotropia

The eyes turn in constantly about 2 months after birth. Both eyes may be esotropic, and abduction is limited in each eye. Cross-fixation is typical, alternation of fixation only occuring on side gaze. This changes as the child grows, and by the age of 2 years, the cross-fixating feature changes so that the child has become a spontaneous alternator with one eye straight and the other eye turned in. Abduction of each eye begins to improve, finally becoming normal. Nystagmus and DVD may become obvious by 2 to 4 years of age. Fusion cannot develop, and the visual adult is left with marked esotropia, which is usually alternating. The overall field of vision is smaller than if the eyes were straightened.[20] The deviating eye provides only the temporal crescent of vision that cannot be seen by the fixing eye.[20] The patient may assume an abnormal head tilt or face turn to improve visual acuity if nystagmus is present. It has been shown that the incidence of DVD and nystagmus is the same in both treated and untreated cases. However, the incidence of amblyopia is less for untreated cases[1,2,6,21] than treated cases. Hence the need for close follow-up postoperatively.

Conditions Misdiagnosed as Congenital Esotropia

Broad Epicanthal Folds

The cover test at near is very important in the differential diagnosis. Cyclopentolate 1% is used not only to assess the refractive state, but also to test for strabismus. After the cycloplegic effect is complete, the child is encouraged to fix an interesting toy at near, that is, about 20 cm away. If an intermittent or small esotropia is present that might be confused with broad epicanthal folds, the esotropia invariably becomes much worse after cycloplegia. Patients with no strabismus tendency do not show an esotropia on near fixation even after cycloplegia.

Unilateral Sixth Nerve Palsy

The congenital strabismus syndrome, which begins in the first 6 months of life, should not be confused with the constant esotropia resulting from sixth nerve palsy possibly acquired from birth trauma. The latter is present at birth but has usually recovered completely by 3 months of age, that is, about the time that congenital esotropia is first seen.

Accommodative Esotropia

A typical acquired accommodative esotropia may occur within the first 6 months of life and is associated with a high plus refractive error. When the refractive error is corrected by glasses, the eyes may straighten completely. This is an unusual condition and does not have the other features of the congenital strabismus syndrome.

High Accommodative Convergence-to-Accommodation Ratio

The infant with a high accommodative convergence-to-accommodation (AC:A) ratio may have straight eyes in the distance but a marked esotropia at near when accommodating. This may be misdiagnosed as a constant congenital esotropia requiring surgery, if the infant is tested at near only (see also Chapter 9).

Diagnostic Tests

The Brückner test, which compares the red reflexes seen in each eye, is useful in uncooperative patients (see Chapter 3).

The Hirschberg test, Krimsky test, or prism and cross-cover test may be used to measure the angle of strabismus, depending on the age and cooperation of the patient. The latter test should be done for distance and near fixation and in different positions of gaze as the age and cooperation of the patient allows. Frequently, it is possible only to get an estimate of the angle at distance and near fixation and in up and down gaze. It is important not to forget to test the child on distance fixation as well as near fixation to avoid misdiagnosing a high AC:A ratio esotropia. Failure to do so could result in unnecessary surgery.

Caution: It is important to ensure that the full deviation in an infant who is crossing both eyes in at the same time, for instance in the nystagmus block syndrome, is measured. In such a case, the fixation light should be lined up along one of the patient's visual axes before the esotropia is measured by the Krimsky or Hirschberg method. Ophthalmologists sometimes have difficulty with this and therefore frequently underestimate the full angle of the strabismus, in some instances only recording about half the manifest deviation. This results in surgical undercorrection.

Park's three-step test, which includes the Bielschowsky head tilt test (see Chapters 12 and 13), should be done if there is a vertical strabismus as well as the esotropia.

Tests for Amblyopia

The fixation pattern is discussed in Chapter 7. Cross-fixation also should be checked during testing to see if the patient can hold fixation with each eye, that is, fixation of the right eye to the left of the patient and fixation of the left eye to the right of the patient.

Eye Movements

Ductions and versions should be tested (see Chapter 5). Deficient abduction, particularly in patients who cross-fixate and those with nystagmus block syndrome, is a typical feature of the congenital strabismus syndrome in an infant.

Refraction and Fundus Examination

Cyclopentolate 1% eye drops or equivalent preparation should be used in each eye for refraction and fundus examination, and the patient tested after the appropriate interval. The fundus is best briefly examined with an indirect ophthalmoscope with the light turned down so it is just bright enough to see the details using a high plus lens, at least a +28 DS.

This allows one to have a quick glance at the optic discs and foveas in children. This method of fundus examination allows visualization of a large field with small magnification and is therefore unreliable in detecting disc pathology. It is most important to examine a child with a direct ophthalmoscope if disc pathology is suspected (e.g., optic nerve dysplasia or cupping).

Tests Used When a Head Tilt or Face Turn Is Present

These are most likely due to micronystagmus. A head tilt or face turn may only be seen after a patient's eyes have been straightened. Sometimes patients who block nystagmus by convergence adopt a face turn or head tilt to take advantage of a null point to improve their visual acuity after their eyes have been straightened.

To confirm nystagmus as the cause of the abnormal head position, the clinician should occlude one the patient's eyes. The patient's head position is not straightened by occlusion of one eye because unilateral occlusion usually increases the nystagmus. If nystagmus is not obvious, the patient's pupils should be dilated with cyclopentolate 1%. The patient's head should be turned or tilted away from the preferred position. Covering one of the patient's eyes will bring out the latent element of the nystagmus. As the patient observes the circle target in an ophthalmoscope or visuscope, small nystagmic movements of the circle can then be seen away from and back to the fovea.

Goals in the Treatment of the Congenital Esotropia Syndrome

The best result in this syndrome is a monofixation syndrome[18,19] (see also Chapter 2). In brief, this is characterized by suppression of one fovea and the surrounding macula but fusion using the paramacular peripheral areas. Some gross stereopsis also may be present.

Stereoacuity is rarely better than 100 seconds of arc with the Titmus test at near, and fusional amplitudes may be anywhere from a few prism diopters to over 30. In order to have a chance of obtaining this monofixation syndrome, it is necessary to straighten the eyes to within 10 prism diopters before the age of 2 years and maintain the eyes in this alignment during visual immaturity. Approximately 50% of the patients whose eyes have remained so aligned will develop a monofixation syndrome, and the remainder will end up without fusion or stereopsis.[9,14,17,19,23] The advantage of obtaining peripheral fusion is that the eyes have some force other than mechanical alignment holding them together to produce a more stable alignment and cosmesis. Gross stereopsis may be some advantage in judging depth.

Treatment

Glasses

In congenital esotropia of 50 prism diopters or more, unless the refractive error under cycloplegia is more than 3.0 diopters, glasses are not prescribed. However, if in the ensuing postoperative months there is some recurrence of the esotropia, the patient should be re-refracted. Any refractive error should be corrected, that is, a +3.00 refractive error should definitely be corrected in such a situation. Half the patients with congenital esotropia will need glasses for treatment sometime before they are 8 years old.[19]

Occlusion

In congenital esotropia where fusion is not possible, the aim of occlusion is to have a dominant eye with slightly better vision than its fellow eye so that the patient is not a true alternator. This avoids the problem of patients spontaneously changing fixation and noticing that the environment appears to "jump" or change position, making reading, driving, or playing ball games difficult. In addition, if DVD is present, it will only become manifest in the nondominant eye. This facilitates treatment.[15]

Surgery

WHEN TO OPERATE

Children with congenital esotropia should undergo surgery at 6 to 18 months of age. Surgery is not indicated before the age of 6 months because some patients improve by this age. Presumably, they have had bilateral sixth nerve pareses that have recovered. Surgery is advised at 6 months to 1 year of age unless one of the following features is present: (1) a variable angle; (2) a refractive error in excess of +3.0 diopters; and (3) a general condition that can affect the tone of the muscles, either hypo- or hypertonicity, or any congenital condition that may make a general anesthetic dangerous at a young age. In these patients it would be better to wait until 18 months to 2 years of age before surgery. This allows one to evaluate the effect of glasses, or these other conditions, on the strabismus. Fusion is less likely to develop if surgery is delayed much past the age of 2 years,[12,13] the chances progressively diminishing as the child gets older. Fusion, if treatment is delayed past 4 years, is rare.

WHAT SHOULD SURGERY ACHIEVE?

Surgery for congenital esotropia should aim to reduce the deviation to less than 10 prism diopters. A recession of up to 7 mm of both medial rectus muscles rather than a recession of the medial rectus and resection of the lateral rectus of one eye is preferred in congenital esotropia because of the frequent presence of the nystagmus block feature. If more correction is required, the addition of a resection of one or both lateral rectus muscles is appropriate according to the principles in Chapter 16. In the surgical plan, calculations should observe the general principle of doing the maximum on one muscle before proceeding to another.

   Example: After bimedial recessions of 7 mm, a resection of up to 10 mm of one lateral rectus should be performed before proceeding to a fourth horizontal muscle. This produces the least scarring if further surgery becomes necessary during infancy or adulthood.

Treatment of Special Features

NYSTAGMUS BLOCK SYNDROME

These patients usually have a huge angle esotropia of 80 to 90 prism diopters. In these patients a large amount of surgery on three muscles must be used. A recession of both medials of 7 mm and a maximum resection of one lateral rectus muscle of 10 mm is required. This amount of surgery will produce an average effect of four prism diopters per millimeter (see Chapter 16). Therefore, in this example, the expected approximate correction should be $7 \times 2 = 14 + 10 = 24 \times 4 = 96$ prism diopters. If a residual esotropia in excess of 15 prism diopters persists for 2 months postoperatively, further surgery should be performed on the unoperated lateral rectus. If still more effect is required, a repeat resection of the previously resected lateral rectus muscle would be the procedure of choice. Although it is unlikely that a resection much in excess of 10 mm can be performed at the first operation, it is easy to resect more at reoperation after an interval of a few months. This may or may not result in some limitation of adduction due to mechanical restriction but is still better than recessing the medial recti further back than 7 mm.

INFERIOR OBLIQUE OVERACTION

If inferior oblique overaction is suspected, a V pattern should be sought to help distinguish this from DVD. If a true pattern exists, then a myectomy of both inferior oblique muscles should be performed (see Fig. 12–3). Occasionally a unilateral superior oblique weakness with overaction of the inferior oblique in a V pattern and a positive Bielshowsky head tilt test is present, but most cases associated with the congenital esotropia syndrome appear to be bilateral. If there is bilateral overaction of the inferior obliques, more so on one side than on the other, or if a V pattern is present, it is usually wise to weaken both inferior obliques at the same time. Only in the event that there is clearly a unilateral superior oblique palsy with a positive Bielshowsky head tilt test and overacting ipsilateral inferior oblique should surgery be confined to that inferior oblique muscle alone. If a V pattern is not present, a weakening procedure on the inferior oblique muscles should not be performed because the vertical is almost certainly due to DVD.

TREATMENT OF DISSOCIATED VERTICAL DIVERGENT STRABISMUS

There is a tendency for this condition to improve slightly as patients grow older, so treatment for DVD at an early age is not recommended. The treatment of DVD should be left until grade school age and even later if cosmesis is acceptable.

Patients with a dominant eye who do not alternate only complain about the DVD in one eye, the nonfixing eye. A recession of the superior rectus or resection of the inferior rectus of the nonfixing eye should be performed to eliminate the vertical deviation. The amount of surgery should be calculated according to principles outlined in Chapter 16. Recession of the superior rectus muscle should not exceed 8 mm because the resultant weakness may cause overaction of the contralateral yoke inferior oblique muscle.[4]

Patients who alternate fixation present much more of a problem. They have equal vision and alternate fixation at times. They usually complain of DVD in just one eye. If this eye is treated surgically and the deviation fully corrected, it usually precipitates the equivalent amount of DVD in the other eye. Some surgeons therefore advise bilateral surgery in such patients.

Results in such cases are not always completely satisfactory. If the superior recti are excessively weakened by recession, overaction of the yoke inferior oblique may be provoked, thus exchanging one type of hypertropia for another.[4] For this reason, if a patient who alternates at times is to undergo surgery to improve the cosmetic appearance of a unilateral DVD, only three fourths of the deviation should be corrected. This leaves the patient with a slight DVD on that side and will not provoke the DVD on the previously less noticeable side. Inferior rectus resection of appropriate amount is particularly useful in such a situation because this brings the lid up to help disguise the remaining uncorrected DVD.

Alternatives to Surgery for the Treatment of DVD

Sometimes DVD is markedly worse fixing one eye versus fixing the other. In such an instance, if the patient can be forced to develop a dominant eye and always fix with the eye that gives the best cosmetic appearance, the problem is solved. These patients characteristically have poor fusion or no fusion; therefore, creating a dominant eye may make no difference to their overall general visual function. Creating a dominant eye is particularly easy to do if the patient wears glasses or contact lenses by simply fogging one lens so that one eye is more blurred than the other eye at all distances. This technique can be used even in those patients who have a dominant eye but no fusion and in whom the DVD is unnoticeable if they fix with the nonfixing weaker eye. This can only be done if the vision is good in the weaker eye (e.g., 6/7.5), when one might blur the vision in the dominant eye to 6/9 or 6/12 and not really interfere much with the visual function of the patient because he or she never had any fusion. Patients vary in their ability to accept fixation with the nondominant eye, and this is to some extent age dependent.

Surgery for Dissociated Vertical Strabismus

Surgery for DVD should be planned, particularly for those patients who have a preferred eye for fixation, or such a situation should be created in those patients who wear glasses or contact lenses. Surgery should be avoided in patients who do not look cosmetically poor if they are alternating and do not wear corrective lenses. Surgery should be postponed as long as possible because the DVD may improve.

Why Do Over Half of the Patients with Congenital Esotropia Fail to Fuse?

Patients with congenital esotropia never achieve bifoveal fusion. Even if ideally treated, only 50% or fewer of these patients whose eyes remain aligned to within 10 prism diopters during visual immaturity achieve some peripheral fusion, and only some of these achieve gross stereopsis.

If peripheral fusion is not developed, ocular alignment is less stable and secondary exotropia is common in teenagers. Evidence is accumulating to support the hypothesis that patients with congenital esotropia are born with a defect in the fusion mechanism.[19] This prevents the development of bifoveal fusion in all cases and peripheral fusion in 50% of cases. At this time we are unable to detect which infants belong to which group, so all should be aligned to within 10 prism diopters before they are 2 years old. Subjective testing of fusion can be done around the age of 4 years. Some children seem to behave differently a few days postoperatively, suddenly standing up, walking, or taking greater interest in objects as if the straightened eyes are functioning better, perhaps because of fusion or because of an increased size of the binocular field of vision. There is no study to show why this happens.

How Does the Patient without Fusion Function?

If the patient does not develop fusion, suppression prevents diplopia. If the patient has a dominant or preferred eye, this eye will contribute both its central and peripheral visual field, which is limited only by the anatomic confines of the nose and orbit, to the binocular field of vision. The nonfixing eye will provide only the peripheral visual field that cannot be seen by the fixing eye because of the obstruction of the nose. This part of the visual field of the deviating eye does not overlap the visual field of the dominant eye, and therefore causes no confusion to the brain. The rest of the visual field of the deviating eye is suppressed.[20] This allows the patient to have a near normal binocular visual field of vision, particularly if a small angle esotropia remains. The larger the remaining esotropia, the smaller the resulting binocular field of vision. A patient with consecutive exotropia resulting from overcorrection of congenital esotropia has a larger binocular field of vision than normal[20] (see Fig. 2–1). All these patients are binocular if one defines binocular vision just as using both eyes. Patients who alternate fixation may change which eye dominates in a specific visual circumstance, but the principle is the same.

Follow-Up Care of the Congenital Esotropia Syndrome

Occlusion, glasses, and more surgery may be necessary. The patient should be checked every 3 months or more frequently if occlusion is included (see Chapter 7). The goal of treatment is to keep the patient's eyes within 10 prism diopters of being straight throughout visual immaturity. At the age of 4 years, tests for fusion and stereopsis can be performed. If fusion is not present at this age, it is most unlikely to develop.

Prescription of Glasses in Follow-Up Cases

Residual esotropia may be reduced to less than 10 prism diopters by the correction of as little a refractive error as +1.00 in the dominant eye. This is an entirely different principle involving the use of glasses for follow-up cases compared with the management of the initial large untreated esotropia.

Occlusion

The aim of occlusion should be to provide near equal vision in both eyes. The occlusion regimen can be arranged by trial and error according to the principles in Chapter 7. In some children, improving the vision may reduce the esotropia to within the 10-prism diopter limit. However, care should be taken not to encourage alternation in patients who do not develop fusion. Alternation is a disadvantage in treating DVD. Alternation may cause subjective symptoms such as objects in the patient's visual environment appearing to jump as they switch fixation[15] (see Chapter 15).

Further Surgery

Residual esotropia (over 15 prism diopters with the full optical correction in place) in a child who is too young to test for fusion (i.e., under the age of 4) and in whom treatment of amblyopia has resulted in clear vision should undergo surgery to reduce the deviation. If the medial recti have already been recessed 7.0 mm, the surgery should be on the lateral recti.

Poor Prognosis for Fusion

Between the ages of 2 and 4 years an unstable alignment may indicate no fusion ability. For example, if the eyes were put approximately straight with surgery, before the age of 2 years, and then a recurrence of the strabismus develops at the age of 2 ½ in the presence of an insignificant refractive error, fusion ability is most unlikely and further surgery is contraindicated. The persistence of asymmetric OKN would add support to the absence of fusion.[11,22,23]

Potential Danger of Good Alignment Under the Age of 2 Years

Congenital esotropia needs correcting before the age of 2 years if the child is to have a chance to develop fusion. Amblyopia occurs in over 50% of cases postoperatively. Children need checks every 3 months, until 8 years of age, to treat or prevent this. The patient may not return for follow-up if good cosmesis is obtained. In areas of the world where ocular trauma is a common cause of blindness, consideration should be given to delaying surgery until visual maturity, when there is no chance of fusion but the incidence of amblyopia is only about 20%.[1, 2, 6]

Follow-Up Care after the Age of 4 Years

At this age, an assessment of visual acuity, fusion, and stereopsis is usually achievable. It is important to remember that less than half the patients who have received treatment will achieve fusion.[19] The group of patients without fusion is identifiable at the age of 4, and future care involves monitoring the development of a dominant eye with vision a line less in the nonfixing eye. Surgery would only be indicated to improve cosmesis. In patients who do not have fusion, postponing further surgery as late as possible, preferably until an age when adjustable strabismus surgery could be performed, may mean less surgery over a lifetime.

Strabismus and Cerebral Palsy

About 50% of children with cerebral palsy have the congenital strabismus syndrome.[10] It is particularly associated with those children who have hypertonicity and spasticity. Just as the muscle tone varies in the skeletal muscles, so it does in the eye muscles. Any type of physical or emotional stress tends to make the spasticity and hypertonicity worse. This exaggerates the strabismus so that virtually straight eyes may become markedly esotropic. Bizarre variability may be noted, sometimes the eyes being exotropic and sometimes esotropic, sometimes with a vertical element, sometimes not.

Management of Strabismus Patients with Cerebral Palsy

Conservative management of these patients usually produces the best long-term results. If they have had a constant strabismus from early infancy, the prognosis for developing fusion is extremely poor and the strabismus should be managed just for cosmetic improvement. Because these patients are likely to get less spastic and less hypertonic as they grow older with no specific treatment, surgery should be delayed as long as possible. The only indication for surgery is when the patient is aware of being teased and demands help. Therefore, surgery in these cases should be delayed until at least 5 or 6 years of age or, unless teasing is an indication at that age, until even later.

Adult Patients Who Have Had Congenital Esotropia

Many patients, particularly those without fusion, will have cosmetically noticeable strabismus in adult age. Commonly, a consecutive exotropia occurs that may require treatment (Chapters 10 and 15).

Spontaneous Alternation

Some visual adults who have had a congenital strabismus but did not develop fusion complain of problems related to spontaneous alternation of fixation.[15] This is particularly disturbing during driving, close work, or sports. An explanation and encouragement to try to develop fixation with a dominant eye will usually resolve the problem. This problem can often be avoided by "deprogramming the patient and parents" when an end point is reached in treatment. The advantages of a dominant eye should be explained, as should the disadvantages of trying to change the sensory status of the eyes.

References

1. Calcutt, C.: The natural history of infantile esotropia. A study of the untreated condition in the visual adult. In: Tillson, G., ed. Advances in Amblyopia and Strabismus. Transactions of the VIIth International Orthoptic Congress, Nuremberg, Germany, 1991:3.
2. Calcutt, C., Murray, A.D.: Untreated essential infantile esotropia: Factors affecting the development of amblyopia. Eye 12(part 2):167, 1998.
3. Ciancia, A.: La esotropia en el lactante, diagnostico y tratamiento. Arch Chil Oftalmol 9:117, 1962.
4. Freeman, R.S., Rosenbaum, A.L.: Residual incomitant D.V.D. following large superior rectus recessions. J Pediatr Ophthalmol Strabismus 26:76, 1989.
5. Friedrich, D., de Decker, W.: Prospective study of the development of strabismus during the first 6 months of life. In: Lenk-Schäfer, M., ed. Orthoptic Horizons. Transactions of the Sixth International Orthoptic Congress, Harrogate, England, 1987:21.
6. Good, W.V., da Sa, L.C.F., Lyons, C.J., Hoyt, C.S.: Monocular visual outcome in untreated early onset esotropia. Br J Ophthalmol 77:492-494, 1993.
7. Guyton, D.L., Cheeseman, E.W. Jr., Ellis, F.J., Straumann, D., Zee, D.S.: Dissociated vertical deviation: An exaggerated normal eye movement used to dampen cyclovertical latent nystagmus. Trans Am Ophthalmol Soc 96:389–424, 1998.
8. Guyton, D.L., Weingarten, P.E.: Sensory torsion as the cause of primary oblique muscle overaction/underaction and A- and V-pattern strabismus. Binocular Vision Eye Muscle Surg Q 9:209–236, 1994.
9. Helveston, E.M.: Dissociated vertical deviation: A clinical and laboratory study. Trans Am Ophthalmol Soc 78:734, 1981.
10. Hiles, D.A., Wallar, P.H., McFarlane, F.: Current concepts in the management of strabismus in children with cerebral palsy. Ann Ophthalmol 7:789, 1975.
11. Hooper, A.: Opticokinetic strabismus and the ages at onset of strabismus. Br Orthoptic J 47:44, 1990.
12. Ing, M.R.: Early surgical alignment for congenital esotropia. J Pediatr Ophthalmol Strabismus 20:11, 1983.
13. Ing, M.R., Costenbader, F.D., Parks, M.M., Albert, D.G.: Early surgery for congenital esotropia. Am J Ophthalmol 61:1419, 1966.
14. Lang, J.: Der Kongenitale oder Fruhkindliche Strabismus. Ophthalmologica 154:201, 1967.
15. Lyons, C.J., Oystreck, D.T.: Presbyopia and strabismus: Old patients, new symptoms. In: Pritchard, C., et al., eds. Orthoptics in Focus—Visions for the New Millennium. Transactions of the IXth International Orthoptic Congress, Stockholm, Sweden. Nuremberg: Berufsverband der Orthoptistinnen Deutschland e.V., 1999:200–204.
16. Nixon, R.B., Helveston, E.M., Miller, K., Archer, S.M., Ellis, F.D.: Incidence of strabismus in neonates. Am J Ophthalmol 100:798, 1985.
17. Noorden, G.K. von: A reassessment of infantile esotropia (XLIV Edward Jackson Memorial Lecture). Am J Ophthalmol 105:1, 1988.
18. Parks, M.M.: The monofixation syndrome. Trans Am Ophthalmol Soc 67:609, 1969.
19. Pratt-Johnson, J.A.: Fusion and suppression: Development and loss. Am J Pediatr Ophthalmol Strabismus 29:4, 1992.
20. Pratt-Johnson, J.A., Tillson, G.: Suppression in strabismus-an update. Br J Ophthalmol 68:174, 1984.

21. Pratt-Johnson, J.A., Tillson, G.: Sensory results following treatment of infantile esotropia. Can J Ophthalmol 18:175–177, 1983.
22. Tychsen, L., Lisberger, S.G.: Maldevelopment of visual motion processing in humans who had strabismus with onset in infancy. J Neurosci 6:2495, 1986.
23. Van Hof-Van Duin, J., Mohn, G.: Stereopsis and opticokinetic nystagmus. In: Lennarstrand, G., ed. Functional Basis of Ocular Motility Disorders. New York: Pergamon, 1982:113.
24. Zak, T.A., Morin, J.D.: Early surgery for infantile esotropia results and influence of age upon results. Can J Ophthalmol 17:213, 1982.

9

Acquired Esotropia

General Features

Acquired Esotropia in a Young Child Is a Daytime Emergency

Children who are born with their eyes straight and develop an esotropia usually do so between 18 months and 3 years of age. This is the age when children start to look for detail. Although they do not read, they nevertheless look with great attention at near objects, toys, etc. This calls into play their accommodation and accommodative reflexes and may precipitate an esotropia, particularly if there is a hypermetropic refractive error and a family history of strabismus. If normal fusion and stereopsis were present prior to the onset of the esotropia and the child is still visually immature, active inhibition of the deviating eye at the cortical level will occur. This may cause a deterioration in visual acuity, fusion, and stereopsis, which can happen in just a few days.

We do not know how quickly the fusion reflexes can be lost irretrievably, but normal vision can drop to 6/60 in a week in a 3-year-old child in cases of acquired esotropia. If an esotropia is acquired within the first 2 years of life, normal central bifoveal fusion is unlikely to be regained if the deviation is present constantly for 2 months or more without treatment. If immediate treatment is undertaken, within a few days of the onset of the esotropia, a cure with perfect bifoveal fusion should be achieved. If treatment is delayed for several months, a monofixation syndrome with one fovea suppressed is likely to occur. If treatment has been neglected for years, eccentric fixation with vision below 6/120 may result.[27]

The interval between the onset of constant esotropia and its treatment, in a child under the age of 3 years, is the factor determining whether the patient will see 6/6 in each eye with perfect fusion or have a legally blind eye and no fusion. Treatment is therefore urgent—indeed, a daytime emergency.

How to Prevent Delay in Treatment

Every ophthalmologist should tackle the problem of trying to see children with acquired esotropia with minimal delay. The following suggestions may help:

1. Secretaries should be alerted to the problem so that referring doctors and patients are questioned to try to elucidate whether or not this is a recently acquired strabismus.

2. Explore the family history. If an infant is seen because there is a positive family history of strabismus but no strabismus is found, inform the parents anyway about the dangers of acquired esotropia and the urgency of immediate treatment.

3. Explain the problem to pediatricians and general practitioners whenever there is a chance to talk to them (e.g., at a hospital meeting).

Treatment of Cases Seen Shortly after Onset

1. Prevent amblyopia by occluding (see Chapter 7). If a case is seen within a week of onset and amblyopia has developed, the amblyopia can usually be cured. This is shown by equal visual acuity or alternate fixation.

2. Prevent loss of fusion by straightening the eyes without delay with glasses, surgery, or both. Glasses should be prescribed for any refractive error to see if the deviation is entirely eliminated when they are worn.

Glasses should be tried for only a short period, such as a day or two, before deciding whether or not the deviation is completely eliminated when they are worn. If the deviation has not been completely eliminated, an immediate return to occlusion until surgery can be done is essential. Surgery should be designed to overcorrect by 10 prism diopters, the residual distance deviation present after wearing the glasses for 2 days.

Occlusion to Eliminate Suppression in Acquired Esotropia

Occlusion of one eye must be maintained at all times. It is important to understand the physiology of suppression and to realize that suppression is only present when both eyes are open.[29,31] Suppression replaces normal fusion and becomes entrenched in visually immature patients.

Unfortunately, no simple test is available to detect whether or not suppression as well as amblyopia has been eliminated by occluding other than by mapping the suppression scotoma with both eyes open. This technique requires a level of cooperation and intelligence that is present only in an adult; therefore, it has little or no place in the management of acquired esotropia in young children when the goal is functional cure. If the patient complains of diplopia, it is obvious that there is no suppression. However, many children tolerate diplopia without complaining. In an esotropia that has been constant for only a few days or a few weeks, alternation or restoration of equal vision should be taken as the signal to eliminate the deviation as quickly as possible. Total occlusion of one eye or the other must be continued until glasses and or surgery have eliminated the motor deviation with minimal delay.

Occlusion amblyopia is avoided in such a regimen by changing the occlusion from one eye to the other as necessary (see Chapter 7). Persisting with glasses alone without occlusion, when the glasses do not completely eliminate the deviation, encourages the immediate return and entrenchment of suppression.

Long-Standing Untreated Acquired Esotropia without Amblyopia

All patients with acquired constant esotropia that developed at an early age (e.g., age 2) will have amblyopia if the esotropia has never been treated and the child is now 4 or 5 years of age. The vision could be 6/60 or less with eccentric fixation. Therefore, if a parent says that a child developed esotropia around the age of 18 months and has never been treated but 6/6 vision is present in each eye, the child probably has an infantile/congenital esotropia that happened to get worse at about the age of 18 months, drawing the parent's attention to the strabismus.

Prognosis for Sensory Cure

In ideal circumstances, when a patient is seen soon after the occurrence of a constant esotropia, a complete functional cure is likely.[27] Energetic treatment of any amblyopia and restoration of visual alignment without delay is needed. The younger the patient is when an esotropia develops and the longer the eye has been crossed without treatment, the less the chance for a complete cure.[27]

Fully Accommodative Esotropia

In the case of a fully accommodative strabismus, wearing the full optical correction, which neutralizes the hypermetropia, straightens the eyes completely.

ETIOLOGY

The etiology of this condition is overconvergence associated with the extra accommodation necessary to overcome an uncorrected hypermetropic refractive error. The condition first appears when the child actively starts to accommodate. This usually occurs at 1 to 3 years of age. However, it is possible for this condition to occur within the first 6 months of life or as late as 5 or 6 years of age.

Treatment

1. Cure the amblyopia by the methods outlined in the treatment of strabismic amblyopia (see Chapter 7).
2. Prescribe the full correction of the refractive error.
3. Monitor the fixation and vision to make sure the amblyopia does not return.
4. Check distance and near measurements with glasses on, using an accommodative fixation target in case there is a high accommodative convergence to accommodation (AC:A) ratio.
5. The patient should be followed frequently, as often as every week, until it is certain the deviation is controlled by the glasses and that amblyopia is not returning. Wearing the glasses at all times is an essential part of treatment.

Will Glasses Be Worn for the Rest of the Child's Life?

This will obviously depend on the amount of hypermetropia present. Generally, children under the age of 3 with hypermetropic spherical errors of less than 3.5 diopters have a good chance of being able to give up their glasses when they are visual adults. There may be a decrease in the hypermetropia as they get older and even if there is none, at about the age of 9 a child may be taught by an orthoptist how to control the strabismus without glasses. In other instances when the hypermetropia exceeds 4 diopters, or where there is a marked astigmatic refractive error, glasses will be necessary for clear vision as well as for keeping the eyes correctly aligned. In these cases the parents should be told it is likely that some sort of optical correction will be necessary throughout the child's life.

Orthoptic Treatment and Fully Accommodative Esotropia

Patients over 8 years of age whose refractive error is less than approximately +3.50 and who have an esotropia that is fully controlled when the glasses are worn may be helped by orthoptic exercises. The aim of this treatment would be to enable the patient to have straight eyes without glasses as well as with glasses. The child must be highly motivated to give up wearing glasses, and the parents must have the time to take the child to the orthoptist for an initial six visits at weekly or 2-weekly intervals. Less frequent visits may then be scheduled. Homework exercises are necessary between all visits. Treatment consists of ensuring that the child appreciates diplopia whenever an esotropia occurs. This is followed by teaching the child to relax accommodation without glasses so that the esotropia is eliminated and the child has blurred but single binocular vision. When the child can maintain this easily, exercises are aimed at establishing clear single binocular vision for distance without glasses and then later for near without glasses. Speed of response to this treatment is individualistic: some children can begin to leave their glasses off and maintain clear binocular vision comfortably after 6 weeks; others require several months to achieve this. Once control of the deviation has been established, the strength of the glasses may be reduced gradually and in some cases eliminated.

Partially Accommodative Esotropia

In this condition the esotropia is reduced for distance and near when glasses are worn but is not completely eliminated.

Prognosis

More judgment and common sense is needed in managing this condition than most types of strabismus. It is unlikely that a complete cure with bifoveal fusion will be achieved in these patients[27] unless:

1. They are diagnosed and treated soon after the onset, i.e., within a few weeks.
2. They are occluded using the principle of making sure the eyes are never open together until they are realigned so that both suppression and amblyopia can be eliminated.
3. The onset is later than usual (i.e., over 3 years of age), so fusion and stereopsis have developed and are fairly strongly established.

Occlusion and Surgery for a Bifoveal Cure

Immediately after the first visit, a regimen of occlusion is instituted that is aimed at eliminating suppression and amblyopia by preventing the eyes from being open together until any glasses prescribed have been obtained and worn. The patient should then return for reexamination. In a partially accommodative esotropia there will be a residual deviation. The deviation should be measured with the glasses on for distance and near fixation as well as side down and up gaze. Time should be allocated to do the surgery within the next few days. Occluding is resumed to prevent the eyes from being open together until after the operation when, hopefully, the eyes will be straight with glasses on. Surgery should be planned to slightly overcorrect the deviation by a few prism diopters with the full optical correction in place because the convergence fusional amplitude potential is much larger than the divergence fusional amplitude. Consequently, the patient can straighten the eyes to obtain fusion without difficulty.

If the eyes are slightly exotropic immediately postoperatively but the deviation later returns to a small angle esotropia, despite all these measures, it is an indication that the end result is going to be a monofixation syndrome with peripheral fusion.[28] Further attempts to eliminate this angle are futile. A small residual angle, within 10 prism diopters of being straight, should be accepted as the best possible result obtainable in this case.

Monofixation Syndrome

If the goal in management is complete cure with bifoveal fixation, it is essential to eliminate any distance angle that is not straightened by glasses. If, on the other hand, it appears to be illogical to pursue a goal of complete cure with bifoveal fusion, because the constant esotropia has been present for several months, the presence of a residual esotropia of up to 10 prism diopters is compatible with the highest quality of monofixation and peripheral fusion.[23] This syndrome is the most common end result in the treatment of all types of esotropia in which some fusion is obtained.

Treatment

Once a monofixation syndrome[24] (with the clinical characteristics described in Chapter 2) is present, it is not possible to upgrade this to bifoveal fusion.[28] Therefore, if a monofixation syndrome is firmly established in a child with partially accommodative esotropia, the goal should be to preserve the monofixation syndrome, not to try to convert this to bifoveal fixation by surgery, prisms, or any other methods. It is also important to understand that the quality of the monofixation syndrome cannot be improved by reducing the angle if it is already less than 10 prism diopters of esotropia at distance with the full optical correction in place.[28] However, esotropia significantly more than 10 prism diopters at distance with the full optical correction in place should be reduced by surgery to under 10 prism diopters. Occasionally, patients who have the fully developed monofixation syndrome may, for some reason, have an increase in the esotropia so that diplopia is experienced. If glasses (or surgery, in the absence of a refractive error) are used to return the strabismus to within 10 prism diopters of being straight, the diplopia is eliminated.

Amblyopia Associated with the Monofixation Syndrome

Usually the monofixation syndrome is associated with amblyopia of the nonfixing eye. The vision may vary from 6/6 in the nonfixing eye (versus 6/5 in the fixing eye) to as little as 6/24 and occasionally worse. The same principle applies here as in the treatment of all amblyopia in that the earlier the treatment is commenced, the better the results.

Nonaccommodative Esotropia

Occasionally, patients are seen in whom there does not appear to be any accommodative factor and in whom the esotropia is not reduced by wearing the glasses or, alternatively, in whom no refractive error is found by cycloplegic refraction.

Treatment

The same principles must be used in establishing the goal of treatment and the same occluding and surgery employed as described for partially accommodative esotropia when glasses do not eliminate the deviation.

Prism Adaptation

Occasionally, a patient with an acquired esotropia and the full optical correction in place may have a much larger angle esotropia on the prism cover test than appears to be present at a casual glance. The patient's esotropia appears to "eat up" the prism, i.e., the prism estimated as needed to neutralize the deviation is inadequate and more and more prism is required.[19,33,35] Such an esotropia may have returned to much the same angle postoperatively as was present preoperatively despite adequate surgery to eliminate the deviation. Such patients are, fortunately, rare. However, in such a situation the following technique may be employed. An increasing strength of prism is used until the esotropia is slightly overcorrected and then the appropriate Fresnel prisms are placed base out over the spectacle lenses. If amblyopia is present, the prism should be placed over the fixing eye because the slight blur produced by it may act as an occluder and therefore may diminish the amblyopia in the other eye. The patient is then seen a few days later and, if necessary, the strength of prism is adjusted. Once the esotropia and amblyopia have been eliminated for a few days, tests for fusion with the prisms in place using either the synoptophore or the Worth four-dot test are necessary. If a fusion response is obtained, surgery should be planned to eliminate this maximum angle of deviation, i.e., the amount of prism needed on the glasses in addition to the full optical correction to eliminate the esotropia. If fusion is not present, surgery should be planned for the minimum amount of deviation obtained using the simultaneous prism introduction test (see Chapter 5) with just the full optical correction in place.

Esotropia with a High AC:A Ratio (Convergence Excess)

This condition is characterized by an overconvergence associated with accommodation. Typically the esotropia at near is more than 20 prism diopters greater than the distance measurement when the full optical correction is worn and the patient is fixing an accommodative target. This condition may be present from a very early age and is frequently seen under the age of 1. Such cases may be incorrectly diagnosed as a large angle congenital esotropia if they are not tested on distance fixation. However, the parents usually report that the child's eyes are straight sometimes.

The average patient with this condition has a cycloplegic refraction of just over +2.00 diopters. Some children have no refractive error and only have an esotropia on near fixation. These children tend to be very bright, highly strung, sensitive individuals in whom the emotions can clearly be seen to play a large part in how severe their strabismus is. The more nervous and uptight they get, the more the eye tends to turn in when any accommodation is invoked. Most of these patients turn one eye in 90 prism diopters once accommodation is triggered.[30,32]

Warning: It is mandatory in cases where the diagnosis of a pure high AC:A ratio is being considered to do a nondissociating cover test for distance fixation with the full optical correction in place as described in Chapter 3. This will avoid a constant esotropia being produced by a prolonged dissociating cross-cover test and a consequent wrong diagnosis of constant esotropia instead of a high AC:A ratio.

Suppression and the High AC:A Ratio

A patient who has fusion at distance with central bifoveal fusion, or peripheral fusion with a monofixation pattern, does not experience double vision when the eyes overconverge at near. This is because the patient has done this habitually from visual immaturity and has therefore learned to suppress when the eyes overconverge. This suppression involves the whole area of the visual field of the deviating eye, which overlaps the visual field of the straight eye.[26]

Management of High AC:A Ratio

These principles only apply in those patients who have a chance of obtaining some fusion because their eyes are straight or within 10 prism diopters of being straight at distance with the full optical correction in place.[30,32] The important principle in treatment is to try to keep the eyes as straight as possible, particularly for distance, while the child is developing during the visually immature years, that is, up to the age of 8.

Because the esotropia is associated with and triggered by accommodation, any uncorrected hypermetropic refractive error in the distance prescription is a fundamental error that must be avoided. This is a case where every bit of hypermetropic refraction, even as little as 1.00 diopters, must be corrected by glasses before considering any other therapy.

The characteristics of this condition make it mandatory to examine all children with esotropia on distance fixation and not just at near fixation with the full optical correction in place so that it is not confused with a constant esotropia of large amount, which would require surgery. Surgery is generally contraindicated in the treatment of the high AC:A ratio in the visually immature age group.

The natural course of this condition is that the overconvergence associated with accommodation tends to lessen as the child grows older and may entirely disappear as the child approaches his or her teens.

Treatment

1. Prescribe the maximum plus that will allow the optimum vision.
2. Eliminate amblyopia.
3. Measure the deviation at distance with the full optical correction in place to determine the next step.

Patients with Fusion Potential

IF THE ESOTROPIA IS LESS THAN 10 PRISM DIOPTERS AT DISTANCE

If the deviation is less than 10 prism diopters at distance with the full optical correction in place, the patient has a chance of developing fusion. If the patient is visually immature, which is typical when first diagnosed, it would be logical to treat this patient with a bifocal add of equal strength in front of each eye (see discussion on bifocals later in this chapter).

IF THE ESOTROPIA IS GREATER THAN 10 PRISM DIOPTERS AT DISTANCE

If an esotropia of more than 10 prism diopters is present at distance with the full optical correction in place, the patient has virtually no chance of developing any fusion unless the deviation is reduced to under 10 prism diopters. If the patient is visually immature, surgical correction to reduce this deviation to within 10 prism diopters should be done. Recession of the medial rectus muscles would be preferred because this tends to decrease the high AC:A ratio. Following this, bifocals may be necessary (see discussion on bifocals later in this chapter).

Patients with No Fusion Potential

Patients may be seen who have had an esotropia at distance from an early age and who are, for example, 4 years of age but no fusion can be found on subjective testing. Some of these patients may have a high AC:A ratio, but there would be little advantage in prescribing bifocal glasses for such patients because they have no fusion at any distance.

Bifocals

Logic

The logic of treating a patient who has a high AC:A ratio with bifocals is that better alignment at near will improve the overall sensory and motor outcome when the child becomes a visual adult. However, there are no data to support this. A study, conducted by us, showed no sensory advantage in bifocal treatment provided the distant deviation was maintained at less than 10 prism diopters of esotropia.[32] The control at distance maintains and builds fusion. When the high

AC:A ratio decreases as the patient approaches his or her teens, the same quality of fusion at near will be found as has been present at distance all along.

Prescription

If bifocals are prescribed, it is advisable to prescribe the +3.00 executive flat-topped type fitted very high so that, with the glasses sitting properly on the nose, the bifocal segments bisect the pupils, or are even slightly higher than this (Fig. 9–1), necessitating a chin-down head position to avoid the bifocal segments when looking in the distance. Precautions need to be taken to keep the frames up on the nose, often by applying a strap or an elastic band round the back of the head to keep the glasses properly positioned. Alternatively, progressive lenses may be used provided they are fitted by an expert, but it is difficult to tell if the near addition is being used correctly. If the full distance correction has been used, +3.00 bifocal additions enable the patient to fix up to a distance of 0.33 m without having to exert accommodation. Once the patient fixes an object closer than this, accommodation will be stimulated and the eyes will overconverge. Children frequently hold interesting toys and small objects closer than 0.33 m, making the bifocals ineffective in preventing overconvergence.

If a Child Will Not Wear Bifocal Glasses

Atropine 1% eye drops to both eyes three times a week can be used so that the bifocal segments provide some obvious visual advantage at near. Once this has encouraged the habit of wearing the glasses, the drops can be discontinued.

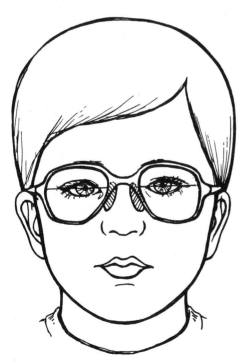

Figure 9–1. Bifocals correctly fitted so that bifocal line splits the pupil and nose pads prevent the glasses from slipping.

How Long Should the Child Use Bifocals?

Bifocal therapy should be continued at least into visual adulthood, up to the age of 8. After this time efforts should be made to try to wean the child out of the bifocals. If this is not done, one will occasionally see patients who are unable to get rid of the bifocals because they experience double vision at near without the bifocal segments and still have a significantly high AC:A ratio.

If the patient does not experience double vision when the eyes overconverge, it is not necessary to wean the patient out of the bifocals gradually. The bifocal adds can just be removed when the patient is about 10 years of age. If a significant hypermetropic (e.g., +6.0) or astigmatic refractive error is present in these children, such that they would have blurred vision if they were not wearing their glasses, an extra +1 diopter may be put into the distance correction and the bifocals removed when the child is over the age of 8. The slight blur in the distance will not be noticed, yet the patient will get better control of the esotropia at near.

Children Who Fail to Use the Bifocal Adds

Some children do not use the bifocal add easily or successfully because most of them see little, if any, visual advantage. Some children actively avoid the bifocal segment even if correctly positioned. Parents may become frustrated in trying to enforce the use of the bifocals even if atropine eye drops are used to blur the near vision without the bifocals. In such a case the bifocal adds should be removed when new glasses are needed. The child should be seen every 3 months to ensure that the distance deviation with the distance correction does not increase (decompensate). Approximately 30% of all cases with a high AC:A ratio will decompensate and require surgery to restore distance alignment with the distance correction.[21]

Why Use Bifocals at All

Our retrospective study showed no advantage in treating this condition with bifocals.[32] To our knowledge, this study is the only one that compares long-term sensory and motor results in two groups of patients with a high AC:A ratio—one group treated with bifocals, the other not. There is a need for a controlled, prospective, randomized, multicenter study to answer, conclusively, whether or not bifocals make any difference in these cases. In the meantime, because the use of bifocals is harmless, it may be safer and more logical to use them in cases with fusion potential if the patients will comply. If the proper use of bifocals does not seem achievable, the patient should be treated with single lens distance correction as needed. Reber summed this up in 1914 when he wrote that "The only claim made is that this proposed addition (bifocals) to our ordinary methods is simple and harmless and offers not only a logical sequence but a reasonable hope that a still greater number of young esotropes may not only escape the scissors but be vouchsafed the blessings of full binocular vision."[34] Unfortunately, we still lack enough evidence to make any greater claim.

Miotics

Phospholine iodide or other miotics have been used in the treatment of this condition in an attempt to reduce the high AC:A ratio.[1,14] Miotics are not as effective as bifocals and are disadvantageous because these potentially powerful drugs would have to be used on a long-term basis (at least 6–8 years). Therefore, the use of miotics is not recommended.

Patients with Straight Eyes for Distance but Markedly Esotropic at Near (Full Optical Correction in Place)

Because the high AC:A ratio tends to decrease as patients grow older and approach their teens, surgery is best left until they are approaching this age group to see whether surgery is really necessary to correct this problem. Surgery should only be considered if the patient has good central fusion or good peripheral fusion. Stereoacuity can be tested for distance by using the American Optical (A/O) Vectograph Slide or by other methods (see Chapter 4) and can be used as an indication of central fusion if stereoacuity of 60 seconds or better is obtained. Fusional amplitudes can be assessed with a synoptophore or in free space, by using a rotary prism or prism bar with distance fixation. Tests are difficult to do at near because the patient tends to overconverge. A 5-mm recession of both medial rectus muscles is indicated in those patients in whom there is no deviation at distance and an esotropia of 20 prism diopters or more at near. This will significantly reduce the high AC:A ratio in most patients.[20,37] If this operation is performed in those cases in which there is very weak fusion or no fusion, the result will be an exotropia at distance and an esotropia at near, hardly a desirable result. Therefore, the vital ingredient is good fusion.

Decompensated High AC:A Ratio (Increased Esotropia at Distance)

Sometimes patients whose eyes were straight for distance fixation will develop a deviation in excess of 10 prism diopters at distance with the full optical correction in place. Surgery is then necessary to restore the distance alignment so that fusion may develop.

Surgery for High AC:A Ratio

An esotropia that measures significantly more on near fixation compared with distance fixation, with the full optical correction in place, warrants surgery on both medial rectus muscles rather than other options if surgical treatment is indicated. As mentioned earlier in this chapter, it is absolutely essential to have all the hypermetropic refractive error corrected prior to an evaluation for surgery in these patients with a high AC:A ratio.

Follow-Up Care

Patients should be followed regularly every 3 months until they are over the age of 8. Parents should be instructed to bring a child for treatment without delay if the eyes become more convergent at distance with the full optical correction in place. The need for such urgent treatment was outlined earlier in this chapter.

Summary of the Management of the High AC:A Ratio Problem

1. If the eyes are straight or within 10 prism diopters of being straight for distance with the full optical correction in place and the patient is under 4 years of age, prescribe bifocal glasses. If the use of bifocals proves difficult, try atropine 1% eye drops to both eyes to encourage use of the bifocals. If this also fails, treat the patient just with the full optical correction needed for distance.
2. Do not use miotics.
3. Follow patients regularly every 3 months until they are 8 years of age to ensure the distance deviation with full correction does not increase. If it does, appropriate surgical correction, preferably on the medial recti, is required.
4. Start to wean the patient out of the bifocals after the age of 8.
5. Do bimedial recessions of 5 mm on teenagers with a persistent high AC:A ratio with the full optical correction in place whose eyes are straight or who have a small angle esotropia with good fusion at distance.

Esotropia without any Fusion Potential

Management

Once a patient has reached an age when subjective testing can be done (approximately 4 years) it is usually possible to determine whether or not the patient has fusion. Once the decision has been reached that fusion is not obtainable, the goal of management changes to one of obtaining the best cosmetic appearance and maintaining the best possible vision. If the strabismus has been present for many years, the child is too old to have therapy that can alter the sensory status. It is important to discuss this end point of management with the patient and parents so that they realize the disadvantages of trying to alter the sensory status.

If a child is teased repeatedly because of an obvious strabismus, surgical correction is advised. If teasing is not a problem or the strabismus is not cosmetically disturbing, no surgery should be performed. It would be logical, in all patients, to suggest waiting until the mid- to late teens, when adjustable strabismus surgery could be performed and the best possible result could be achieved. This would eliminate many operations and give the overall best appearance for the adult life of the patient. However, this is a somewhat inhumane approach in patients who have a cosmetically disturbing strabismus during school age. These factors should be taken into account before advising surgery.

Aim of Surgery in Patients with Esotropia without Fusion

The aim of surgery should be to leave an esotropia of 5 to 10 prism diopters. The logic for this is that there is a tendency for the eyes to diverge as the patients grow older. It is important to assess the angle kappa (see Chapter 5). If a positive angle kappa gives a divergent appearance, the eyes can be left with an esotropia of 10 prism diopters or more to protect from future divergence and yet still appear straight.

Emotional Esotropia

The emotional state of a patient may affect the amount of esotropia present.[25] This is commonly seen in our society with much social upheaval at the family level. A child under emotional stress may suddenly exhibit an increase in the esotropia. An esotropia that was in satisfactory cosmetic alignment may suddenly go out of alignment and look unattractive and even give rise to double vision, if the patient has fusion ability, purely on the basis of an increased emotional tone. It is essential to be aware of this in order to avoid unnecessary treatment and even surgery. The effect of the emotions is particularly likely to be exhibited in patients with a high AC:A ratio, but all types of esotropia may be increased by the emotions.

Malingering and Esotropia

A visual adult who has learned the trick of asymmetric convergence can create a situation very similar to an acquired strabismus of 30 prism diopters.

Giveaway Features of Voluntarily Produced Esotropia

1. Pupils: Always closely examine the pupils when the patient has a manifest esotropia that is suspected of being produced voluntarily because it is impossible to voluntarily converge the eyes without producing a miosis of the pupil. Some patients may complain of intermittent esotropia, but while talking they relax and their eyes straighten. The pupils can be seen to dilate under these circumstances.
2. Measurements: It is also important, if this condition is suspected, to check the measurements in side gaze. It is difficult to maintain an esotropia in side gaze voluntarily.
3. Retinoscopy: Retinoscopy also can be used to show an accommodative myopic shift in the refraction during the esotropic phase.

Esotropia Following Recovered Sixth Nerve Palsy

Patients develop a marked esotropia of the ipsilateral eye following a sixth nerve palsy. If occlusion of the unaffected eye is performed to prevent contracture of the medial rectus of the paretic eye and an apparent recovery of the lateral rectus restores full eye movement of the involved eye, a residual esotropia of 30 to 40 prism diopters frequently remains. This residual esotropia may be concomitant, showing the same measurements in side gaze to right and left and fixing either eye. If the patient is a visual adult at the onset of the palsy, good fusion potential is demonstrable. In a visually immature patient, suppression and amblyopia may occur, demanding urgent treatment. The correction of the esotropia may be achieved with adjustable strabismus surgery. Note that the timely administration of botulinum toxin to the medial rectus of the affected eye may prevent this sequela (see Chapter 13).

Acute Concomitant Esotropia

Acquired esotropia commonly appears in children 2 to 3 years of age. The onset may be sudden and is often associated with hypermetropia.There is often a family history of strabismus. At this age, children are very susceptible to suppression and amblyopia of the deviated eye. If the deviation is constant, it requires urgent treatment. One of us (JPJ) has seen the vision in a 3-year-old decrease to 6/60 in a week.

Acute esotropia occurs occasionally in a visual adult, but no suppression occurs and the deviation is concomitant. This concomitancy excludes an etiology associated with paresis or paralysis of an extraocular muscle. The strabismus is seldom associated with hypermetropia. Usually the cause remains a mystery.[5,6,11,12] Most cases are idiopathic, and the patients respond very well to surgery. The amount of surgery is calculated in the usual manner (see Chapter 16) and results in normal single binocular vision. We have only seen this idiopathic type which has an excellent prognosis and outcome. However, there is always the alarming possibility that this type of esotropia in children or adults may have resulted from a tumor of the central nervous system.[2,3,9,10,17,18,38,40,42] Tumors presumed to have caused the acute concomitant esotropia have been reported in the cerebellum, pons, corpus callosum, and hypothalamic region, but the actual mechanism remains elusive. Lyons et al.[22] reported a particularly disturbing case of a 4 and a half year old child who presented with an acute esotropia concomitant in side gaze and with a V pattern in the vertical positions of gaze. She complained of diplopia. She had no refractive error and the rest of her examination was normal. The clinical neurologic examination was normal, but neuroimaging revealed a very large midline cerebellar tumor. This case clearly demonstrates that every case of concomitant acquired esotropia should have neuroimaging in addition to a clinical neurologic examination. The youngest child (18 months) presenting with acute concomitant esotropia was reported by Jafaar et al. in 1995.[18] Wasserman reported a case of acute-onset concomitant esotropia in an 11-year-old boy, which was the presenting sign of demyelinating disease of the central nervous system. The lesion was neuroimaged in the periaqueductal gray area of the mid-brain and pons.[41]

Diagnostic Features of Acute Esotropia

The strabismus is usually large (30-60 prism diopters) and remains the same in all directions of gaze, looking up, down, side gaze, at distance, and at near. There is no difference in the deviation fixing right eye or fixing left eye. A Hess chart shows exactly comparable squares displaced equally from the center for each eye. These patients can fuse if the angle of deviation is eliminated with prisms or on a synoptophore. It is most unlikely in such a case that an acquired neurologic condition is present because there are no features of paretic strabismus. However, if this acute onset esotropia cannot be explained on the basis of a decompensated esophoria, if there is no significant hypermetropia, and if there is no family history of strabismus, a neurologic examination is necessary. Because this type of strabismus may be caused by a supranuclear acquired lesion, especially neoplasms, this possibility must be eliminated before embarking on treatment. Sometimes, these patients may have a hypermetropic refractive error, but the elimination of the strabismus with glasses is rare. Alignment of the visual axes can only be restored with surgery. The results are excellent in the absence of any neurologic disease.

Cyclic Esotropia

Cyclic strabismus may be of any type. The most common type is cyclic esotropia.[7,8,13,15,36,43] These patients characteristically have an esotropia of 30 to 40 prism diopters one day and perfectly normal straight eyes the following day. The cycles may vary in length but are usually 24 hours. This is a strange condition and not well understood. If left untreated it tends to become constant within 6 months.

Treatment

This condition frequently affects older children in whom fusion has been firmly established. They appreciate diplopia on the days when the strabismus is present and have single binocular vision with normal fusional amplitudes when the eyes are straight. A full strabismic examination should be completed in such a patient with particular attention to the correction of any refractive error.

   If the cyclic esotropia has persisted for many months, it is obviously not going to get better spontaneously and surgery should be recommended. The amount of surgery is calculated to correct the esotropia present during the strabismic cycle. Results are excellent. It does not result in a divergent strabismus one day and straight eyes the next but usually eliminates the whole strabismic problem.

Occlusion Esotropia

Occasionally an esotropia may be precipitated, in a patient who has never had any strabismus, following the interruption of binocular vision by occlusion of one eye. This is especially likely if there is an uncorrected hypermetropic refractive error and a family history of strabismus. In some of these patients the refractive error may be minimal. It is a distressing and alarming development in a patient who has never had any strabismus and is being treated for another ocular condition involving covering one eye for several days. This may occur in the treatment of unilateral corneal ulcer,[16] postoperative ptosis, or occlusion after lid surgery[4] or a swollen lid from trauma,[23] and occasionally in the treatment of anisometropic amblyopia.[39]

Treatment

Occlusion for the amblyopia may be necessary. The prescription of glasses to correct any refractive error may restore alignment and fusion. Surgery is often necessary in addition to the correction of any refractive error. The sudden appearance of this strabismus while treating another condition and the measures that are necessary to restore alignment are a shock to the patient and an embarrassment to the ophthalmologist.

Secondary Esotropia

Acquired esotropia may follow loss of fixation due to an organic lesion at the fovea. Careful examination of the fovea of the deviating eye is mandatory to exclude such lesions as retinoblastoma, toxoplasmosis, or foveal damage from trauma.

For further discussion on esotropia associated with divergence paralysis, see Chapter 13; for consecutive esotropia, see Chapter 10; and for adult esotropia, see Chapter 15.

References

1. Abraham, S.V.: The use of miotics in the treatment of convergent strabismus and anisometropia: A preliminary report. Am J Ophthalmol 32:233, 1949.
2. Anderson, D.W., Lubow, M.: Astrocytoma of the corpus callosum presenting with acute comitant esotropia. Am J Ophthalmol 69:594–598, 1970.
3. Astle, W.F., Miller, S.J.: Acute comitant esotropia: A sign of intracranial disease. Can J Ophthalmol 29:151–154, 1994.
4. Bielschowsky, A.: Lectures on Motor Anomalies. Hanover, NH: Dartmouth College Publications, 1943 (reprinted 1956).
5. Burian, H.M.: Motility clinic: Sudden onset of comitant convergent strabismus. Am J Ophthalmol 28:407, 1945.
6. Burian, H.M., Miller, J.E.: Comitant convergent strabismus with acute onset. Am J Ophthalmol 45:55, 1958.
7. Chamberlain, W.: Cyclic esotropia. Am Orthopt J 18:31, 1968.
8. Costenbader, F.D., Mousel, D.K.: Cyclic esotropia. Arch Ophthalmol 71:80, 1964.
9. De Young Smith M., Baker, J.D.: Esotropia as the presenting sign of brain tumour. Am Orthopt J 40:72–75, 1990.
10. Flynn, J.T.: Problems in strabismus management. Transactions of the New Orleans Academy of Ophthalmology, New York: Raven, 1986:456.
11. Franceschetti, A.: Le strabisme concomitant aigu. Ophthalmologica 123:219, 1952.
12. Franceschetti, A.: Bischler, V.: Strabisme convergent concomitant aigu chez l'adulte. Confin Neurol 8:830, 1947/1948.
13. Friendly, D.S., Manson, R.A., Albert, D.G.: Cyclic strabismus—Case study. Doc Ophthalmol 34:189, 1973.
14. Goldstein, J.H.: The role of miotics in strabismus. Surv Ophthalmol 13:31, 1968.
15. Helveston, E.M.: Cyclic strabismus. Am Orthopt J 23:48, 1973.
16. Holland, G.: Über den akuten strabismus convergens concomitans. Klin Monatsbl Augenheilkd 140:373, 1962.
17. Hoyt, C.S., Good, W.V.: Acute onset concomitant esotropia: When is it a sign of serious neurological disease? Br J Ophthalmol 79:498–501, 1995.
18. Jafaar, M.S., Collins, M.Z.L., Rabinowitz, A.I.: Cerebellar astrocytome presenting as acquired comitant esotropia at 18 and 27 months. In: Update on Strabismus and Pediatric Ophthalmology. Boca Raton, FL: CRC Press, 1995:597–600.

19. Jampolsky, A.: A simplified approach to strabismus diagnosis. In: Symposium on Strabismus. Transactions of the New Orleans Academy of Ophthalmology. St. Louis: Mosby, 1971:3.
20. Kushner, B.J., Preslam, M.W., Morton, G.V.: Treatment of partly accommodative esotropia with a high accommodative convergence-accommodation ratio. Arch Ophthalmol 105:815–818, 1987.
21. Ludwig, I.H., Parks, M.M., Getson, P.R., Kammerman, L.A.: Rate of deterioration in accommodative esotropia correlated to the AC:A relationship. J Pediatr Ophthalmol Strabismus 25:8, 1988.
22. Lyons, C.J., Tiffin, P.A.C., Oystreck, D.: Acute acquired comitant esotropia: A prospective study. Eye 13:617–620, 1999.
23. Noorden, G.K. von.: Binocular Vision and Ocular Motility. St. Louis: Mosby, 1990:308.
24. Parks, M.M.: The monofixational syndrome. Trans Am Ophthalmol Soc 67:609, 1969.
25. Pratt-Johnson, J.A.: Emotional factors in strabismus. Can J Ophthalmol 12:258, 1977.
26. Pratt-Johnson, J.A.: Suppression associated with esotropia with convergence excess (high AC:A ratio). Doc Ophthalmol 58:119–123, 1984.
27. Pratt-Johnson, J.A., Barlow, J.M.: Binocular function and acquired esotropia. Am Orthopt J 23:52, 1973.
28. Pratt-Johnson, J.A., Barlow, J.M.: Stereoacuity and fusional amplitude in foveal suppression. Can J Ophthalmol 10:1, 1975.
29. Pratt-Johnson, J.A., Tillson, G., Pop, A.: Suppression in strabismus and the hemiretinal trigger mechanism. Arch Ophthalmol 101:218–224, 1983.
30. Pratt-Johnson, J.A., Tillson, G.: Sensory outcome with nonsurgical management of esotropia with convergence excess (a high accommodative convergence/accommodation ratio). Can J Ophthalmol 19:220–223, 1984.
31. Pratt-Johnson, J.A., Tillson, G.: Suppression in strabismus-An update. Br J Ophthalmol 68:174–178, 1984.
32. Pratt-Johnson, J.A., Tillson, G.: The management of esotropia with high AC:A ratio (convergence excess). J Pediatr Ophthalmol Strabismus 22:238–242, 1985.
33. Prism Adaptation Study Research Group: Efficacy of prism adaptation in the surgical management of acquired esotropia. Arch Ophthalmol 108:1248, 1990.
34. Reber, W.: Concerning the use of invisible bifocals in the treatment of convergent strabismus (esotropia) in little children. Ophthalmol Rec 23:612–616, 1914.
35. Repka, M.X., Connett, J.E., Baker, J.D., Rosenbaum, A.L.: Surgery in the prism adaptation study: Accuracy and dose response. J Pediatr Ophthalmol 29:150, 1992.
36. Roper-Hall, M.J., Yapp, J.M.S.: Alternate day squint. In: The First International Congress of Orthoptists. London: Henry Kimpton, 1968:262.
37. Rosenbaum, A.L., Jampolsky, A., Scott, A.B.: Bimedial recession in high AC:A esotropia. Arch Ophthalmol 91:251–253, 1974.
38. Simon, J.W., Waldman, J.B., Couture, K.C.: Cerebellar astrocytoma: Manifesting as isolated comitant esotropia in childhood. Am J Ophthalmol 121:584–586, 1996.
39. Swan, K.C.: Esotropia following occlusion. Arch Ophthalmol 37:444, 1947.
40. Timms, C., Taylor, D.: Intracranial pathology in children presenting as comitant strabismus. In: Update on Strabismus and Pediatric Ophthalmology. Boca Raton, FL: CRC Press, 1995:593–596.
41. Wasserman, B.N.: Letter to the editor. Br J Opthalmol 83:1205–1206, 1999.
42. Williams, A.S., Hoyt, C.S.: Acute comitant esotropia in children with brain tumors. Arch Ophthalmol 107:376–378, 1989.
43. Windsor, C.E., Berg, E.F.: Circadian heterotropia. Am J Ophthalmol 67:656, 1969.

10

Exotropia

Congenital Exotropia

Congenital exotropia is much less common than congenital esotropia. It has the same general features as the congenital esotropia syndrome except that the apparent limitation of abduction and cross-fixation that occurs in some cases of congenital esotropia are not present. Whether constant exotropia is present at birth or whether it develops at about 3 months of age like congenital esotropia is not known because of the obvious difficulty in compiling data on this relatively rare condition. In this book the term *congenital exotropia* will be used.

General Features of Congenital Exotropia

Commonly, a large constant exotropia of 30 to 50 prism diopters is present. The patient's fixation usually alternates; therefore, strabismic amblyopia is rare. Dissociated vertical divergent strabismus and micronystagmus occur in some cases.

Congenital Exotropia Associated with Neurologic Problems and Syndromes

In some cases congenital exotropia is associated with other neurologic syndromes and defects, which should be sought in all cases. Hence, referral to a pediatrician is advised.

Differentiating Between Congenital Exotropia and Intermittent Exotropia

Congenital exotropia is present at all distances. The eyes are never correctly aligned. In sharp contrast, in cases of intermittent exotropia the eyes are aligned some of the time, usually at near fixation. It is therefore important to make the patient fix an interesting object at near to rule out a large intermittent exotropia with poor control. In the latter case, the eyes are intermittently aligned, especially at near fixation.

Treatment of Congenital Exotropia

PRESCRIPTION OF GLASSES

Glasses are seldom indicated before surgery. They may be indicated after surgical alignment of the eyes in cases where there is more than 1 diopter of anisometropia or astigmatism of more than 1 diopter. Hypermetropia in excess of 3 diopters or myopia in excess of 2 diopters requires spectacle correction before surgery.

OCCLUSION

Occlusion should be planned to achieve equal visual acuity unless fusion is absent on sensory testing of a cooperative patient, in which case a dominant eye with vision one line better than the nonfixing eye is the goal to prevent symptomatic alternation in adult life (see Chapter 15).

SURGERY

Surgery should be planned to align the eyes to less than 10 prism diopters of eso- or exotropia. The principles for treating micronystagmus and dissociated vertical divergent strabismus are the same as when these occur in the congenital esotropia syndrome (see Chapter 8).

Prognosis and Management Goal

The goal in management is to straighten the eyes to within 10 prism diopters before the age of 2. If this is achieved, it is possible that some peripheral fusion may be obtained.

Intermittent Exotropia

History

Intermittent exotropia usually starts before 18 months of age.[1] The condition is characterized by one eye becoming intermittently divergent. The patient is unaware of this and, because there is suppression, does not appreciate diplopia. Relatives often report that they see one of the patient's eyes drift out, particularly when the patient is sick, tired, or under emotional stress. A characteristic feature of the syndrome is the closure of the eye that diverges in bright light. Sunshine is a common stimulus. The patients do not report double vision even then but complain of discomfort.

   If the parents have seen one of the child's eyes drifting outward but the results of the examination appear normal, occluding one of the child's eyes for a prolonged period may help in detecting the exodeviation.

Etiology

There is often a family history of strabismus, but not necessarily of intermittent exotropia. The tendency toward an exodeviation is probably present from birth. Patients with a deviation of less than 20 prism diopters can usually control the deviation and so grow up with an exophoria, excellent control, and diplopia if the eyes ever do diverge. These patients are rarely seen with a frank exotropia. In contrast, if the deviation exceeds 20 prism diopters, it is likely that the patient will be unable to control the deviation all the time and so the eye is frequently divergent. Because this starts from a very early age, suppression occurs when the eye is divergent.

Suppression and Intermittent Exotropia

If diplopia is appreciated when the eye is manifestly divergent, there is a decompensating exophoria without suppression. If there is no diplopia with manifest divergence, the diagnosis is intermittent exotropia and suppression.[7,9,10]

In intermittent exotropia, suppression occurs when the eye is divergent, whether there are 2 prism diopters of exotropia or 50 prism diopters of exotropia. If the deviation is made esotropic by prisms or surgery, the patient will experience diplopia. This diplopia occurs whether the esodeviation measures as little as 2 prism diopters or as much as 50 prism diopters. Patients who are able to align their eyes perfectly intermittently are able to fuse and obtain 40 seconds of arc stereoacuity. Once suppression has been triggered by the eye drifting out, all the visual field of the deviating eye that overlaps that of the fixing eye is suppressed, that is, both nasal and temporal sides of the retina are suppressed. The only part of the visual field of the deviating eye that is not suppressed is that part that does not overlap the visual field of the fixing eye. This always includes the monocular temporal crescent. Any concept of hemiretinal suppression is incorrect. Exotropic patients have a larger binocular peripheral visual field than normal patients because of the exodeviation of the eyes. They are able to see "around the corner" more on the side of the deviating eye. If a patient with intermittent exotropia is made esotropic, in any position of gaze diplopia will be experienced, the objects being duplicated wherever the visual fields of the two eyes overlap. Crossing the vertical hemiretinal line determines whether suppression or double vision occurs everywhere the two visual fields overlap. This phenomenon is called the hemiretinal trigger mechanism[10] (see Chapter 2).

Symptoms

Occasionally, patients report that as one eye diverges, their eyes feel uncomfortable or that they close one eye, particularly in bright light. Treatment is unlikely to relieve these symptoms in adult patients with intermittent exotropia. Frequently, however, patients are unable to tell whether or not their eyes are straight. Intermittent exotropia does not usually cause headache, asthenopic symptoms, or reading problems unless there is also a convergence weakness.

Why Don't the Patients Notice the Loss of Stereopsis?

Typical cases of intermittent exotropia have 40 seconds of arc stereoacuity at near with the Titmus test. The fact that they do not seem to be aware of suddenly losing stereopsis when their eyes diverge supports the suggestion that stereopsis is probably important only at near fixation. This is where most patients with intermittent exotropia control their deviation.

Types of Intermittent Exotropia

Divergence Excess Type

This is the most common type. The deviation with the full optical correction in place is greater at distance than near fixation. The deviation may increase further at infinity with fixation on a far distant object. This deviation should be measured and recorded.

Simulated Divergence Excess (+3.0 Lenses at Near)

This term is used to describe those cases with greater exotropia at distance in whom the exotropia at near approximates that at distance when measured with the patient looking through +3.00 diopter sphere (DS) lenses. We do not routinely measure intermittent exotropias at near with +3.0 lenses in nonpresbyopic patients in addition to any distance optical correction because we wish to see the deviation as it would be in the everyday environment when accommodation is used at near. Our treatment is based on these findings. What happens to the exodeviation at near with the use of +3.0 lenses (which neutralizes accommodation) does not influence our recommendations concerning treatment. However, the findings are interesting and may help in the overall etiologic considerations.

Convergence Weakness (Convergence Insufficiency) Type of Intermittent Exotropia

This type of intermittent exotropia is characterized by the exotropia being greater at near fixation with the full optical correction in place (without the addition of +3.0 DS lenses).

Convergence weakness (convergence insufficiency) type of intermittent exotropia has all the usual signs, symptoms, and suppression of intermittent exotropia. This syndrome must not be confused with the entirely different entity of isolated convergence insufficiency (convergence weakness), in which there is diplopia when convergence "breaks," because there is no suppression (see Chapter 6). This isolated weakness of convergence usually responds well to orthoptic exercises.

Caution: Do not confuse either of these conditions with convergence paralysis, in which there is no convergence. However, confusion may arise if convergence is not assessed specifically. The patient will require approximately 25 prism diopters base-in to avoid diplopia because of the inability to converge and because of the angle subtended between the two eyes at the near fixation distance (see also Chapters 6 and 13).

Basic Type

In these cases the measurements with the full optical correction in place are similar at distance and at near.

Diagnostic Tests

Sensory tests should include assessment of vision, fusion, and stereopsis.

Tests for Suppression to Differentiate Between Exophoria and Intermittent Exotropia

The patient fixes a small light at the end of the examination room. Many intermittent exotropic deviations will become manifest spontaneously. A cover test can be used to make the deviation manifest if necessary. The patient is asked how many lights are seen at the end of the room while the eyes are divergent. If one light is seen, suppression is confirmed and intermittent exotropia is diagnosed. In contrast, an exophoria is usually well controlled under these circumstances and a divergent position of the eyes can only be obtained by a prolonged dissociating cover test. The patient must be instructed not to blink or try to control the deviation as the cover is removed from the eye. The patient with an exophoria will see two lights any time the eyes diverge. This shows the absence of suppression.

Motor Tests

A full strabismus workup is indicated, paying particular attention to the deviation for far distance (to bring out the maximum angle) as well as the deviation at 6 m and at near fixation. It is not always possible to get detailed measurements in patients at the age of 2 when surgery may be indicated. However, if repeatable measurements are obtained for infinity, at 6 m, and at near fixation in the primary position, and ductions and versions are normal, there should be sufficient information on which to base surgery.

Patients with a typical history of intermittent exotropia but in whom the condition cannot be detected can have an eye occluded for half an hour or even as long as one day and then return to the office with the occluder on. The patient fixes with the unoccluded eye, the occluder is carefully removed, and the eye behind the occluder is observed as the occluder is removed to see if it is exotropic (divergent). However, if the deviation is so well controlled that it is only manifest under these conditions it is most unlikely that treatment is indicated and the patient should be reviewed in a few months.

Stereopsis and the Monofixation Intermittent Exotropia Syndrome

If a child is old enough, special attention should be focused on stereopsis at near. Patients with the divergence excess type of intermittent exotropia should have perfect stereopsis (40 seconds of arc using the Titmus test). In a cooperative patient, stereopsis of 100 seconds or worse should make one suspicious that the patient has a monofixation intermittent exotropia. Monofixation intermittent exotropia is similar to typical intermittent exotropia except that there is imperfect stereopsis and a constant flick exotropia with the cover-uncover test when the deviation appears to be controlled. Most patients with typical intermittent exotropia control perfectly at near and show no tropia with a cover-uncover test.

Intermittent Exotropia and Unilateral Superior Oblique Palsy

A patient with superior oblique palsy and intermittent exotropia frequently does not have a head tilt because there is suppression when the eye diverges, so diplopia is not experienced. These patients present with intermittent exotropia with a vertical element, which has all the typical features of a superior oblique palsy, increasing on head tilt to the same side and on horizontal gaze to the opposite side. Some of these patients with the divergence excess type of intermittent exotropia may show a head tilt for near, where they usually control if their control of the deviation is disturbed by intermittent vertical diplopia. This may be seen in patients who have always had an intermittent exotropia and acquire a vertical strabismus in visual adulthood.

How Important Is Lateral or Side Gaze Incomitance?

Side gaze measurements often reveal less exotropia than in the primary position at the same fixation distance. Some of this may be artifactual[11] and some real. This lateral incomitance can be ignored in children under the age of 8 years, and it seems to disappear after surgery to correct the deviation in the primary position. In adults, however, it frequently persists and may be a cause for overcorrection in side gaze with resultant diplopia postoperatively (see section on Exotropia in Chapter 15).

Management and Goals of Treatment in Intermittent Exotropia

The aim of treatment is to eradicate the suppression that is characteristic of this condition and reduce or eliminate the exotropia. The only method that currently appears to be successful in eliminating suppression is to operate when the child is young, preferably under 4 years of age, and prevent any recurrence of the exotropia that stimulates the suppression. It must be remembered that an exotropia of as little as 5 prism diopters is all that is necessary to trigger suppression. Under ideal conditions, one would be able to produce a small esophoria so that when the patient was tired or relaxed his or her fusion, the eyes would not become divergent but in fact would become slightly convergent. One can seldom get reliable repeatable measurements from a patient before the age of 2 years, so, if possible, surgery should be postponed until then. Patients who undergo surgery before the age of 4 have a better prognosis than those who undergo surgery when they are 6 years of age or older, when the suppression is more entrenched.[6]

Which Patients Require Treatment?

If intermittent exotropia is first diagnosed in a patient under the age of 2 years, arrangements should be made to review the child around the age of 2 years.

At this time the parents are asked to answer four questions:

1. How frequently does the child's eye diverge when looking at distance?
2. How frequently does the child close one eye in the sunshine?
3. How frequently does the child's eye diverge when daydreaming, or when sick or tired?
4. If the parents, as adults, had the same condition as their child has at present, would they have it corrected purely from a cosmetic standpoint?

The parents should be given several months to evaluate their child so that they can feel comfortable in answering these questions. When they return, the answers usually differentiate between patients who will require treatment because their control of the deviation is poor and those who control the deviation most of the time, allowing surgery to be postponed and the patient reassessed 6 months later. It is important to realize that the control of intermittent exotropia fluctuates from one week to another. It also varies with fixation distance, lighting, and the patient's general well-being. This is why it is necessary to allow several months for the parents to evaluate the child at home. Parents who see a manifest divergence as frequently as 30 or 40 times a day (or almost always when the child looks in the distance) and who notice that the child always closes one eye in sunshine usually conclude that, if they had this condition, they would like to have it corrected purely from a cosmetic standpoint.

Treatment Options

No Treatment

Left untreated, the deviation is likely to remain approximately the same all the patient's life. Occasionally, patients have an increase in the exotropia and some patients a decrease, but in the majority of patients it remains about the same all their lives. These patients never develop strabismic amblyopia because the divergence is intermittent and, for the same reason, they will always retain their excellent stereopsis at near fixation.

Optical Treatment

In the rare cases in which the intermittent exotropia measures less than 20 prism diopters at distance fixation, prism glasses to fully neutralize the distance deviation may be prescribed, combined with -1.00 lenses to stimulate accommodative convergence. Because the prisms are base-in, the thick part of the prism is not too obvious cosmetically as it is adjacent to the nose. Plastic, not Fresnel, prisms should be prescribed for long-term use.

Comment: This method of treatment is rarely successful unless the patient is myopic and needs glasses anyway in order to see clearly. Patients who have a normal refraction cannot see any obvious advantage in wearing the glasses and will rarely use them. It is absolutely essential for the exotropia to be eliminated by the glasses and for the patient to use the glasses all the time in order to change the strabismus from an intermittent exotropia with suppression to an exophoria without suppression.

Orthoptic Treatment

ROLE OF THE ORTHOPTIST

In addition to performing a full evaluation of the motor and sensory aspects of the exotropia, as well as performing follow-up checks, the orthoptist may be able to treat some cases of small angle exotropia (primary or remaining postoperatively) if the deviation is intermittent and the patient is a visual adult. Orthoptic exercises are only of help in a small group of patients. In the past orthoptic treatment has been unfairly neglected because of the large number of treatment sessions given to poorly selected or poorly instructed patients. In our experience, in the circumstances described below, orthoptic treatment can be of benefit.

SELECTION OF PATIENTS FOR ORTHOPTIC TREATMENT

1. The deviation must be intermittent and fusion must be demonstrable.

2. The deviation should not be greater than 20 prism diopters.

3. Patient should be mature enough to understand the exercises. It is rare for patients under the age of 8 years to be mature enough to complete more than the initial stages of treatment. It is better to delay starting orthoptic treatment until the complete course can be performed.

4. Patient should be motivated. Patients who have not completed a course of exercises will often decide that orthoptic exercises will never help them. This is particularly so if the patient has been told before to do "pen push-ups" to try to improve their control of an intermittent exotropia of the convergence weakness type. Usually these patients are rechecked in several months, by which time they have become disillusioned. Pen push-ups are just the beginning of treatment. If the patient is properly instructed and really follows instructions, convergence should be markedly improved after 1 or 2 weeks, and the patient will be ready to progress to the next group of exercises. Unless the patient is really keen to try exercises, progress will be limited at best.

5. Patients should be able to attend treatment sessions lasting half an hour once a week for 6 weeks initially. At the end of this time, the patients should notice an improvement in their ability to keep their eyes aligned. If further treatment is indicated, the interval between sessions can be increased because the patient will have a greater understanding of the process and will be motivated to continue. It is unusual for a patient to require more than an additional six sessions. If there has been no progress after the initial six sessions with good patient compliance, further exercises are not indicated.

Orthoptic exercises may be of help if the patient has divergence excess type or convergence weakness type.

AIM OF ORTHOPTIC TREATMENT

1. To teach the patient to recognize when one eye begins to diverge.

2. To teach the patient how to quickly regain control of the exotropia.

3. To increase the patient's fusional amplitude and improve the near point of convergence to avoid possible symptoms from struggling to keep the eyes aligned.

Provided the cases meet the criteria already described, orthoptic treatment principles are the same as for symptomatic exophoria and convergence insufficiency, which are discussed in detail in Chapter 6.

Surgery

Surgery is the only treatment that can eliminate consistently the exotropia. The aim is to achieve a small esophoria. This change in alignment is necessary to eliminate suppression. If the angle is under 20 prism diopters and is cosmetically reasonable, surgery is usually contraindicated, but orthoptic treatment may be advised.

SURGERY IN PATIENTS UNDER THE AGE OF 3 YEARS

Because these patients are in the amblyogenic age group and it is not possible to assess them in detail subjectively, surgery should be designed to eliminate the deviation but not overcorrect it.

For divergence excess type, a bilateral lateral rectus recession is planned to fully eliminate the deviation at distance (infinity). The amount of surgery is planned according to the principles described in Chapter 16. This will inevitably produce an overcorrection at near with double vision, which should disappear within a few days of surgery. These young patients should be followed carefully in the postoperative period to make sure that the esotropia does not persist because of the risk of amblyopia developing. If a persistent esotropia is present after more than a week, base-out prism glasses should be prescribed to eliminate the deviation. The esotropia may reduce and disappear after a few weeks or months, in which case the prisms can be discontinued. If the exotropia recurs, base-in prisms are used in an attempt to prevent the return of suppression.

If the deviation is the same for distance and near, surgery should be limited to the deviating eye (recession of the lateral rectus, resection of the medial rectus). For guidelines in planning of surgery, see Chapter 16.

SURGERY IN PATIENTS OVER THE AGE OF 3 YEARS

Once the patient is old enough to cooperate with subjective testing for vision and stereopsis, surgery should be planned to produce an overcorrection of 10 prism diopters of esotropia for distance. This overcorrection usually disappears over the first 10 days after the operation and results in a higher number of cures. Patients should be followed in case the esotropia does not disappear as expected.

Treatment of Persistent Postoperative Esotropia

CONSTANT ESOTROPIA

If a constant esotropia is present for more than 1 week after surgery, alternate occlusion should be used, occluding one eye one day and the other eye the next day for a period of a further week.

If esotropia is still present at all distances after occlusion for a week, prisms should be used in patients under the age of 3 to prevent possible amblyopia. If the patient's eyes are straight at near or at distance, no treatment is needed. An older patient can be followed on a weekly basis assessing the vision. Base-out prisms are used to relieve the patient's diplopia, and then it is possible to wait another 2 months for the esotropia to subside. Provided the patient is fusing with the prisms and wears the glasses, further treatment is not urgent. Patients who remain esotropic whenever the prism glasses are removed are likely to loose the suppression, which is characteristic of intermittent exotropia after several months. Surgery in such cases is best delayed. If surgical treatment is then required for the persistent esotropia, a complete cure is likely.

CONSECUTIVE ESOTROPIA UTILIZING THE BLIND SPOT

Occasionally, an esotropia of 10 or 15 prism diopters 1 week postoperatively may increase to as much as 30 prism diopters. The reason for this is that the patient has learned to get rid of the diplopia by increasing the esotropia to use the blind spot.[4]

These patients should have a cycloplegic refraction to make sure there is no underlying hypermetropic refractive error. Glasses should be prescribed that correct any refractive error and a 15-prism diopter base-out Fresnel prism applied over each lens. Most of these patients "relax out" of the blind spot syndrome after a period of 2 months with the help of the prisms. When the patients are able to hold their eyes straight without the prisms some of the time, the prisms can be removed from one lens; after another 2 months, the prisms can be removed from the other lens. Patients who refuse to wear the glasses will need surgery to eliminate the consecutive esotropia. This rare occurrence must not discourage planning for surgical overcorrection where appropriate.

SURGERY FOR PERSISTENT ESOTROPIA THAT DOES NOT RESPOND TO PRISMS

The patient should be evaluated like a new case, with measurements in all positions of gaze. Surgery should then be planned on the measurements found and not on the previous surgery performed. For example, if a patient had intermittent divergent strabismus with a divergence excess type measuring 25 prism diopters at distance and 10 prism diopters at near, initial surgery would be a recession of both lateral rectus muscles of 6 mm. If a persistent esotropia of 20 prism diopters remained at both distance and near with the full optical correction in place after 6 months, a recession of the medial rectus of 4 mm and an advancement of the lateral rectus of 4 mm would be planned for one eye.

BOTULINUM TOXIN FOR PERSISTENT CONSECUTIVE ESOTROPIA PRESENT AFTER 1 MONTH

Persistent consecutive esotropia in a patient with good fusion potential and normal ductions may be treated with an injection of botulinum toxin into one medial rectus muscle. This is rarely considered before at least 1 month postoperatively. We have not had personal experience in using this form of treatment, but it seems logical.

Treatment for Recurrence of Intermittent Exotropia

If the exotropia has recurred, base-in prisms can be used[2] with minus lenses[8] to help the patient maintain fusion as much of the time as possible. Base-in prisms that neutralize the full distant deviation can be combined with −1.0 lenses to stimulate some accommodative convergence. This is very acceptable if the patient is already myopic or wearing glasses, an addition of −1.0 simply being added to the prescription as well as the prisms. This can be used as a temporary measure to stimulate fusion for a few months or, if the angle is under 20 prism diopters, may be continued for years. Some patients may finally achieve a cure.[2,8] Although base-in prisms of up to 10 prism diopters over each eye are cosmetically acceptable because the thick part of the glasses is adjacent to the nose, compliance with full-time wear of the glasses is unlikely if the child does not need glasses ordinarily to see.

More surgery should be considered after a few months if the patient is under the age of 8 years, unless the prism therapy is working well and the patient is wearing the glasses constantly.

If the patient is a visual adult, a sensory cure is unlikely and the decision to reoperate should be based on cosmesis. The patient is fully evaluated. If divergence excess is still present, the lateral recti can be recessed as far as 10 mm from the insertion without seriously reducing abduction, particularly if some months have elapsed since the previous surgery to allow the previously recessed lateral rectus to "take up the slack." If more correction is required, a resection of one or both medial recti should be included. Calculation would be based on the method outlined in Chapter 16.

If the recurrence of the intermittent exotropia measures approximately the same at distance and near, a resection of both medial rectus muscles should be done. The amount should be calculated according to the principles in Chapter 16.

Problem of the Small-Angle Intermittent Exotropia Under 20 Prism Diopters

This is unusual because most patients, with this small of an angle, do not have the suppression characteristics associated with intermittent exotropia but have an exophoria. If stereopsis at near is below normal, consider a monofixation intermittent exotropia. However, one sometimes sees patients with a small intermittent exotropia with all the typical features. When considering surgery, it is important to remember that patients with broad epicanthal folds may well complain of looking cross-eyed, when the eyes are perfectly aligned postoperatively. Empirically these patients are difficult to cure and recurrence is common. One should be reluctant to operate on them if their cosmesis is reasonably satisfactory. The orthoptic treatment discussed earlier this chapter should be considered.

Criteria for Cure of Intermittent Exotropia

When a patient who has had treatment for intermittent exotropia is being evaluated, the appropriate corrective lenses should be worn by the patient if there is a significant refractive error.

The patient is cured if the following criteria are met[5]:

1. There is no manifest deviation in any position of gaze or at any distance.

2. There is no winking or closing of one eye in sunshine or bright light.

3. There is stereopsis of 60 seconds of arc or better using the American Optical Vectograph or other test at distance.

4. There are convergent and divergent fusional amplitudes and diplopia when these are exceeded.

5. There is a near point of convergence of better than 8 cm.

6. There is central fusion with amplitudes using a major amblyoscope such as a synoptophore and fusion slides that have central controls and subtend a visual angle less than 5°.

The presence of these criteria confirms that the suppression originally present when the exodeviation was manifest has been removed by treatment. It is important that these criteria are maintained for at least a year after treatment. Recurrence after 1 year is possible but most unusual. However, recurrence in the first 6 months postoperatively is, unfortunately, common.

All cases of intermittent exotropia (except the uncommon monofixation exotropia) have fusion with 40 seconds of arc using the Titmus stereotest at near before any treatment is commenced. Using this as part of the criteria for cure is fallacious.

Treatment of the Closure of One Eye in Sunshine

This is often the most refractory symptom and sign to cure. Commonly patients meet all other criteria for cure but this problem still persists. It is alleviated by wearing sunglasses whenever the problem occurs.

Monofixation Intermittent Exotropia

This syndrome may be present before treatment has started. The diagnosis is usually missed unless the patient is old enough to do the Titmus stereotest reliably at reading distance. This will show imperfect stereopsis of 100 seconds or worse, in contrast to patients with intermittent exotropia who record stereopsis of 40 seconds of arc before any treatment. In addition, whereas a quick relatively nondissociating cover-uncover test at near fixation reveals no tropia in the typical case of intermittent exotropia, an exotropic flick is present in cases of monofixation intermittent exotropia. Usually a slight degree of amblyopia (of half or one line Snellen acuity) is present in the nondominant eye. Some peripheral convergence and divergence fusional amplitudes are present. The patient may not close one eye in sunshine.

Because these differences can usually only be detected in a cooperative child who is over 4 years of age, patients who undergo surgery before this age may have had this undetected syndrome preoperatively. It is also possible that the persistence of a consecutive esotropia following surgery in a patient under 6 years of age may have caused the suppression of one fovea, but for the reasons outlined above this is difficult to prove and is probably rare. In any event, eso- or exotropia of less than 10 prism diopters with the monofixation syndrome is still a satisfactory end result because this is a stable situation with some convergence and divergence fusional amplitudes. Many of the patients with the monofixation intermittent exotropia do not close or wink one eye in sunshine.

This good result in the monofixation syndrome with peripheral fusion should not be confused with the limited improvement associated with a reduction of the angle of the manifest exodeviation in typical intermittent exotropia. In the latter case, suppression will persist if any exotropia remains, as will the unattractive closure of one eye in sunshine. The manifest intermittent exodeviation may increase in some of these patients to near preoperative findings 1 year after surgery.

It is impossible to assess the results of the treatment of strabismus if the only criteria given for a so-called satisfactory result is motor alignment to within 10 prism diopters and no sensory information is provided.

Prognosis for Intermittent Exotropia

Surgical alignment of the eyes, under the age of 4 years should give a complete cure in over 50% of cases.[6]

Convergence Paralysis

This usually presents as an exodeviation of 25 to 30 prism diopters at near with straight eyes at distance (see also Chapters 6 and 13).

Consecutive Constant Exotropia (Following an Esotropia)

1. If the patient has good fusion potential, an esotropia is often best treated by surgical overcorrection of up to 10 prism diopters. If an exotropia is present in the immediate postoperative period, even if up to 30 prism diopters, it may not be a permanent problem provided that adduction is normal or is only slightly weak in each eye. Sometimes a strange condition of "muscle shock" appears to exist. This seems to recover a month or so after the operation and result in an excellent alignment of the eyes (see Chapter 17). It is therefore wise, provided that adduction is normal, to wait 2 months before reoperating, provided the patient is older than 4 years, when vision can be monitored and a permanent change of fusion is most unlikely. During this period active duction and convergence exercises can be performed but no other treatment is required.

2. If the patient is under the age of 2 years and has fusion potential, and if a consecutive exotropia of more than 10 prism diopters is constantly present, surgery should be undertaken to realign the eyes to within 10 prism diopters of orthotropia and give the child a chance of developing peripheral fusion. A decision about what surgery to do should be based on a thorough reassessment of the strabismus, refraction, etc. These results, rather than what surgery was done before, determine what to do.

3. Patients with onset before 6 years of age and with no fusion potential usually had congenital esotropia with overcorrection postoperatively. If adduction is near normal, the decision of whether or not to perform more surgery should be based purely on the desire for improved cosmesis. At least 2 months should be allowed to elapse following the previous surgery before further surgery is considered.

4. In visually adult patients with no fusion potential, the patient who develops a consecutive exotropia over the age of 8 years may experience diplopia (see Chapter 19). Should this persist, surgery may be needed to restore esotropia and eliminate the diplopia.

Large Angle Consecutive Exotropia

If an unexpected 70-prism diopter exotropia follows surgery for esotropia, the possibility of a slipped medial rectus should be ruled out by making sure the suspect eye can adduct well past the straight ahead midline position (see also Chapters 16 and 17).

Treatment of Consecutive Exotropia

It is important to assess the deviation in every direction of gaze. It is also important to do a cycloplegic refraction, particularly if a patient with consecutive exotropia has been treated elsewhere.

Some of these patients may have had their hypermetropic glasses removed in an effort to control the exotropia. If, for instance, glasses to correct a +4.0 refractive error are needed, it is important to be able to assess the effect of such glasses on the position of the eyes before deciding what treatment is appropriate. Some patients who have developed consecutive exotropia under the age of 6 lose the suppression associated with their original esotropia and develop suppression associated with the consecutive exotropia. These patients will appreciate diplopia if their eyes are put back on the esotropic side of being straight, so the aim of surgery is to cosmetically straighten the eyes but leave them with an exotropic flick. It is important to check for this phenomenon by simulating esotropia with a base-in prism preoperatively.

A, V, and X Patterns and Exotropia

An A, V, or X pattern may be combined with an exotropia. Details of diagnosis and treatment of these patterns are provided in Chapter 11.

Exotropia in Adults

Exotropia in adults has special features that require special attention (see Chapter 15).

Secondary Exotropia

This is usually defined as an exotropia secondary to loss of fixation in an eye from an organic cause. Examples include a cataract or an organic amblyopia from a lesion in the retina, such as a retinoblastoma.

Management

The fundus should be examined to detect treatable or organic causes of loss of fixation. Ductions and versions and the full motility examination should be done, and if visual acuity is good enough, a sensory evaluation should also be done. If there is no treatable foveal condition and no evidence of retinoblastoma, the angle kappa of the fixing eye should be assessed (see Chapter 5). Surgery should be planned to leave the patient with a small angle esotropia without diplopia, particularly if they have a positive angle kappa. An adjustable suture technique should be used if the patient is old enough.

References

1. Costenbader, F.D.: The physiology and management of divergent strabismus. In: Allen, J.H., ed. Strabismic Ophthalmic Symposium 1. St. Louis: Mosby, 1950:353.
2. Hardesty, H.H.: Management of intermittent exotropia. Binocular Vision Q 5:145, 1990
3. Noorden, G.K. von.: Binocular vision and ocular motility. St. Louis: Mosby, 1990:324.
4. Pratt-Johnson, J.A.: Prisms in the management of surgically overcorrected strabismus. Am Orthopt J 26:7, 1976.
5. Pratt-Johnson, J.A.: Intermittent exotropia: What constitutes a cure? Am Orthopt J 42:72, 1992.
6. Pratt-Johnson, J.A., Barlow, J.M., Tillson, G.: Early surgery in intermittent exotropia. Am J Ophthalmol 84:689, 1977.
7. Pratt-Johnson, J.A., Pop, A., Tillson, G.: The complexities of suppression in intermittent exotropia. In: Mein, J., Moore, S., eds. Orthoptics Research and Practice. London: Kimpton, 1979:172.
8. Pratt-Johnson, J.A., Tillson, G.: Prismotherapy in intermittent exotropia: A preliminary report. Can J Ophthalmol 14:243, 1979.
9. Pratt-Johnson, J.A., Tillson, G.: Suppression in strabismus: An update. Br J Ophthalmol 68:174, 1984.
10. Pratt-Johnson, J.A., Tillson, G., Pop, A.: Suppression in strabismus and the hemiretinal trigger mechanism. Arch Ophthalmol 101:218, 1983.
11. Repka, M.X., Kyle, A.A.: Lateral incomitance in exotropia: Fact or artifact? J Pedriatr Ophthalmol Strabismus 28:125, 1991.

11

A, V, Y, and X Pattern Strabismus

The letters A, V, or X are used to indicate a changing pattern of horizontal strabismus when looking up and looking down. Some strabismologists distinguish between the V and Y patterns, the Y pattern being used for eyes that go out in up gaze but maintain approximately straight alignment in the primary and down gaze positions. We include the Y under the V pattern in this book. The letters may be used to describe a pattern in an esotropia or an exotropia. It is essential that the examiner has completed the workup for strabismus as outlined in Chapter 3 and, where indicated, the workup for paretic strabismus as indicated in Chapter 13 in order to detect the presence of one of these patterns. The presence of one of these patterns may influence the planned treatment.

Specific Precautions in Testing

1. Is a chin-up or chin-down head position present? If so, this could be a clue to the presence of nystagmus or an A, V, or X pattern. A reduction in the deviation with the preferred head position would allow the patient to fuse (see Chapter 18).

2. The full optical correction should be worn and the deviation measured in the primary position at 6 m, chin down with the patient looking up, as far as possible and, then, with the chin up looking down below the horizontal meridian at 6 m to simulate the reading position and that needed to negotiate stairs, to ski, etc. The fixation test object remains stationary at 6 m and the patient either tilts the chin approximately 20° up or 30° down. If the patient is wearing glasses, the up and down gaze positions may be limited by the edges of the spectacle lenses (frames). Measurements with fixation at 6 m are important to avoid a misdiagnosis that may result from accommodative influences on the deviation at the reading distance.

3. If the patient wears glasses, once the diagnosis has been made on the basis of measurement at a distance of 6 m with the glasses on, it may be useful to remove the glasses to see what sort of pattern results at near and at distance, when the patient looks up as far as possible and then down as far as possible.

This may provide additional information but it must never be used on its own as the criteria for determining what or how much surgery to perform.

4. If a V pattern is present, the versions must be checked for overaction of both inferior oblique muscles, presumably due to weakness of both superior oblique muscles.

5. If an A pattern is present, the versions must be checked for overaction of both superior oblique muscles, which may be associated with weakness of both inferior oblique muscles.

6. In intermittent exotropia, the possibility that the appearance of an A or V may be due to the patient controlling the deviation more easily in the primary position than up gaze (giving an imitation of a V or in down gaze simulating an A pattern) must be excluded. This variation in control may be just part of the intermittency of the exotropia that happens to be worse in looking up or looking down rather than the influence of an A or V syndrome. It is an easy trap to fall into and is best avoided by relying on the measurements of the prism and cross-cover test in the primary position at 6 m and on up and down gaze with the full optical correction in place.

When Is It Necessary to Treat the Pattern?

To Improve Head Position

Often a patient is disturbed by a chin-up or chin-down head position adopted for fusion. This is a common reason for treating the V esotropia present in bilateral superior oblique palsy, where the patient can usually only obtain fusion in up gaze (see Fig. 12–5A). The most important practical positions for comfortable fusion are straight ahead and down gaze.

To Achieve Fusion

If the patient has fusion potential, treating the pattern allows the patient to achieve fusion over a wider field of vision.

Caution: A tenotomy of both superior obliques may be contraindicated in A exotropia if the patient has fusion because a vertical element may be induced (see also the section on Surgery for the A/V Syndrome later in this chapter).

Cosmetic Improvement in V Exotropia

In the absence of fusion, cosmetic improvement is most often needed in a V exotropia with obvious overaction of both inferior obliques. This V pattern may be more cosmetically disturbing than an A pattern exotropia because in the latter the diverging eyes will be largely covered by the upper lids in down gaze. A myectomy of both inferior obliques is indicated for the V pattern exotropia (see the section on Surgery for the A/V Syndrome later in this chapter).

To Prevent Recurrence of A Exotropia without Fusion

If an exotropia of 35 prism diopters or more is present in the primary position, superior oblique overactions should always be sought specifically. The long-standing exodeviation may have resulted in some contracture of the superior oblique with resultant overaction and an A pattern. If overaction is present and the 35-prism diopter deviation increases by more than 20 prism diopters in down gaze, both superior obliques should be weakened by a tenotomy in addition to the horizontal surgery necessary to improve the exotropia in the primary position. If this A pattern is ignored, recurrence of the exotropia in the primary position is likely. Horizontal rectus muscle surgery should be planned to allow for the additional 10-prism diopter esotropic effect in the primary position and 20- to 30-prism diopter esotropic effect in down gaze from the tenotomy of both superior obliques (see ensuing section on Surgery for the A/V Syndrome).

Surgery for the A/V Syndrome

The V Pattern with Bilateral Inferior Oblique Overaction

MYECTOMY OF BOTH INFERIOR OBLIQUE MUSCLES

This operation involves excising a small ±5 mm section of the inferior oblique between the inferior rectus and lateral rectus muscles (see Fig. 12–3). The effect of bilateral inferior oblique myectomies on the horizontal alignment is as follows:

1. Twenty prism diopters of esotropia in up gaze, thereby reducing an exotropia in upgaze by 20 prism diopters.
2. No effect on the deviation in the primary or down gaze positions.
3. Sometimes a small vertical strabismus may result immediately after a bilateral inferior oblique myectomy but this rarely persists for more than a week or two.

The A Pattern with Bilateral Superior Oblique Overaction

TENOTOMY OF BOTH SUPERIOR OBLIQUE MUSCLES

The tendon should be isolated under direct vision between the trochlea and the medial border of the superior rectus (see Fig. 14–3). The tendon and sheath should then be cut through with a cautery. It is important not to dissect widely or strip the sheath off. This produces the desired weakening effect but usually does not result in a paralysis of the superior oblique muscle because the many fascial connections in and around this part of the superior oblique tendon allow some recovery of action of the superior oblique. The effect of bilateral superior oblique tenotomies is as follows:

1. The effect on horizontal alignment is to produce approximately 0 to 10 prism diopters of esotropia in the primary position and 20 to 40 prism diopters esotropia in down gaze relative to the amount of overaction present. This therefore reduces an exotropia in down gaze by 20 to 40 prism diopters.
2. There is no effect on the horizontal alignment in up gaze.
3. Sometimes a significant vertical strabismus may result, which is disturbing to a patient with fusion ability and may result in a head tilt to preserve fusion. This operation cannot be reversed. For these reasons such surgery is seldom in-

dicated if the patient has good fusion. Instead, a silicone expander can be used to weaken the tendon of the superior oblique as first described by Wright.[1] He maintains that it is possible to relocate the tendon if another adjustment is required.

HORIZONTAL RECTUS MUSCLE TRANSPOSITION IN ABSENCE OF OBLIQUE DYSFUNCTION

Rules:

1. The medial rectus muscles should be moved vertically half a tendon width in the direction of greatest esotropia (or least exotropia) that is up in the A pattern and down in the V pattern (Fig. 11–1).

2. The lateral rectus muscles should be moved vertically half a tendon width in the direction of greatest exotropia (or least esotropia) that is up in the V pattern and down in the A pattern (Fig. 11–1). The approximate effect on the pattern is a reduction of the pattern by about 10 to 15 prism diopters.

3. This effect can be increased by recessing the upper or lower margin of the appropriate transposed horizontal muscle insertion 2 mm more in the direction that more weakening is required, for example, V esotropia in bilateral superior oblique palsy (see Fig. 12–7).

The X Pattern

Occasionally a patient is seen with both superior and inferior oblique overaction resulting in a combination of an A and V pattern. No treatment in these cases is indicated because the patients are usually fusing in the primary position and it is usually impossible to enlarge their field of single binocular vision.

Tight Lateral Rectus Syndrome

Sometimes tight lateral rectus muscles from previous surgery or a congenital anomaly may produce an X pattern. These patients rarely require treatment because most of them fuse in the primary position. The usual techniques of helping to alleviate an A or V pattern do not work if it is due to a tight lateral rectus muscle. Slackening off the lateral rectus muscles and doing whatever else is necessary to remedy the resultant effect may improve the muscle balance.

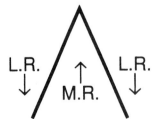 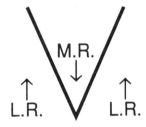

Figure 11–1.   Directions to move horizontal recti for treatment of A and V syndromes.

Summary of Management of A and V Patterns

1. Observe the special precautions in testing outlined in this chapter.
2. Consider if it is necessary to treat the pattern.
3. Operate on the inferior oblique muscles if they are overacting in V patterns.
4. Operate on the superior obliques if they are overacting in A patterns, except when fusion is present; in these cases, consider using Wright's silicone expander.[1]
5. Transpose the horizontal recti in all other cases.

Reference

1. Wright, K.W.: Superior oblique silicone expander for Brown's syndrome and superior oblique overaction. J Paediatr Ophthalmol Strabismus 28:101–107, 1991.

12

The Patient with a Vertical Strabismus

The Four Golden Rules

1. A vertical strabismus is caused by a superior oblique palsy until proved otherwise. In many clinician's experience it is the most common cause of a vertical deviation.[15]

2. A superior oblique palsy is congenital until proved otherwise. In many clinician's experience it is the most common cause of a vertical deviation.[15] It may not be obvious that the palsy is congenital in origin. The patient may deny having noticed anything wrong with his or her eyes or experiencing diplopia until recently when the palsy began decompensating. The patient usually has a compensatory head posture but may not be aware of it. However, friends and family may comment that they had always noticed it. The patient should be asked for early childhood photographs in an effort to document a consistent head tilt and prove the early presence of the paresis. Sometimes, a patient may have noticed double vision over many years for a few moments on first awakening after a night's sleep or after an alcoholic drink but not at any other time. Some patients with a pronounced head tilt due to congenital superior oblique palsy may have facial asymmetry, the larger half being on the side of the hypertropia caused by the weak superior oblique. Torsion is seldom a symptom in patients with congenital cases, in contrast to acquired cases, who complain of torsion.

3. A superior oblique palsy is traumatic if not congenital. A head injury is involved. However, it need not be a serious head injury. It is not necessary for the patient to lose consciousness for a head injury to cause a superior oblique palsy.

4. If the superior oblique palsy is not congenital, decompensated congenital, or traumatic in origin, a neurologic consultation to exclude intracranial neoplasm and other acquired lesions is essential.

Unilateral Superior Oblique Palsy

Classic Features of a Superior Oblique Palsy

1. There is a head tilt to the opposite shoulder (Fig. 12–1A).
2. The affected eye is hypertropic when the head is straight (Fig. 12–1B).

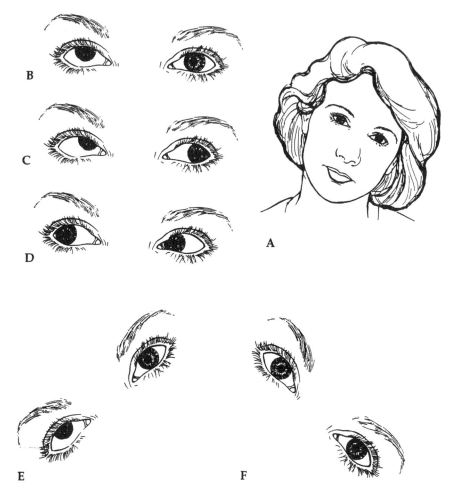

Figure 12–1. Right superior oblique palsy fixing with normal left eye. (*A*) Head tilt to left shoulder, no vertical imbalance. (*B*) Right hypertropia with head straight. (*C*) Right hypertropia increases on gaze left. (*D*) Right hypertropia disappears in gaze right. (*E*) Right hypertropia increases on tilt right. (*F*) Right hypertropia disappears on tilt left.

3. There is an overaction of the inferior oblique in the affected eye. This results in an increase of the deviation in gaze to the same side as the head tilt, i.e., away from the affected side (Fig. 12–1C).
4. There is a positive Bielschowsky head tilt test with resultant increase of the hypertropia in tilting the head to the affected side (Fig. 12–1E).

Unusual Presentation of a Superior Oblique Palsy

The patient will present with a hypotropia of the unaffected eye instead of the expected hypertropia of the affected eye in a classic superior oblique palsy (Fig. 12–2B) The patient has all the features of a superior oblique palsy, including the head tilt (Fig. 12–2A), except that the patient prefers to fix with the affected eye, the eye with the superior oblique palsy.

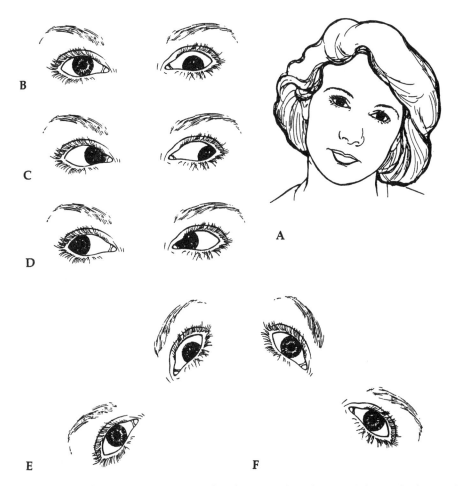

Figure 12–2.   Right superior oblique palsy fixing with right eye. (*A*) Head tilt to left shoulder, no vertical imbalance. (*B*) Left hypertropia with head straight. (*C*) Left hypertropia increases on gaze left. (*D*) Left hypertropia disappears in gaze right. (*E*) Left hypertropia increases on tilt right. (*F*) Left hypertropia disappears on head tilt left.

Example: The patient with a right superior oblique palsy whose right eye is dominant will present with a left hypotropia that becomes more marked in left gaze and in head tilt to the right (Figs. 12–2C and E). The classic features of a right superior oblique palsy can be seen immediately if the Parks' three-step test is applied or if the patient is forced to fix with the left eye (Fig. 12–1).

Diagnosis

A standard complete assessment and measurement of the strabismus in all positions of gaze should be performed, with particular emphasis on the following.

DOES THE PATIENT TILT THE HEAD TO OBTAIN FUSION AND AVOID DIPLOPIA?

If the patient tilts the head to obtain fusion and avoid diplopia:

1. The patient's head should straighten if one eye is occluded. However, it might not straighten completely if the patient is an adult.

2. The patient should be able to fuse with the preferred head position and unable to fuse with the head in the opposite position.

3. The cover test should show no manifest vertical deviation with the head in the preferred position but, when the head is held straight or in the opposite position, a manifest or increased latent vertical strabismus is present. Occasionally, in those patients who have only peripheral fusion, a small manifest vertical or horizontal deviation may be present even with the head in the preferred position. In addition, the patient with peripheral fusion is less bothered by diplopia when fusion is disrupted and may only complain of blurring of the vision.

4. If the patient is old enough, subjective assessment of diplopia using a red filter in front of one of the patient's eyes and a light as a fixation target should be done in the nine positions of gaze to find out where the vertical separation of the images is maximal. This may be particularly valuable in assessing a patient who has already had some corrective surgery and may help in determining the next procedure.

TESTS FOR TORSION

These include the double Maddox rod, the Bagolini striated glasses, or a major amblyoscope such as the synoptophore. A person with normal fusion is able to adapt to at least 10° of torsion. The cortical sensory system allows this. Therefore, there are no compensatory cyclovergence movements on the synoptophore when the fusion target presented to one eye is torted.

Double Maddox Rod Test. Two Maddox rods, preferably a red and a white, in a trial frame are used. The red one is placed in front of one eye and the white one in front of the other eye in such a way that the cylinders are vertical in front of each eye and the patient sees two lines horizontally through the light. The patient is then asked to make the two lines parallel by rotating one Maddox rod in the frame, which is marked in degrees.

Interpretation of test: It is important to remember the diplopia rules in the interpretation of diplopia reported by the patient. The "diplopic" image seen by the deviated eye will always be projected in the opposite direction to the deviation of the eye; e.g., if an eye is up (hypertropic) the image will be down, if the eye is in (esotropic) the image will be out (uncrossed). The patient will see the horizontal line tilted inward with the inner end of the line tilted down toward the nose if there is excyclotorsion. In order to make the lines parallel, the patient will rotate the lever on the Maddox rod downward on the temporal side, in other words, rotating the lever in an excyclo fashion. To interpret the result, note the direction in which the patient has to move the lever to make the lines parallel; if this is outward, there is an excyclotorsion. The measurement can be read in degrees from the dial.

Bagolini Striated Glasses in a Trial Frame to Measure Torsion. These are used in a similar fashion to the double Maddox rods. The test allows the examination of torsion in a more natural environment, whereas the double Maddox rod disrupts fusion and measures torsion without any fusional influence.

The Synoptophore. Although not readily available in every office, this is the most accurate way to measure torsion in each eye. Specially designed dissimilar slides are used, and the patient is asked to try to superimpose them (see Fig. 4–4B). The synoptophore arm in front of the deviating eye is adjusted horizontally, vertically, and torsionally until both images are superimposed and upright. Here again the patient sees the image on the slide tilted in the opposite direction to the torsion. The angle and type of deviation can be read off a scale for each type of deviation. The synoptophore can be used to measure the deviation in any direction of gaze with either eye fixing. It is particularly useful for measurements in the primary position and on 25° of down gaze where the torsion effects are usually greatest.

The Hess Chart. Unless the test is specially adapted, the amount of torsion cannot be calculated.

TORSION

Humans use the torsional muscles of the eye to keep torsion within tolerable limits during the complex eye movements to all gaze positions. Torsion suddenly becomes apparent when the fusion target is torted somewhat in excess of 10°. Torsion usually is not noticed by patients with a congenital superior oblique palsy because they have adapted to it. If torsion is a prominent subjective symptom, it means that the superior oblique palsy is acquired. Torsion is only noticed by a patient with an acquired superior oblique palsy when fusion is disrupted, resulting in diplopia. Once the patient fuses, torsion is no longer noticed. If torsion exceeds 15° it may be a barrier to fusion.

If patients with excyclotorsion cannot fuse when the horizontal and vertical alignment have been neutralized by prisms in free space or on a synoptophore, the conclusion is that the excyclotorsion by itself is a factor preventing fusion.[22] In our experience, this is indicative of a bilateral superior oblique palsy. In such cases, treatment needs to be chosen that will alleviate the torsion as well as the other features of the strabismus.[22]

The superior oblique muscle is a primary intorter of the eye, particularly when the eye is looking down. If a weakness of the superior oblique muscle is suspected, it is important to test the patient for excyclotorsion, particularly in down gaze. This can be done, as already described, by using the double Maddox rod, the Bagolini striated glasses, or the synoptophore. The synoptophore is the easiest and most accurate way to test torsion in down gaze, and unlike the Maddox rod or Bagolini glasses, it can determine whether or not torsion is a barrier to fusion.

Treatment of Unilateral Superior Oblique Palsy

PRISMS

Occasionally the measurements in a superior oblique paresis of long-standing may be sufficiently concomitant to warrant a trial of prisms, especially if the patient already wears glasses all the time. This set of circumstances is unusual.

SURGERY: GENERAL PRINCIPLES

In long-standing cases the aim is to undercorrect the vertical deviation because the patient has built up the fusional amplitude over the years to cope with the hypertropia of the affected eye and will have no vertical fusional amplitude if this eye is hypotropic after surgery.

In large vertical deviations it is always safer to proceed one muscle at a time, waiting to assess the effect of this for 2 months after surgery before reassessing the patient and considering a further procedure.

Caution: Great respect for the inferior rectus muscle is necessary. It is unforgiving. If possible, and if proper indications are present, an inferior oblique myectomy or superior rectus recession rather than a recession of the inferior rectus should be performed. However, one should not shy away from surgery on the inferior rectus muscle if it appears to be the correct and best procedure. It is important, however, to undercorrect the deviation.

Ipsilateral Inferior Oblique Weakening Procedures. If an overaction of the antagonist inferior oblique is present as well as a hypertropia of 5 prism diopters or more in the primary position with the head straight, the treatment of choice is a myectomy of the inferior oblique muscle. Approximately 5 mm of muscle between the inferior rectus and lateral rectus muscles should be cut out (Fig. 12–3). Alternative surgery is a recession of the inferior oblique muscle. This is more difficult to perform and offers no particular advantage.

A standard myectomy of the inferior oblique is easy to perform. The conjunctiva is incised in the inferior fornix between the inferior and lateral rectus muscles approximately 6 mm from the limbus. The assistant surgeon places a strabismus hook around the inferior and lateral rectus muscles, and the eye is pulled up. These strabismus hooks are used not only for traction and exposure but also for identification so that the surgeon is certain that the myectomy is performed on the inferior oblique muscle and not, inadvertently, on the inferior or lateral rectus muscles.[20] With the eye held up, a good light is directed into the depths of the wound to visualize directly the inferior oblique around which a third strabismus hook is passed by the surgeon (Fig. 12–3A). The assistant now removes the hooks from the inferior and lateral recti. A second strabismus hook is placed under the inferior oblique muscle. It is essential that both hooks pass around the whole belly of the inferior oblique muscle (Fig. 12–3B). If a small slip of the muscle is missed (Fig. 12–3C), the muscle will join up again, rendering the procedure ineffective. The two strabismus hooks around the inferior oblique muscle are separated by approximately 5 mm and mosquito clamps placed across the muscle adjacent to each hook. The hooks are removed and the muscle between the mosquito clamps is excised. The ends are cauterized and allowed to retract into the lower fornix.

The inferior oblique muscle is very forgiving and usually achieves just the right amount of correction. The maximum effect seldom exceeds 20 prism diopters of hypertropia in the primary position with the head straight. If hypertropia in excess of 20 prism diopters is present, only a myectomy of the inferior oblique should be performed and the patient completely reevaluated 2 months after this surgery. Frequently, a smaller residual deviation can be controlled comfortably by the patient, in which case no further treatment is indicated. The same procedure is performed for vertical deviations of 5 to 20 prism diopters, the muscle amazingly growing onto the eyeball again in just the correct position for the requisite amount of weakening. Inferior oblique action has usually returned 3 weeks after surgery.

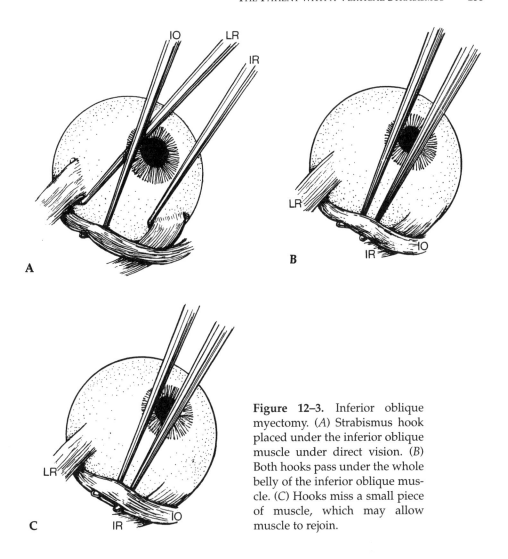

Figure 12–3. Inferior oblique myectomy. (*A*) Strabismus hook placed under the inferior oblique muscle under direct vision. (*B*) Both hooks pass under the whole belly of the inferior oblique muscle. (*C*) Hooks miss a small piece of muscle, which may allow muscle to rejoin.

Recession of the Contralateral Inferior Rectus Muscle. If the inferior oblique muscle is not overacting, recession of the contralateral inferior rectus muscle (the yoke muscle) should be considered. The hypertropia should be greater in down gaze, particularly in the field of action of the paretic superior oblique muscle. The inferior rectus muscle is an unforgiving muscle in contrast to the inferior oblique, and very precise surgery must be performed, aiming to undercorrect the deviation in primary and down gaze. If more than 3 mm of recession or resection of this muscle is performed, the lower lid height will be affected. An adjustable suture on the inferior rectus should be used if the patient is old enough to cooperate. In the adjustment it is important to make sure that the deviation is undercorrected by a few prism diopters in the primary position, particularly in down gaze. As a guideline, a correction of 3 prism diopters per millimeter in the primary position and 5 prism diopters per millimeter in down gaze should be calculated.

Example: If there is a right hypertropia of 14 prism diopters in the primary position increasing to 25 prism diopters in down gaze, a recession of the left inferior rectus muscle of 4 mm should correct 12 prism diopters of right hypertropia in the primary position and 20 prism diopters in down gaze. Hopefully, this will leave the deviation slightly undercorrected, which is the preferred result. Recession of the inferior rectus of more than 6.0 mm is not recommended. Reassessment of the patient should be delayed for 2 months after surgery before deciding if further surgery is warranted.

Recession of the Ipsilateral Superior Rectus Muscle. Some cases of superior oblique palsy that have been present for many years become surprisingly concomitant so that the hypertropia is approximately the same in side gaze to the left and right as well as on head tilting. In such a situation and particularly if there is minimal increase of hypertropia in down gaze, the safest procedure is a recession of the ipsilateral superior rectus muscle of up to 6 mm. If a larger recession is performed, subsequent overaction of the yoke inferior oblique muscle may result. The recession is best performed with an adjustable suture if the patient is old enough. It is a much safer operation than recessing the contralateral inferior rectus muscle because any overcorrection in the field of action of the muscle is in up gaze, which is the least practical position of gaze. In contrast, the inferior rectus muscle, a totally unforgiving muscle, has its field of action in down gaze, which is essential for reading, going up and down stairs, hiking, skiing, etc. The inferior rectus muscle should only be recessed if there is a marked increase of the hypertropia in down gaze. In some cases of long-standing superior oblique palsy associated with hypertropia of more than 10 prism diopters, a contraction of the ipsilateral superior rectus may result.[9,23] Clinically the hypertropia increases in down gaze when the eye is slightly abducted. In these cases, the appropriate surgical procedure is a recession of the superior rectus muscle of the hypertropic eye.

Tuck of the Ipsilateral Superior Oblique Tendon (the Paretic Muscle) for Torsion. In an occasional case of unilateral superior oblique palsy, torsion exceeding 10° interfering with fusion may be present. In such a case a tuck of the ipsilateral superior oblique is indicated as an initial procedure. However, it is important to first search for other signs of bilateral superior oblique palsy because torsion exceeding 10° is common in this condition but rare in unilateral cases.

Tuck of the Ipsilateral Superior Oblique Tendon (the Paretic Muscle) for the Hypertropia. This is occasionally indicated in patients with a hypertropia in the primary position of 10 to 15 prism diopters remaining after a recession of the yoke inferior rectus muscle. The hypertropia increases to double this amount in down gaze, particularly in the field of action of the paretic superior oblique. As mentioned previously, the contralateral inferior rectus muscle should not be recessed more than 6.0 mm for a unilateral superior oblique palsy. Even if the inferior rectus has only been recessed 4.0 mm, a tuck of the ipsilateral superior oblique should be considered because this may be preferable to reoperation on the inferior rectus muscle because the inferior orbit is prone to scarring. A tuck of the superior oblique tendon is difficult to titrate and may result in an iatrogenic Brown's syndrome.[17] The tendon is tucked until the slack is taken up, usually a total of about 8.0 mm, i.e, 4 mm on either side of the clamp or hook.

It is also important to perform the tuck as temporal as possible, pulling the superior oblique tendon under the belly of the superior rectus muscle to the temporal side (Fig. 12–4). This minimizes the likelihood of inducing a Brown's syndrome. Helveston has described slackness in the tendon of the superior oblique in some cases of apparent congenital superior oblique palsy.[6] This slackness seems responsible for the classical signs and symptoms of superior oblique palsy. This can be confirmed at the time of operation by performing a superior oblique traction test (forced duction). It is important to stress this muscle's tendon by pushing the eye being evaluated back into the orbit before moving the eye into the field of action of the superior oblique muscle (see also Chapter 13). In such cases we still recommend following the treatment principles described previously in this chapter. If the clinical signs suggest that a tuck of the ipsilateral superior oblique tendon is the best treatment, the tendon should be tucked only until the slackness has been taken up to avoid an iatrogenic Brown's syndrome. A traction test at the end of the operation, with the surgeon moving the eye into the field of action of the ipsilateral inferior oblique muscle will check this.

UNILATERAL SUPERIOR OBLIQUE PALSY IN PATIENTS UNDER THE AGE OF 4 YEARS

Congenital unilateral superior oblique palsy may result in a noticeable head tilt from the age the child sits up or starts walking. Young children are difficult to examine, particularly because they cry as soon as you touch their head. The following procedures are helpful. The Bielschowsky head tilt test is especially valuable.

1. Establish whether or not the child is fusing with the preferred head position by performing a nondissociating quick cover test on each eye while the child is interested in a fixation object. The parent is then asked to tilt the child's head to the opposite shoulder while the examiner observes the child's eyes and, hopefully, the child is still fixing the target. If there is a positive Bielschowsky head tilt test, the eye with the affected muscle reveals more hypertropia when the head is tilted to the same side. This usually indicates a superior oblique palsy.

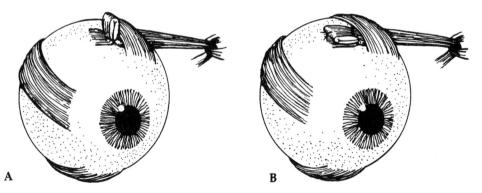

Figure 12–4. Superior oblique tuck. (*A*) Tuck of right superior oblique temporal to the right superior rectus. (*B*) Tendon protrusion resulting from tuck anchored with suture to sclera temporal to superior rectus.

An overaction of the antagonist inferior oblique muscle should also be sought. The compensatory head tilt should disappear with patching of either eye. If all of these findings are present, including the overaction of the inferior oblique and hypertropia of the affected eye with the head straight, an inferior oblique myectomy is indicated even in the absence of detailed measurements in a young child.

2. If there is definitely no overaction of the inferior oblique muscle, it would be safer and wiser to wait until the child is old enough for all the necessary diagnostic tests. These can usually be performed satisfactorily when the child is about the age of 6 years. The unforgiving nature of a recession of an inferior rectus muscle necessitates having accurate measurements of the deviation in all positions of gaze and with the head tilted to either side. Likewise, a tuck of the affected superior oblique muscle or a recession of the ipsilateral superior rectus muscle requires very special indications that can only be detected after a detailed and careful assessment.

CONGENITAL ABSENCE OF THE SUPERIOR OBLIQUE MUSCLE

Congenital absence of the superior oblique muscle presents with signs indistinquishable from other cases of congenital superior oblique palsy, except that no muscle or tendon can be seen by high-quality coronal magnetic resonance imaging or computerized tomography scan.[1] Treatment follows the same general principles.

Superior Oblique Palsy and Acquired Brown's Syndrome

Penetrating trauma in the region of the trochlea such as a dog bite,[12] knife wound, or surgical trauma[16] may produce a superior oblique palsy as well as mechanical restriction to elevation in adduction.

Bilateral Superior Oblique Palsies

This condition may occur as a congenital anomaly, although it is more common as an acquired palsy associated with severe head trauma. The clinical features include:

1. Chin-down head position for fusion on up gaze (Fig. 12–5A).
2. A small vertical deviation in the primary position that is easy to overlook (Fig. 12–5B).
3. There is a left hypertropia on gaze right and a right hypertropia on gaze left (Fig. 12–5C,D).
4. An esotropia on down gaze exceeding the measurements in the primary position by at least 10 prism diopters (V pattern) (Fig. 12–5E).
5. An excyclotorsion that is often bilateral and exceeding 10° in the primary position with a marked increase of excyclotorsion on down gaze to as much as 30°. The extent of the excyclotorsion in the primary and down positions can be used as an indicator as to whether the deviation is unilateral or bilateral. Unilateral

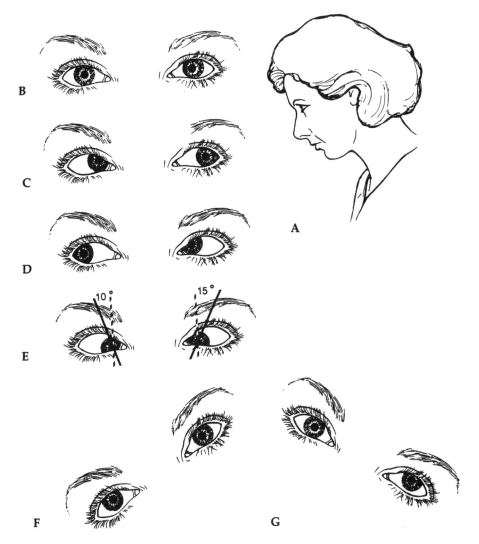

Figure 12–5.   Bilateral superior oblique palsies. (*A*) Chin-down head position to fuse. (*B*) Minimal vertical in primary position. (*C*) Small right hypertropia in gaze left. (*D*) Small left hypertropia in gaze right. (*E*) Obvious esotropia in down gaze with bilateral excyclotorsion. (*F*) Small right hypertropia in head tilt right. (*G*) Small left hypertropia in head tilt left.

superior oblique palsies rarely have an excyclotorsion in excess of 10°, whereas bilateral superior oblique palsies commonly do. Excyclotorsion can be seen in the fundus viewed by either a direct or indirect ophthalmoscope. The fovea normally has a horizontal relationship to the lower half of the optic disc (Fig. 12–6).

6. There is a left hypertropia on head tilt left and a right hypertropia on head tilt right (bilateral positive Bielschowsky head tilt test) (Fig. 12–5F and G).

7. A reversal of the vertical in gaze right and left and head tilt left and right may not always be present, but the V esotropia and the excyclotorsion is always

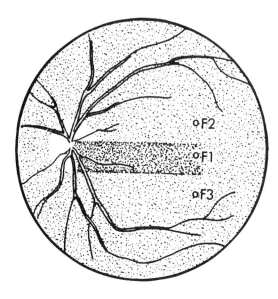

Figure 12–6. Objective assessment of torsion. The shaded area represents the normal variation in the relationship of fovea F1 and optic disc in the left fundus. F2 foveal position would be incyclotorsion and F3 excyclotorsion viewed with a direct ophthalmoscope.

present in bilateral superior oblique palsies. The presence of the V pattern and the marked amount of excyclotorsion present should alert one to the diagnosis of a bilateral superior oblique palsy.

Is the Correction of the Torsion Essential in the Treatment?

In order to evaluate this question, the deviation should be assessed in the reading position, looking down, where the excyclotorsion associated with bilateral superior oblique palsies is maximized. In this position the deviation should be neutralized with horizontal and vertical prisms to see if the patient is able to fuse when this is done. If the patient is unable to fuse, particularly if the images are seen as tilted, surgery must be planned to address the excyclotorsion in addition to the other aspects of the strabismus. This can be assessed more easily with the help of an orthoptist using a synoptophore.

Masked Bilateral Superior Oblique Palsy

Sometimes, a bilateral superior oblique palsy is not obvious until after surgery for what appears to be a typical unilateral superior oblique palsy.[7,8,13]

Example: After a left inferior oblique myectomy for a left superior oblique palsy, all the features of a right superior oblique palsy with a right hypertropia and overaction of the right inferior oblique appear.

These features were undetected initially and appear to have been uncovered or unmasked by the treatment of the presumed left superior oblique palsy. In such a situation, a myectomy of the now overacting right inferior oblique muscle is indicated and usually gives a good result. Certainly the presence of a V esotropia in down gaze or the presence of marked excyclotorsion should alert one to the likelihood of bilateral superior oblique palsies even in the absence of other features of a bilateral superior oblique palsy. Likewise, the reversal of the vertical in any gaze or tilt position is indicative of its presence.

Treatment of Bilateral Superior Oblique Palsies

Diplopia is experienced everywhere the patient looks except in up gaze, which is most distressing to the patient.

Goal of Management

The goal of management is to obtain single binocular vision in the practical positions of gaze looking straight ahead and looking down.

Surgical Principles

First of all it must be determined whether or not torsion is preventing fusion. If it is, surgery specifically to alleviate the torsion must be performed before addressing the other features resulting from the bilateral superior oblique palsies. If, prior to any surgery, the patient can fuse when just the vertical and horizontal elements of the deviation are neutralized, it is possible to ignore the torsion when planning treatment.

1. If excyclotorsion exceeds 15° in down gaze, torsion by itself may be a barrier to fusion. This is indicated if neutralization of the horizontal and vertical deviations with prisms or with a synoptophore does not allow the patient to fuse. The patient is able to fuse only when torsion is neutralized. This can only be done by the synoptophore. Bilateral superior oblique tucks that take up all the slack (usually about 8 mm) are needed as the primary procedure. If a significant hypertropia is present, tuck the superior oblique of the hypertropic eye more. Nothing else should be done until the effect of this is evaluated a month after surgery. Bilateral tucks may produce some correction of the esotropia in down gaze as well as correction of the excyclotorsion to within an adaptable range.

2. If both inferior oblique muscles are overacting and if there is a hypertropia of 10 prism diopters or more in the primary position a weakening procedure such as an inferior oblique myectomy or recession of the inferior oblique of the hypertropic eye only should be performed. If this results in a marked overaction of the other inferior oblique muscle when assessed 2 months after surgery, an inferior oblique myectomy or recession is indicated on the second inferior oblique. If both inferior obliques are obviously overacting and there is a vertical strabismus of less than 6 prism diopters, a myectomy of both inferior oblique muscles should be performed initially.

3. If there is esotropia in down gaze, this problem should be tackled last because surgery on the oblique muscles, particularly the superior oblique tucks, may help to reduce the esotropia in down gaze.

Both the medial recti should be recessed and infraplaced and the insertion angled as follows: infraplace the tendon half the width of the tendon insertion downward. The upper border should be recessed to produce an exophoria of approximately 6 prism diopters in the primary position using the standard calculation of 2 1/2 prism diopters per millimeter.

The lower border should be recessed an additional 2 mm from a straight line drawn down from the normal insertion (Fig. 12–7). This slants the insertion and together with the infraplacement should neutralize the V pattern esotropia in down gaze, which usually exceeds the primary deviation by at least 10 prism diopters.

Persistent Excyclotorsion Preventing Fusion in Down Gaze

The significance of the torsion preventing fusion per se may have been missed in the initial examination, or the patient may have already had some surgery elsewhere. If previous surgery has largely taken care of the vertical and V pattern esotropia, a modified[4] bilateral Harada Ito procedure[5] may help in alleviating much of the torsion without disrupting the vertical balance, thereby restoring fusion if the superior oblique tendons had not been operated on previously. A conjunctival incision is made on the temporal aspect of the superior rectus 8 mm from the limbus. The speculum is removed, and a Desmarres retractor is used to expose the superior oblique insertion while a strabismus hook is placed under the superior rectus muscle and the eye pulled straight down (see Fig. 14–3A). The strabismus hook is then placed underneath the fibers of the superior oblique insertion on the temporal side of the superior rectus and brought up half way across the tendon so that the anterior half of the superior oblique can be transposed temporally and anteriorly. This is done by inserting a double-arm 6.0 Vicryl suture into the tendon near the insertion, cutting it from the sclera and pulling it up so it is adjacent to the insertion of the superior rectus muscle. It is then pulled temporally until it is firm and attached to the sclera in this position (Fig. 12–8). This operation is only indicated if the excyclotorsion is a problem preventing fusion. This torsion is usually in excess of 15° in down gaze. In such an instance a maximum procedure to achieve overcorrection of the torsion in the immediate postoperative period is indicated. It is not possible to operate again on such patients because the transposed anterior position of the superior oblique tendon blends inseparably with the

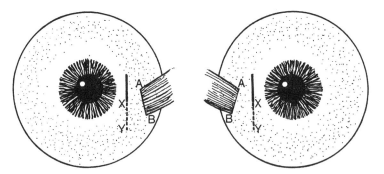

Figure 12–7. Bilateral medial rectus infraplacement and angulation for V esotropia. AB: new medial rectus insertion; XY: straight line drawn down from original insertion.

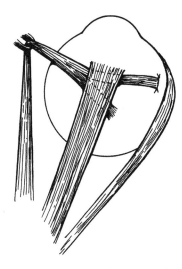

Figure 12–8.   Anterior half of right superior oblique muscle transposed anteriorly and laterally until it is tight.

sclera, so it is important to do the maximum amount first. Temporary overcorrection for a few days is common and desired. We have not encountered permanent overcorrection 2 months after surgery.

Bilateral Superior Oblique Palsies and Central Fusion Disruption

Severe head injuries resulting in bilateral superior oblique palsies also may cause a traumatic central disruption of fusion.[19,22] These patients are unable to fuse even if all aspects of the strabismus, including torsion, are eliminated. This combination is not common but does occur. If marked excyclotorsion is present and appears to prevent fusion, examination on an amblyoscope such as the synoptophore is essential.[22] If necessary, a referral should be made to an orthoptist specifically for this test to see whether the problem is due purely to the marked torsion, relievable by the correct surgical treatment, or due to central fusion disruption, which is incurable and for which surgery is pointless except for cosmetic improvement.

Referral to a Strabismologist

The treatment of bilateral superior oblique palsies is one of the more complicated problems in strabismology and it may be prudent to refer such a patient to a strabismologist for management if it is feasible. Alternatively, a consultation may be arranged with an expert (see also the section on Telemedicine and Treatment of Strabismus and Amblyopia in Chapter 22). It is essential to have all the information for such a consultation, including the measurements in up, down, and side gaze, and head tilt to right or left presence or absence of inferior oblique overaction, and the significance of the torsion, particularly in down gaze as well as an assessment of the patient's fusion potential.

When the Vertical Is Not Due to Superior Oblique Palsy

Consider the following conditions:

Incomitant Vertical Strabismus

This may be due to a cyclovertical muscle restriction or paresis, other than the superior oblique. Refer to Chapter 13 for diagnosis and special tests, particularly the Park's three-step test.

Skew Deviation: Concomitant Acquired Vertical Strabismus

This is generally an acquired lesion in older people and is usually caused by a presumed vascular insult in the mid-brain area.[10] It is a supranuclear lesion and is usually associated with normal ductions. The deviation may be similar in up, down, and side gaze as well as on head tilting.

TREATMENT

Consider prisms if the patient wears glasses or if the strabismus is mainly concomitant, measuring less than 8 prism diopters. The superior rectus in the hypertropic eye should be recessed, calculating 3 prism diopters per millimeter, up to a maximum of 8 mm for larger deviations.

Brown's Syndrome or Inferior Oblique Palsy

The parent or patient usually complains that one eye shoots upward (see also Chapter 14). This is the unaffected eye. It should be kept in mind that primary overactions do not occur; therefore, a Brown's syndrome or inferior oblique palsy in the other eye should be sought. Treatment is only indicated for a Brown's syndrome in which there is a hypotropia of the affected eye of 10 to 15 prism diopters with the head straight and the patient has some fusion ability. Otherwise, treatment is not recommended because the problem is not cosmetically noticeable when patients are fully grown. Brown's syndrome is particularly noticeable in infants and children because most people are taller than they are so they have to look up at them. Some surgeons recommend a more aggressive approach.[2,18]

Mechanical Restriction

This is most common in the inferior part of the orbit. Mechanical restriction in the inferior part of the orbit usually results in a noticeable vertical strabismus in up gaze. This may be associated with the restriction of the inferior rectus muscle, thyroid ophthalmopathy (orbitopathy), blow out fracture, or congenital abnormalities (see also Chapter 14). Initially, the patient will often complain of one eye shooting upward under the upper lid on up gaze. This is due to Hering's Law affecting the normal eye. This is not confusing if it is remembered that primary overaction does not occur and the other eye is examined. Forced duction tests, under local anesthetic, should be used to confirm the diagnosis if the patient is sufficiently cooperative.

Congenital Double Elevator Palsy (Monocular Elevation Deficit)

Again, the patient or parents will frequently complain about one eye shooting up and disappearing under the lid when in fact that is the normal eye (Fig. 12–9). A patient with fusion may adopt the chin-up head position with a hypotropia of 10 to 20 prism diopters of the affected eye. Pseudoptosis is usually present

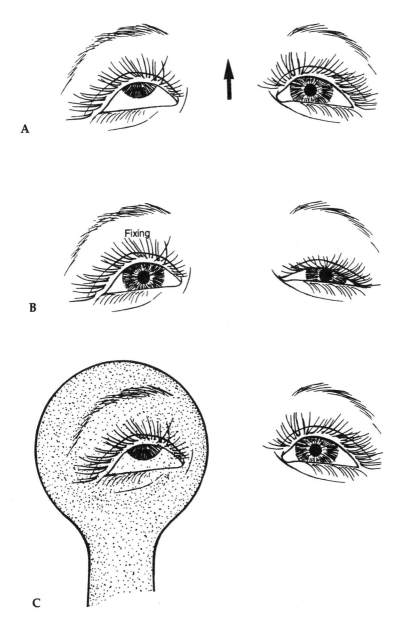

Figure 12–9.   Left double elevator palsy. (*A*) Up gaze, head straight. (*B*) Fixing normal right eye with pseudoptosis of left eye and slight chin-up position. (*C*) Absent elevation of left eye, but pseudoptosis is gone with left eye fixing, head straight.

(Fig. 12–9B) and may be more noticeable to the patient than the hypertropia. Pseudoptosis is readily distinguished from true ptosis by getting the patient to fix with the eye under the drooping lid. The upper lid remains at the same level in true ptosis but elevates to the normal position in pseudoptosis provided the eye comes up approximately to the primary position, as is the case with double elevator palsy (Fig. 12–9C).

DIAGNOSIS

1. Ductions usually show complete inability to raise the eye above the primary horizontal straight ahead position.
2. The forced duction test is normal, excluding mechanical restriction in the inferior orbit.
3. Bell's phenomenon is normal because double elevator palsy is a supranuclear lesion. This distinguishes it from an infranuclear palsy of the superior rectus muscle.

TREATMENT

Knapp's operation[11] transposing the horizontal recti to the superior rectus in the involved eye improves the alignment in the primary position but rarely results in any upward movement (Fig. 12–10).

Double Depressor Palsy

This congenital condition is rare.

DIAGNOSIS

1. The patient has a complete inability to depress the eye below the horizontal primary position.

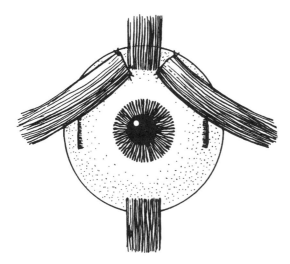

Figure 12–10. Transposition of horizontal recti to superior rectus insertion for double elevator palsy.

2. A forced duction test is performed to exclude mechanical restriction in the upper orbit.

TREATMENT

The horizontal recti in the involved eye should be transferred to the insertion of the inferior rectus muscle.

Dissociated Vertical Divergent Strabismus

Dissociated vertical strabismus is the big imitator in strabismus but should not be confused with these other causes of vertical strabismus. It occurs in the congenital strabismus syndrome (see Chapter 8). When the patient fixes with the hypertropic eye there is no corresponding hypotropia of the opposite eye.

Heimann Bielschowsky Phenomenon

A peculiar slow up-and-down movement of one eye may occur in patients with poor vision (hand movements) in that eye.[14] The reason is unknown. It is sometimes cosmetically disturbing. A recession of the superior rectus muscle may improve cosmesis.

Superior Oblique Myokymia

See Chapter 14.

Horizontal Muscle Surgery for Vertical Strabismus

Surgically raising both medial and lateral rectus tendons in the same eye raises that eye relative to the other eye slightly, and lowering them has the opposite effect. Plan on 1 prism diopter of vertical correction for each millimeter that both tendons are raised or lowered to a maximum of about 6 prism diopters. The technique allows some vertical correction of a concomitant deviation while not involving surgery on a third rectus muscle in the same eye (see also Chapter 16).

Surgical Correction of Vertical Strabismus Remaining in Down Gaze

This usually is a problem remaining after one or more operations have been performed for a vertical strabismus. If further conventional cyclovertical muscle surgery would not alleviate the problem, consider the following procedures:

1. Posterior fixation suture[3] on the inferior rectus muscle. This is placed as far back as possible on the inferior rectus muscle of the eye that is hypotropic in down gaze (see Fig. 16–5). This will weaken the inferior rectus in down gaze, thereby reducing the hypotropia in down gaze by up to 10 prism diopters in our experience. It may be helpful and is seldom harmful. Care should be used in inserting the sutures to anchor the inferior rectus muscle to the sclera as well as avoiding the vortex veins in the area.

2. Adjustable recession of both vertical recti in the hypotropic eye.[21] The remaining muscle imbalance in positions other than down gaze including head tilting should be concomitant within 5 prism diopters. The inferior rectus is recessed on an adjustable suture, calculating an effect of 3 prism diopters per millimeter in the primary position and 5 prism diopters in down gaze. Then the superior rectus is recessed on an adjustable suture to neutralize the resultant hypertropia in the primary position (see also Chapter 16).

References

1. Chan, T.K., Demer, J.L.: Clinical features of congenital absence of the superior oblique muscle as demonstrated by orbital imaging. J AAPOS 3:143–150, 1999.
2. Crawford, J.S.: Surgical treatment of true Brown's syndrome. Am J Ophthalmol 81:289, 1976.
3. Cüppers, C.: The so-called "Fadenoperation." II Kongr. I.S.A. Marseille, 1974. Paris-Marseille: Diff Gen Libr 5: 395, 1976.
4. Fells, P.: Management of paralytic strabismus. Br J Ophthalmol 58:255, 1974.
5. Harada, M., Ito, Y.: Surgical correction of cyclotropia. Jpn J Ophthalmol 8:88, 1964.
6. Helveston, E.M.: The Eighth Bielschowsky Lecture: The influence of superior oblique anatomy on function and treatment. In: Lennerstrand, G., ed. Advances in Strabismology. Buren, The Netherlands: Aelous Press Science, 1999:lxiii–lxiv.
7. Hermann, J.S.: Masked bilateral superior oblique paresis. J Pediatr Ophthalmol Strabismus 18:43, 1981.
8. Hugonnier, R., Maynard, P.: Paralysies a bascule du grand oblique. Bull Soc Ophthalmol Fr 69:587, 1969.
9. Jampolsky, A.: Vertical strabismus surgery. Transactions of the New Orleans Academy of Ophthalmology. St. Louis: Mosby-Year Book, 1971:366–385.
10. Keane, J.R.: Ocular skew deviation. Arch Neurol 32:185, 1975.
11. Knapp, P.: The surgical treatment of double elevator paralysis. Trans Am Ophthalmol Soc 67:304, 1969.
12. Knapp, P., Moore, S.: Diagnosis and surgical operations in superior oblique surgery. Int Ophthalmol Clin 16:137, 1976.
13. Kraft, S.P., Scott, W.E.: Masked bilateral superior oblique palsy. Clinical features and diagnosis. J Pediatr Ophthalmol Strabismus 23:264, 1986.
14. Lawton-Smith, J., Flynn, J.T., Spiro, H.J.: Monocular vertical oscillations of amblyopia—The Heimann Bielschowsky Phenomenon. J Clin Neuroophthalmol 2:85, 1982.
15. Noorden, G.K. von: Binocular Vision and Ocular Motility. St. Louis: Mosby, 1990:384.
16. Noorden, G.K. von: Binocular Vision and Ocular Motility. St. Louis: Mosby, 1990:386.
17. Noorden, G.K. von: Binocular Vision and Ocular Motility. St. Louis: Mosby, 1990:407.
18. Parks, M.M., Eustis, H.S.: Simultaneous superior oblique tenectomy and inferior oblique recession in Brown's syndrome. Ophthalmology. 94:1043, 1987.
19. Pratt-Johnson, J.A.: Central disruption of fusional amplitude. Br J Ophthalmol 57: 347–350, 1973.
20. Pratt-Johnson, J.A.: Management of strabismus failure. Trans Pacific Coast Otoophthalmol Soc 63:197, 1982.
21. Pratt-Johnson, J.A.: Complicated strabismus and adjustable sutures. Aust N Z J Ophthalmol 16:87–92, 1988.
22. Pratt-Johnson, J.A., Tillson, G.: The investigation and management of torsion preventing fusion in bilateral superior oblique palsies. J Pediatr Ophthalmol Strabismus 24:145, 1987.
23. Souza-Diaz, C.: Surgical management of superior obliques. In: Moore, S., Mein, J., eds. Orthoptics, Past, Present, Future. Miami: Symposia Specialists, 1976:379–391.

13

Paralytic and Paretic Strabismus

Similar features are present in both paralytic and paretic strabismus, the difference being one of degree. Paretic strabismus is caused by a partial paralysis of one or more of the extraocular muscles. The investigation is the same in both cases.

General Features

If an extraocular muscle is paralyzed, a deviation will result from the unbalanced pull of the direct antagonist muscle. The greatest deviation is produced when the patient looks in the direction in which the affected muscle normally works. The patient may turn the face or head in that direction to preserve binocular vision and to minimize the necessity for using the weak muscle. When this is not possible, the resultant manifest deviation may cause a visual adult to become aware of diplopia and a child to develop suppression and amblyopia.

Amblyopia

Strabismic amblyopia is an immediate danger if a strabismus of any type is acquired in the visually immature years (0–8 years). The younger the patient, the greater the danger, but urgent steps should be taken in all young patients to prevent amblyopia.

Onset in the Visually Mature Patient

DIPLOPIA

Diplopia is the presenting symptom with an acquired paretic strabismus in the visually mature years.

Diplopia results from an image of the fixation object falling on an extra foveal area (the diplopia point) in the deviating eye and on the fovea in the straight eye. These are noncorresponding retinal points; therefore, the brain cannot fuse the images and diplopia is apparent to the patient. Visual adults cannot suppress the second image, which is very annoying for them.

CONFUSION

This is said to occur in a recent strabismus in a visual adult and results from the fovea of each eye seeing a different object and superimposing one on the other. If retinal correspondence is normal, what each fovea sees will be seen superimposed in the same position in space no matter how the eyes themselves are aligned.

However, if each fovea sees a different object that cannot be fused, retinal rivalry occurs and the fovea of the straight eye, which is looking at the object of conscious desired attention, is dominant. All conscious attention is focused on what the fovea of the straight eye is looking at, and the other image is immediately suppressed. For this reason, the patient is rarely aware of this type of confusion.

Importance of Hering's Law

A thorough understanding of Hering's law of equal innervation of the yoke muscles in the two eyes is essential to comprehend the investigation and treatment of paretic strabismus. For example, if the left lateral rectus is paretic, increased innervation will flow to the left lateral rectus to keep the eye straight and, particularly, to move it to the left in abduction. This increased innervation will also go to the right medial rectus (yoke muscle). This will result in a greater esotropia when fixing with the left eye, particularly in left gaze. This type of effect is graphically recorded in a Hess chart when the secondary deviation with the paretic eye fixing is greater than the primary deviation with the normal eye fixing (see also Chapter 5 and Fig. 5–9).

Precisely the same type of effect will result if there is mechanical restriction to abduction of the left eye caused by a contracted fibrosed medial rectus or by scarring on the medial side of the orbit. The forced duction test may help to differentiate between mechanical restriction and paresis in severe cases, but it may be difficult in less severe cases. Saccadic velocities may give some help in this situation. In patients with a severe mechanical restriction preventing a movement or in those with a complete paralysis of a rectus muscle, weakening the yoke muscle is ineffective in significantly improving the muscle balance because of the inevitable effect of Hering's law. For example, if the inferior rectus muscle is paralyzed as a result of an orbital floor fracture, the resultant muscle imbalance is not helped significantly by a tenotomy of the yoke superior oblique or by recessing the antagonist superior rectus. However, some improvement can be obtained by transposing the horizontal recti adjacent to the insertion of the paralyzed inferior rectus muscle because this will help to reduce the effect of Hering's law. Strangely, in the case of the superior oblique paralysis, this does not apply in the same way, because weakening the direct antagonist or yoke is often effective in improving the muscle balance. A possible explanation may be that a complete paralysis is rare or that some of its action is taken over by other cyclovertical muscles in the involved eye.

Measurement of the deviation and assessment of versions in the various gaze positions are necessary to evaluate the effects of Hering's law on any particular paretic strabismus. Hering's law is the logical basis for obtaining measurements of the deviation fixing each eye. The secondary deviation, when the paretic eye is fixing, is greater than the primary deviation when the normal eye is fixing. It is the physiologic basis of the Parks' three-step test.[16]

There is a tendency for a smoothing out of the muscle imbalance to take place as the years pass, so that a paretic strabismus of long standing tends to be more comitant than one of recent onset.

Investigation of Paretic Strabismus

In addition to all the tests mentioned in the normal workup in Chapters 3, 4, and 5, particular emphasis must be placed on the following:

1. Diplopia test. It is important to make sure that diplopia is on the basis of a binocular imbalance and not monocular diplopia due to astigmatism, lens opacities, or other pathologic conditions. A useful test to make sure that binocular diplopia is actually present and is not imagined by the patient is to ask the patient to describe where the two images are located. If the patient replies "one on the left and one on the right," then ask the patient to look first at the left one and then at the right one. The eyes will move if the patient has double vision from a manifest deviation and the diplopia is binocular (see also Chapter 19).

2. Head tilt or face turn. If a head tilt or face turn is present because of an ocular motor muscle imbalance caused by paretic strabismus, it is almost always due to the fact that fusion is obtained by assuming the particular head position, thus avoiding diplopia. This compensatory head posture (CHP) should be sought prior to taking visual acuity and disrupting the fusion. If it is present then without changing the CHP check, by a brief nondissociating cover-uncover test, that the eyes are straight and presumably the patient is fusing with the aid of the CHP. Following this, the head should be moved to the opposite side to see if fusion is lost and diplopia provoked (see also Chapter 18).

3. Measurements fixing with the right eye and fixing with the left eye will be different, the deviation being greater when the eye with the paretic muscle is fixing (Hering's law). This information is important in the diagnosis of cyclovertical muscle paresis. It is important to be constantly aware which eye is fixing. If vision is equal, the patient usually fixes with the normal eye. However, if the eye with the muscle weakness has better vision, the patient will often fix with this eye.

4. Side gaze measurements need particular attention if a horizontal muscle is involved.

5. Parks' three-step test[16]:

Step I	Which eye is higher?
Step II	Measure the vertical deviation in horizontal gaze left and horizontal gaze right. Which is greater?
Step III	Measure the vertical deviation in head tilt to left and head tilt to right. Which is greater? This is the Bielschowsky head tilt test.

The conclusion as to which cyclovertical muscle is paretic is obtained by referring to Table 13–1. This table and its conclusions are not infallible but are very helpful in arriving at a diagnosis.

6. Subjective Parks' three-step test for cyclovertical muscle imbalance. Place a red glass in front of the right eye and a green glass in front of the left eye. Ask the

Table 13-1.   The Parks' 3-Step Test to Determine Which Is the Paretic Muscle

Step 1 (Which eye is higher?)	Step 2 (Is vertical deviation greater on gaze right or gaze left?)	Step 3 (Is the vertical deviation greater on head tilt right or head tilt left?)	Paretic Muscle*
Right eye	Gaze right	Tilt right	LIO
		Tilt left	RIR
	Gaze left	Tilt right	RSO
		Tilt left	LSR
Left eye	Gaze right	Tilt right	RSR
		Tilt left	LSO
	Gaze left	Tilt right	LIR
		Tilt left	RIO

* RIR: right inferior rectus; LSR: left superior rectus; LIO: left inferior oblique; RSO: right superior oblique; LSO: left superior oblique; RIO: right inferior oblique; RSR: right superior rectus; LIR: left inferior rectus.

patient to fixate a muscle light at 6 m and to identify if the red or green image is higher. The higher eye will see the lower image. Repeat the question when the patient's eyes are turned to the left with the face turned to the right, or when the eyes turned to the right with the face turned to the left. Third, ask the patient if the vertical separation of the images increases with a head tilt to the left shoulder, or to the right shoulder. This test can also be performed at 1/3 m.

7.   The subjective diplopia test in the nine diagnostic positions of gaze. This test is performed using the same red and green glasses, as described in the previous test, and asking the patient to fix a small fixation light held 1 m away in each of the nine diagnostic positions in turn. The patient is asked to identify where the two images are most widely separated and where they are less widely separated or fused. This same test can be performed using a red filter in front of one eye, which does not have the disadvantage of the restriction caused by the red/green glass frames. The widest separation of images occurs when the patient is looking in the field of action of the paretic muscle. This is even more exaggerated if the patient fixes with the involved eye due to Hering's law.

8.   Objective assessment. Measuring the deviation in each of the diagnostic positions of gaze with prisms is more difficult and time consuming. It is only indicated in complicated cyclovertical deviations when the diagnosis is uncertain or when testing aphasic patients.

9.   The Hess chart. The Hess chart can be plotted using a Hess screen or a Lees screen. It is one of the best subjective repeatable charted documentations of the effect of paretic strabismus on all the extraocular muscles of both eyes. It can only be done if the patient has some fusion because otherwise suppression or alternation will occur when attempting to superimpose. It has particular value in comparing pre- and postoperative muscle balance and in recording progressive changes because the conditions of the test are repeatable and consistent. The results of either test are recorded on a Hess chart.

10.   The forced duction test. The forced duction test should be used to distinguish between defective movement of an eye from mechanical restriction and that due

to weakness of the muscle primarily responsible for the movement of the eye to that gaze position. This test can be performed with topical anesthesia (e.g., tetracaine 0.5% drops) in adult patients and in some cooperative youngsters. This test also can be performed on patients under general anesthesia to eliminate the possibility of mechanical restriction just before commencing strabismus surgery. The eye should be pulled forward if testing rectus muscles and pushed back if testing oblique muscles.[6] This takes up any possible slack in the muscles putting them on stretch. The forced duction test in general is only reliable if it is markedly positive and a mechanical restriction is obvious.

Ocular muscle tone initially increases when succinyl choline is administered for intubation in general anesthesia. The forced duction test may be slightly influenced by this effect. However, the test is only useful for detecting obvious mechanical restrictions and is unaffected, from a practical standpoint, by the use of succinyl choline. The anesthetist need not be discouraged from using it.

11. Active force generation test.[18] This test is most useful in testing the action of the rectus muscles. The eye is grasped with forceps after instilling topical anesthesia, as for a forced duction test, and the action of the muscle being tested is felt by the hold of the forceps. This is a test to see if the rectus muscle being assessed can work properly or is completely paralyzed. It is particularly useful in an old sixth nerve palsy with secondary contraction of the ipsilateral medial rectus, where a constant esotropia is present with active abduction being unable to straighten the eye more than 25 prism diopters of esotropia. This test will differentiate between the lateral rectus being completely paralyzed or the presence of some lateral rectus function that is being disguised by the contracture of the ipsilateral medial rectus muscle. The eye should be grasped near the limbus adjacent to the medial rectus, and with the eye adducted 50 prism diopters the patient is asked to try to straighten the eye. Can any active pull of the eye out to abduction be detected, or does the eye move to the 25 prism diopters of esotropia by passive relaxation of the medial rectus, yielding a negative test result?

A scleral suction cup with a rubber plunger attached in the middle can be used for evaluation of forced duction and active force generation.[1] The plunger can be seen protruding forward between the lids and moves with the patient's eye. Forced ductions can be tested by gently pushing the plunger in the appropriate direction with one finger. An example is a right lateral rectus palsy with constant esotropia of 25 prism diopters where the plunger is used to push the eye into abduction. Resistance to movement can be detected. Active force generations are tested with the eye adducted 50 prism diopters and the plunger gently held over by one finger while the patient tries to bring the eye to the 25-prism diopter esotropic position. Active muscle movement can be detected more easily by this method than by using forceps.

12. Saccadic velocities (these are involuntary and cannot be altered on a voluntary basis). Saccadic velocities can be measured by sophisticated machinery but they seldom give any more information than can be seen clinically by getting the patient to change fixation between two fixation targets 20° to 30° apart in the appropriate gaze position to evaluate the suspected weak muscle. The eye with a weak muscle may show slowing of the saccade when compared with the normal side.

Neurologic Investigation of Patients with Ocular Motor Palsy

If the etiology is not obvious, such as following severe trauma or if the patient has an isolated acquired weakness of the medial or vertical recti, the patient should be referred to a neurologist for evaluation to help exclude such conditions as myasthenia gravis and multiple sclerosis.

Treatment

Prisms in the Treatment of Paralytic Strabismus

Prisms are not commonly useful in the treatment of paralytic strabismus because of incomitance. However, if it allows single vision in the most important directions of gaze, a temporary membrane (Fresnel) prism may be helpful for some patients.

Urgency of Treatment

Occlusion of the unaffected eye to prevent amblyopia should be started immediately if the patient is too young for reliable subjective visual acuity monitoring and has not spontaneously adopted a compensatory head fracture that preserves fusion. Contracture of the antagonist muscle is only a problem in acquired sixth nerve palsy.

   In cases of sixth nerve palsy, the following two techniques are used:

1.   Occlusion of the normal eye followed by injection of botulinum toxin (Botox) into the medial rectus of the affected eye may be indicated in the absence of any signs of recovery after a month. If botulinum toxin is not available, surgical correction should be considered if there is no sign of any recovery after 3 months. Treatment should be delayed as long as gradual recovery can be documented. In contrast, an acquired cyclovertical muscle palsy, such as a superior oblique, is rarely associated with contractures causing treatment problems, and surgical treatment can be delayed 6 months or longer without adversely affecting the result of later surgical treatment.

2.   Active duction and version exercises. Active duction exercises may be useful in restoring strength in a recovering paretic eye muscle similar to a physiotherapist building recovery in skeletal muscles. The patient covers the "normal" eye and tries to move the affected eye as far as possible into the field of action of the paretic muscle. This is repeated for a few minutes several times a day. In addition, version exercises also may be advised. The patient is instructed to find a head or eye position in which fusion is regained and then make efforts to extend the limits of this fused vision by slowly moving the head or eyes away from that position while maintaining single vision.

Surgical Treatment Options

These become clear once the affected muscle has been diagnosed. The general rules for surgery to produce the most beneficial improvement in all gaze positions are as follows:

1. Weakening either the antagonist or the yoke muscle of the involved paretic muscle is physiologically sound and should result in the best improvement when all fields of gaze are taken into consideration. The choice of which of these two muscles to treat surgically may be influenced by the predictability of surgery on one in comparison with the other. For example, in an inferior rectus weakness, the yoke muscle is the contralateral superior oblique muscle and the direct antagonist is the ipsilateral superior rectus. It would be easier to weaken the superior rectus in a graduated procedure or with an adjustable suture than it would be to weaken the superior oblique in such a predictable fashion.

2. Attempted strengthening of a totally paralyzed muscle itself is usually ineffective. Attempted strengthening of this muscle will have no effect on the total ocular motor muscle balance between the two eyes as determined by Hering's law, which ultimately governs the deviation. However, muscle transposition may be considered.

3. In the unusual circumstance where the deviation has become concomitant, choice of surgery is not determined by the above rules. In concomitant vertical deviations, surgery should be confined to the vertical rectus muscles. Because the inferior rectus muscle is unforgiving after surgery, affecting the all-important reading position, as well as the cosmetic height of the lower lid, surgery should be confined to the superior rectus muscle for correction of up to 20 prism diopters. This would involve 6 to 7 mm of surgery. If more correction is required, then surgery on the inferior rectus muscle can be included. The adjustable suture technique should be used if possible. In horizontal deviations that have become concomitant, surgery may be confined to the affected eye. Such an example is an acquired paresis of the lateral rectus, which recovers completely but leaves the patient with a concomitant esotropia of 35 prism diopters, which measures the same fixing right or left eyes even in left and right gaze. Here a recession of the medial rectus and a resection of the lateral rectus on an adjustable suture on the originally involved eye should restore good muscle balance and alignment.

In some instances a large recession of the medial rectus and resection of the lateral rectus on the same eye also may produce the best result in a patient with sixth nerve paresis who has any evidence of lateral rectus function.

Acquired Sixth Nerve Palsy (Lateral Rectus Palsy)

Occlusion may be used for two purposes: (1) to prevent amblyopia in the visually immature years in the presence of an acquired paretic strabismus; and (2) to prevent contractures of the antagonist muscles from developing. For instance, in the event of a sixth nerve palsy in a visual adult, occlusion of the good eye is preferred to occlusion of the paretic eye because the former will prevent contracture of the antagonist medial rectus muscle from developing. A patient with a sixth nerve palsy usually presents with an esotropia of 60 prism diopters. If the good eye is covered, the patient can bring the other eye straight by complete inhibition of the medial rectus muscle. This prevents contracture of the ipsilateral medial rectus so commonly seen in an eye with a paralyzed lateral rectus muscle. This contracture of the medial rectus may contribute to an inferior result in long-standing complete sixth nerve palsies after treatment.

Botulinum toxin injection for acquired sixth nerve palsy may be necessary, and these cases should be referred to a strabismologist with expertise in its use. Botulinum toxin injection may be indicated in adults who show no improvement after a month. A child who develops an acquired sixth nerve palsy from trauma should be treated in the following fashion. The child may be able to maintain fusion with the help of a compensatory face turn. This is sometimes possible if the deviation is not too great. In the event that a head turn preserves vision and fusion, no other treatment is required for a month. The use of botulinum toxin in the management of acquired sixth nerve palsies in children who are visually immature may be useful if the child is unable to achieve fusion with a compensatory face turn. However, alternate patching should be introduced to prevent amblyopia. The patient should be encouraged to obtain fusion with a face turn if possible. If this can be achieved, then occlusion of the normal eye should be continued part time to prevent any contracture of the medial rectus of the affected eye. If no recovery appears to be taking place after a month, botulinum toxin should be injected into the antagonist medial rectus muscle. This will usually allow the eye to become straight and the patient to regain fusion, if necessary, with a slight face turn. The effects of botulinum toxin wear off in approximately 2 months, but the sixth nerve palsy should have recovered by that time. The great advantage of this treatment is that it allows a temporary return of the eye to a straighter position so that fusion can be resumed. This prevents the secondary effects of an interruption of fusion in children for a month if fusion cannot be achieved by a face turn. Some clinicians advocate botulinum toxin in the visually immature under the age of 6 years if no recovery of fusion is present after a week. The danger, however, is that the possible side effects of an induced ptosis or a vertical strabismus may cause an additional barrier to fusion.

Surgery for Acquired Sixth Nerve Palsy

If some action of the lateral rectus muscle can be shown by the results of an active force generation test, by the presence of any active abduction past the straight ahead midline position, or by the presence of any abduction after the injection of botulinum toxin into the medial rectus, an adjustable recession of the medial rectus and resection of the lateral rectus should be performed to eliminate the deviation in the primary position. If absolutely no action in the lateral rectus is evident and it is a "dead" muscle, two options are available, depending on whether or not botulinum toxin is to be used in the treatment.

1. Surgery without using botulinum toxin, Jensen's procedure.[8] This is a good operation but, in order to achieve a satisfactory result, with the eye approximately straight in the primary position and fusion away from the site of the palsied muscle, attention must be directed to the following details.

The rare complication of anterior segment necrosis in patients over the age of 50 must be remembered.[4] The vertical recti should be divided in half, making sure that one intact artery remains in the half of the vertical rectus muscle not involved in the operation. The anterior ciliary arteries should be preserved if possible when recessing the medial rectus[5,14] (Fig. 13–1A,B).

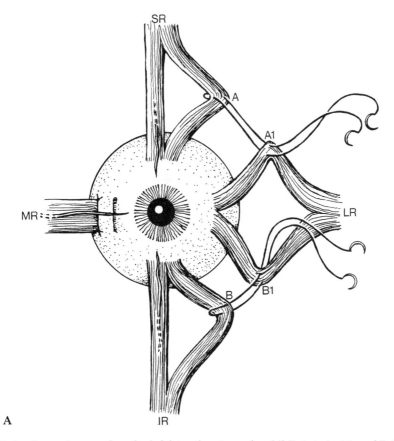

Figure 13–1. Jensen's procedure for left lateral rectus palsy. (*A*) Points A, A1, and B, B1 are 6 mm from each insertion. (*Figure continued on next page.*)

The ipsilateral medial rectus, antagonist to the paralytic lateral rectus muscle, should be recessed 6 mm.

Non-absorbable 5.0 white Dacron sutures should be used to tie, permanently and securely, the loops from the vertical recti and the lateral rectus 6 mm from the insertion (Fig. 13–1A). The sutures should be placed 6 mm from the insertion in the outer half of the vertical rectus muscle and the adjacent half of the paralytic lateral rectus muscle so they are joined up 6 mm from the insertion (Fig. 13–1B). The eye should be abducted by an assistant to facilitate tying the sutures to bring together the loops from the vertical recti and lateral rectus (Fig. 13–1B): the loops of muscle must be firmly sewn together 6 mm from the insertion using several nonabsorbable sutures. This must create an exotropia of approximately 25 to 30 prism diopters at the end of surgery. There must be a positive forced duction test so that one is unable to pull the eyes straighter than the 25 prism diopters of exotropia.

Postoperatively, the patient will assume fusion with a face turn opposite to the preoperative face turn, but within 2 months the overcorrected position of the eye with the lateral rectus palsy will reduce and give a good functional result. If there

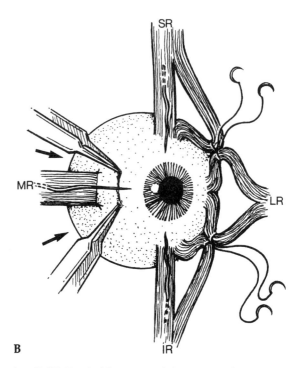

Figure 13–1. (*Continued*) (*B*) Eye held over in abduction so that sutures can be drawn up tight.

is not an overcorrection of 25 prism diopters of exotropia and a positive forced duction test at the end of surgery, there will be an undercorrection. It is virtually impossible to go back and operate or do any more. This is a situation in which there is only one chance to achieve a good result, and that is the first time the operation is performed. It is important to make sure it is done right the first time. It is therefore essential to get this type of result the first time.

2. Surgery can be combined with botulinum toxin. If the surgeon is experienced in the use of botulinum toxin, the following operations can be performed, both of which are effective in straightening the eye.

The injection of the ipsilateral medial rectus (antagonist to the paralytic muscle) with botulinum toxin 1 week before surgery will allow the paralysis of the medial rectus muscle, which usually takes up to 5 days, to have taken effect prior to the surgery. Then, a Jensen's procedure with precautions detailed above but omitting the recession of the medial rectus muscle should be performed. Alternatively, the injection of the ipsilateral medial rectus adjacent to the paralyzed lateral rectus should be performed 1 week before surgery for the reasons stated above. Then the whole of the vertical recti should be transposed to the insertion of the paralyzed lateral rectus, sewing each transposed tendon down to the sclera adjacent to the insertion of the lateral rectus muscle.[17] Finally, if there is some abduction of the eye following temporary paralysis of the direct antagonist medial rectus, a large adjustable recession of the medial rectus and resection of the lateral rectus in the involved eye should be combined with an adjustable recession of the contralateral medial rectus (yoke muscle), when the effects of the botulinum toxin have worn

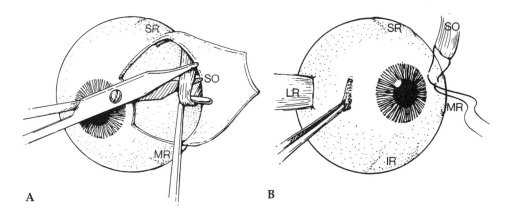

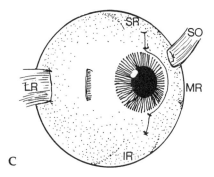

Figure 13–2. Superior oblique transposition for right third nerve palsy. (*A*) Superior oblique tendon cut. (*B*) Superior oblique tendon shortened to make it tight when sutured adjacent to paralyzed medial rectus. (*C*) Eye pulled over into adduction to facilitate tightening shortened superior oblique adjacent to medial rectus.

off. This would be preferred to transposition surgery, provided the involved lateral rectus muscle has some life and action.

All of these procedures are reasonably effective. It is just a question of choosing the one most suitable for the surgeon and the patient.

WHAT CAN BE EXPECTED FROM THE SURGICAL TREATMENT OF UNILATERAL SIXTH
NERVE PALSY WITH THE JENSEN TYPE PROCEDURE ON A "DEAD" MUSCLE?

1. The affected eye will be within 10° of being straight and the patient will be able to obtain some fusion with amplitude away from the site of the paralyzed muscle.

2. Some pseudoabduction up to 20° may be present due to the elastic band effect of the transposed muscle, which is mechanically tight. However, the patient rarely fuses looking past the midline toward the side of the paralytic muscle because of Hering's law. Instead, the patient usually fuses looking from straight ahead and in gaze away from the side of the palsy, hence the importance of not recessing and weakening the ipsilateral medial rectus muscle more than 6 mm.

3. A vertical strabismus may result as a secondary effect of surgery. Any second surgery for this or for residual esotropia is best treated with surgery on the normal eye. Reoperation on the affected eye is difficult, messy, and usually unproductive.

VERTICAL MUSCLE TRANSFER TO LATERAL RECTUS INSERTION WITH
CHEMODENERVATION OF THE MEDIAL RECTUS WITH BOTULINUM TOXIN

The whole of the inferior and superior recti may be transferred to the site of insertion of the paralyzed rectus muscle 1 week after botulinum toxin has been injected into the medial rectus muscle. We do not advise recession of the medial rectus as an alternative unless the anterior ciliary vessels are spared[5,14] or the patient is a child because of the danger of anterior segment ischemia.[4] Our experience is limited with this procedure, but results in our practice are inferior to those with Jensen's procedure when dealing with a totally paralyzed dead lateral rectus muscle. However, good results have been reported, and for some surgeons this has become the procedure of choice.[3,17]

Bilateral Sixth Nerve Palsy

A person with bilateral complete sixth nerve palsy will have a maximum esotropia that will alternate depending on which eye is fixing. Alternate patching should be performed to prevent medial rectus contracture. The various operations mentioned in the treatment of unilateral sixth nerve palsy are options for use on both eyes in this condition. However, it is extremely difficult to produce a satisfactory result because of the tremendous innervation going to the medial rectus muscle of whichever eye is not fixing (Hering's law). The main benefit, noticed by most patients postoperatively, is slightly increased mobility of the fixing eye, particularly if there was any contracture of the medial rectus with a fixed mechanical esotropia prior to surgery. However, it is impossible to produce straight eyes or any fusion with muscle surgery, and a significant esotropia of 50 prism diopters usually remains because of the effect of Hering's law. Repeated injections of botulinum toxin into each medial rectus every few months is a possibility that is logical and may help temporarily, but we have no personal experience of this.

Third Nerve Palsy

A complete congenital or acquired third nerve palsy is a difficult condition in which to produce a cosmetically satisfactory result. The eye, characteristically, is down 15 to 20 prism diopters and exotropic about 70 prism diopters. Complete ptosis is always present unless some aberrant regeneration has occurred.

Special Diagnostic Test

Is the superior oblique muscle functioning on the side of the third nerve palsy? The horizontal conjunctival vessels or other markings on the eye are observed when the patient attempts to look down. If this attempt to look down produces incyclotorsion of the eye, the superior oblique muscle is working.

Goal of Treatment

The goal of treatment is to prevent amblyopia by occlusion if necessary in a child in the amblyogenic age group. Good vision in both eyes is a "spare tire" precaution in this situation. The aim of surgery for all age groups is to improve cosmesis as much as possible. It is unrealistic to hope that alignment will be good enough to achieve any useful fusion.

Treatment of a Total Paralysis of the Third Nerve

A maximum recession of the ipsilateral lateral rectus muscle is essential. Neither an adjustable suture nor a hang-back technique should be used because the muscle is likely to creep forward and reattach itself to the scleral closer to the limbus. Scleral sutures should be placed approximately 12 mm from the insertion and sewn down to the sclera at that position. This will still allow a little abduction.

Transposition of the superior oblique tendon can be done provided the superior oblique is working and a significant hypotropia of more than 20 prism diopters is present. The superior oblique tendon is cut between the trochlea and the medial border of the superior rectus muscle (Fig. 13–2A) and the end of the superior oblique tendon is straightened out so it comes to lie along the belly of the paralyzed medial rectus muscle. The tendon therefore comes straight from the trochlea to the insertion of the medial rectus muscle.[19] Enough of the tendon should be resected so that it is tight and will hold the eye in 20 prism diopters of adduction. At the end of surgery, under the anesthetic, the eye is 15 to 20 prism diopters esotropic, with a positive forced duction test preventing the eye from drifting out into the exotropic position. This overcorrected position soon disappears, and the permanent result, usually apparent 2 months after surgery, is a recurrence of the exotropia of about 15 prism diopters, which is a marked cosmetic improvement.

If the hypotropia is less than 15 prism diopters, the trochlea should be dislocated from the frontal bone with smooth curved mosquito clamps. Then the tendon of the superior oblique should be cut between the trochlea and the medial border of the superior rectus muscle and brought up tightly beside the medial rectus muscle (Fig. 13–2B). It will now lie parallel to the medial rectus muscle. It is most important to resect as much of the transposed tendon as necessary to create an esotropia at the end of surgery of 20 prism diopters with a positive forced duction test preventing the eye from going into the exotropic position. This is facilitated by the assistant holding the eye over in the adducted position while the surgeon sutures the transposed superior oblique muscle tightly in position (Figs. 13–2C). Once again, this will not persist past a month or two, and the patient will usually end up with a marked cosmetic improvement and a small exotropia in the primary position.

Treatment of the Ptosis

If a complete ptosis is still present in the absence of any aberrant regeneration, a frontalis sling procedure is performed. Because Bell's phenomenon is absent, there is a definite danger of exposure keratitis, and for this reason monofilament nylon suture should be used on long ski-shaped needles for the initial sling. This is easy to remove under local anesthetic if one runs into any problem with exposure. It is safer to undercorrect this ptosis rather than fully correct it, but if no exposure occurs and cosmesis is not good, another sling can easily be placed in the lid without removing the original one. If the sling proves troublesome in any way or the lid droops again, the patient's autologous fascia lata can then be used, but it is better not to use this initially in case it has to be removed because of exposure.

Precaution: If Supramid is being used, at least three or four knots should be used to secure the suture and then the ends cut off flush with the knot complex. It is important to be sure to bury the knot complex well beneath the skin and suture the skin carefully to prevent any exposure of any ends of the suture. If any exposure occurs, then a granuloma will persist that will only be relieved by removal of the suture and the sling.

Partial Recovery and Aberrant Regeneration of the Third Nerve

Some recovery of function following paralysis of this nerve usually involves aberrant regeneration.[9] If any aberrant regeneration is present, it has been our experience that the elevation of the upper lid on the affected side is always present even to a small degree.

Cosmetic appearance can often be improved by surgery on the recti in the affected eye or the normal eye. However, functional improvement is rare if significant aberrant regeneration is present because this is a motor barrier to fusion, binocular motor cooperation being impossible in different fields of gaze.

Fourth Nerve Palsy

This is the most common palsy of the cranial nerves supplying the eye muscles and is addressed in detail in Chapter 12.

Congenital Paralysis of the Inferior Oblique Muscle

This condition is described in Chapter 14 because it is indistinguishable from Brown's syndrome unless a forced duction test is performed. Treatment involves a tenotomy of the ipsilateral (direct antagonist) superior oblique tendon, which is also described in Chapter 14.

Congenital Palsy of the Superior Rectus Muscle

This may be seen as a paresis or paralysis of the superior rectus and is associated with ptosis. The affected eye is hypotropic, and the patient may occasionally preserve fusion with a chin-up position. The absence of a Bell's phenomenon in this infranuclear condition distinguishes it from a double elevator palsy (supranuclear). A normal forced duction test upward excludes tethering in the inferior rectus area.

Ptosis: Real or Pseudo

The ptosis may be caused by the eyelid following the hypotropia, in which case the lid will become open normally if the patient fixes with the affected eye, which will then come up to the primary position even if the superior rectus is totally paralyzed. If the lid still droops in this situation, a true ptosis is involved, the paresis involving the whole superior division of the third nerve. It is not possible to assess the levator function in detail because the patient cannot elevate the eye.

Treatment

1. Inferior rectus recession 6.0 mm with preservation of the anterior ciliary vessels.[5,14]

2. Transposition of the horizontal recti to the insertion of the paretic superior rectus (Knapp[10] procedure).

Congenital Paralysis of the Inferior Rectus Muscle

This is uncommon in our experience and when it occurs is usually a weakness rather than a complete paralysis. There is usually some degree of lid lag (often small) on the affected side.

A complete examination involving measurements in all positions of gaze, a subjective and objective 3 step test and a diplopia test in the 9 diagnostic positions of gaze will be essential for proper analysis. A Hess or Lees screen examination and an orthoptic examination on a synoptophore measuring fusion and torsion may be useful in determining the correct course of treatment. Prisms may be useful if the imbalance has become reasonably concomitant, although separate readers and distance prism glasses may be needed. Surgery on the direct antagonist superior rectus, the paretic muscle itself, or the yoke superior oblique may be indicated, depending on the results of the examination.

Acquired Traumatic Paralysis of the Inferior Rectus Muscle

Occasionally, a blow-out fracture involving the floor of the orbit may cause a permanent paralysis of the inferior rectus muscle, presumably by the fractured edge of bone irreparably damaging or severing the nerve. The 10- to 15-prism diopter hypertropia that should result from this complete paralysis may be disguised by the tethering of the muscle in the fracture area. However, once this has been relieved by the usual blow-out fracture surgery, the hypertropia will be manifested. The diagnosis can only be reached after showing that passive depression of the eye in the field of action of the involved inferior rectus is normal in the absence of inferior rectus function.

It is disappointing how little improvement is obtained from a tenotomy of the contralateral superior oblique (yoke muscle) or recession of the ipsilateral superior rectus. The only operation that will produce significant improvement is a transposition of the whole of the horizontal recti to the insertion of the paralyzed inferior rectus muscle.

Lost Medial Rectus Muscle Simulating a Paralysis

There is always the history of previous surgery on this muscle. We have seen patients in whom the muscle became detached spontaneously 1 month after surgery (see Chapter 16).

Acquired Nontraumatic Paresis of Vertical or Medial Recti

This type of strange weakness of an isolated muscle supplied by the third nerve should make one consider the possibility of myasthenia gravis or multiple sclerosis. Consequently, the patient must be referred to a neurologist for an evaluation.

Convergence Palsy

Congenital

This condition may not be diagnosed until the patient complains of diplopia for reading and at close fixation. Many patients do not complain until they have been in school for several years. Cosmetically, they look excellent and the diagnosis may be missed.

SIGNS

The patients are orthophoric at distance, becoming increasingly exotropic at near, fixation measuring about 25 prism diopters at 33 cm. Accommodation is also usually involved but can be spared. Partial congenital paralysis of convergence and accommodation may be seen and may be mistaken for functional convergence weakness or insufficiency, which would respond well to orthoptic therapy. Partial congenital paralysis of convergence and accommodation is not improved by orthoptic exercises.

TREATMENT

Surgery is not helpful. Bifocal glasses with appropriate base-in prisms in the reading segments or separate readers with prisms incorporated offer some relief.

Acquired

The most common cause of this is head trauma. We have seen one 30-year-old woman with a permanent complete paralysis of convergence that resulted from a whiplash type of injury sustained in a motor vehicle accident in which she did not lose consciousness. Acquired lesions affecting the mid-brain area can cause convergence palsy. Multiple sclerosis, encephalitis tabes, and mushroom poisoning also have been documented as etiologic factors.

INVESTIGATION

A neurologic assessment is needed.

TREATMENT

Surgery is of no avail. Appropriate bifocal glasses with base-in prisms in the reading portion or separate readers with prisms incorporated offer some relief.

Divergence Paralysis

This is a rare condition. The features of divergence paralysis are an esotropia of 10 to 20 prism diopters on distance fixation, fusion at about 1 m with orthophoria, and normal ductions and versions. The esotropia measured at distance remains the same in all positions of gaze at distance fixation. These findings distinguish the condition from bilateral sixth nerve paresis. The patient has fusion at near with convergence fusional amplitudes but has no fusional divergence amplitudes.

This rare condition of divergence paralysis may be congenital or acquired. If acquired, a neurologic examination is necessary if the etiology is not obviously head trauma. "Divergence cells" have been demonstrated in the monkey's mid-brain,[13] and it is likely that a small lesion affecting this area just rostral to the third nerve nucleus may be involved. Some patients get better spontaneously if the condition is milder and can be considered a divergence insufficiency.

Example: Two patients with divergence paralysis, one congenital and one acquired, which appeared to be permanent and not associated with any demonstrable etiology, underwent surgery. A resection of both lateral recti planned to overcorrect the distance esotropia by 10 prism diopters was performed in both cases. Relief was only temporary, the condition recurring within a year. The literature mentions influenza, increased intracranial pressure, encephalitis, multiple sclerosis, vascular lesions, and neoplasms in addition to head trauma as causes of acquired divergence palsy.[15]

Congenital Absence of an Oblique or Rectus Muscle

Congenital absence of each of the recti and each oblique muscle has been recorded in the literature for over 100 years.[2] More recent reports substantiate the functional and surgical evidence with appropriate imaging of the orbit.[7,11,12] The realization that a muscle imbalance results from congenital absence of a muscle in the affected eye is seldom reached before meticulous surgical exposure and subsequent imaging have been performed.

References

1. del Monte, M.: Personal demonstration. 1991.
2. Duke-Elder, S.: In: Systems of Ophthalmology, Vol. VI:32. London: Henry Kimpton, 1973:736.
3. Fitzsimmons, R., Lee, J.P., Elston, J.: Treatment of sixth nerve palsy in adults with combined botulinum toxin chemodenervation and surgery. Ophthalmology 95:1535, 1988.
4. France, T.D., Simon, J.W.: Anterior segment ischemic syndrome following muscle surgery: The A.A.P.O.S. Experience. J Pediatr Ophthalmol Strabismus 23:87, 1986.
5. Freedman, H.L., Waltmann, D.D., Patterson, J.H.: Preservation of anterior ciliary vessels during strabismus surgery: A non-microscopic technique. J Pediatr Ophthalmol Strabismus 29:38, 1992.

6. Guyton, D.L.: Exaggerated traction test for the oblique muscles. Ophthalmology 88:1035, 1981.

7. Helveston, E.M., Giangiacomo, J.G., Ellis, F.D.: Congenital absence of the superior oblique tendon. Trans Am Ophthalmol Soc 79:123, 1981.

8. Jensen, C.D.F.: Rectus muscle union: A new operation for paralysis of the rectus muscle. Trans Pacific Coast Otoophthalmol Soc 45:359, 1964.

9. Johnston, A.C., Pratt-Johnson, J.A.: The ocular sequelae of third cranial nerve palsy. Can Med Assoc J 89:871, 1963.

10. Knapp, P.: The surgical treatment of double elevator paralysis. Trans Am Ophthalmol Soc 67:304, 1969.

11. Mather, T.R., Saunders, R.A.: Congenital absence of the superior rectus: A case report. J Pediatr Ophthalmol Strabismus 24:291, 1987.

12. Matsuo, T., Ohtsuk, H., Sogabe, Y., Konishi, H., Takenawa, K., Watanabe, Y.: Vertical abnormal retinal correspondence in three patients with congenital absence of the superior oblique muscle. Am J Ophthalmol 106:341, 1988.

13. Mays, L.E.: Neural control of vergence eye movements: Convergence and divergence neurons in the midbrain. J Neurophysiol 51:1091, 1984.

14. McKeown, C.A., Lambert, M., Shore, J.W.: Preservation of anterior ciliary vessels during extraocular muscle surgery. Ophthalmology 96:498, 1989.

15. Noorden, G.K. von: Binocular vision and ocular motility. St. Louis: Mosby, 1990:432.

16. Parks, M.M.: Isolated cyclovertical muscle palsy. Arch Ophthalmol 60:1027, 1958.

17. Rosenbaum, A.: Vertical rectus muscle transposition and botulinum toxin (Oculinum) to medial rectus for abducens palsy. Arch Ophthalmol 107:820, 1989.

18. Scott, A.B.: Active force tests in lateral rectus paralysis. Arch Ophthalmol 85:397, 1971.

19. Scott, A.B.: Transposition of the superior oblique. Symposium. Incomitant strabismus. Am Orthopt J 27:11, 1977.

14

Mechanical Restrictions and Syndromes

Duane's Retraction Syndrome

In 1905, Duane published his paper on "Congenital Deficiency of Abduction Associated with Impairment of Adduction, Contraction of the Palpebral Fissures, Retraction Movements and Oblique Movements of the Eye."[10] It is now recognized that there is more than one type of Duane's syndrome.

Huber's Classification

Huber classified Duane's retraction syndrome into three types[17]:

- Type I: Marked limitation or absence of abduction, normal or slightly defective adduction, narrowing of the palpebral fissure on adduction, and widening of the palpebral fissure on attempted abduction.
- Type II: Limitation or absence of adduction. Normal or slightly limited abduction. Narrowing of the palpebral fissure and retraction on attempted adduction.
- Type III: Limitation or absence of both adduction and abduction as well as narrowing of the palpebral fissure and retraction of the globe on attempted adduction.

In any of the three types, the duction restriction may not be complete, resulting in limited rather than absent movements.

Patients with Duane's retraction syndrome usually have a strabismus, more commonly esotropia in type I and exotropia in type II if the head is held straight. In type III, the eyes are usually straight or exotropic in the primary position. Duane's retraction syndrome is more common in females and in the left eye.[19,22,26,31] Type I Duane's retraction syndrome is by far the most common type

In a possible fourth type of Duane's syndrome, synergistic divergence is characterized by limitation of adduction and simultaneous abduction of both eyes on attempted adduction in the affected eye. The condition may be bilateral. The eyes are always exotropic.[5,8,9,11,12,14,20,40,43,44,46] Because this rare condition appears to be an innervational anomaly with simultaneous cocontraction of the lateral recti, it would appear reasonable to classify it as Duane's syndrome type IV.

Associated Syndromes

Many syndromes have been described as being associated with Duane's retraction syndrome.[23,32] It is advisable to assess any child with Duane's syndrome for defects of hearing, spinal or skeletal abnormalities, and features of Goldenhars' syndrome.[43]

Etiology

Congenital anomalous innervation causing cocontraction of the medial and lateral rectus muscles in the same eye is thought to explain most cases.[4,18,39] However, fibrosis of and in the region of the lateral[29,41] or medial[31] rectus muscles may play a part in explaining a few cases. This congenital anomaly has frequently been reported in infants delivered from mothers who received thalidomide during early pregnancy,[2,26,28] the teratogenic insult being crucial about 3 weeks after conception. There is pathologic evidence of coinnervation of the medial and lateral rectus muscles by branches of the third nerve where the sixth nerve and sixth nerve nucleus were absent.[15]

Typically only a small strabismus is present in association with this condition in contrast to what one would expect with a lateral rectus palsy when a significant esotropia of 50 prism diopters or more would be present.

The most common presentation of this syndrome is type I with a small esotropia and a compensatory face turn to the side of the affected eye to preserve fusion. In the primary position with the head perfectly straight there is a small esotropia, usually 15 to 20 prism diopters, corresponding to the size of the face turn.

Characteristics of Type I Duane's Retraction Syndrome

The condition is usually unilateral. The patient is unable to abduct the affected eye past the straight ahead midline position. On adduction there is some retraction of the eye into the orbit with a consequent pseudoptosis. The lid, therefore, is seen to droop on adduction and open widely on attempted abduction.

Some patients may have an upshoot of the affected eye on attempted adduction when they look slightly above the horizontal meridian and a downshoot of the affected eye on attempted adduction when looking slightly below the horizontal meridian.[38] This is sometimes called pseudoinferior and pseudosuperior oblique overaction, respectively, because it mimics these conditions.

Typical Findings in Type I

1.   Vision 6/6 in each eye.

2.   Central fusion with 40 seconds of arc stereopsis using the Titmus test at near with a compensatory face turn in the direction of the affected eye. The patient has preserved fusion since infancy by assuming this slight face turn.

3.   When the head is straight, an esotropia is present in the primary position of 10 to 30 prism diopters.

4.   If the patient attempts to abduct the affected eye there will be increasing esotropia and diplopia.

5.   The lid is seen to droop on adduction and open widely on attempted abduction.

Type I Duane's syndrome is rarely a threat to the normal development of fusion and vision; therefore, treatment in the younger age groups is not indicated. The face turn may first become a problem in grade school from a functional and cosmetic standpoint.

Presentation of Type I Duane's Syndrome in Infancy

Most parents of infants will notice the esotropia when the child attempts to look to the same side as the affected lateral rectus. It is important to recognize that the parents usually interpret this as the child being "cross-eyed," and rarely have they noticed that the main problem is an inability to abduct one eye with consequent esotropia when the normal eye moves in that direction (Fig. 14–1). This emphasizes the importance of checking the versions in young children, in whom a 15-prism diopter face turn position may be easily missed.

Treatment

TREATMENT TO ERADICATE THE COMPENSATORY FACE TURN

This should be delayed until the child is over the age of 6 years and in school, when the functional and cosmetic aspects can be evaluated to see if surgery is indicated. A recession of the antagonist medial rectus muscle 6 mm should be performed. This will take care of approximately 15 prism diopters of face turn or an esotropia of approximately 15 prism diopters with the head straight. If it is necessary to correct 30 prism diopters, it is essential to perform a further recession on the medial rectus muscle of the other eye, preferably using an adjustable suture. It is important to recognize that the patient will have fusion straight ahead and away from the affected side; i.e., after surgery in a left type I Duane's syndrome, the patient will fuse straight ahead when looking toward the right from this position.

A recession of the antagonist muscle greater than 6 mm will straighten the eye more than 15 prism diopters but will also take away from the fusional amplitude on right gaze. This is the reason for operating, where necessary, on the medial rectus muscle of the other eye (i.e., in the same example, on the right eye in the case

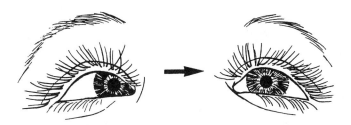

Figure 14–1.   Type I left Duane's syndrome in left gaze.

of a left type I Duane's syndrome). It does not matter how much the right medial rectus is recessed in a left type I Duane's syndrome because it will affect the alignment in primary gaze and looking left. The patient will never have fusion on looking to the left of the straight ahead position. It is never possible to provide normal abduction in the case of type I Duane's retraction syndrome. The aim of treatment, should be to eradicate the face turn or the esotropia that is present in the primary position with the head straight.

TREATMENT OF THE UPSHOOT AND DOWNSHOOT IN ADDUCTION

The upshoot or downshoot on adduction are caused in marked adduction by the tight lateral rectus muscle slipping over the globe . The upshoot and downshoot can be minimized by a posterior fixation suture after a 6-mm recession of the affected lateral rectus muscle. The posterior fixation suture (Faden) should be inserted as far back as possible along the lateral rectus muscle to anchor it to the sclera in this position. An alternative procedure is to fan out the lateral rectus insertion in the shape of a Y and suture the ends down to the sclera in this position after recessing the muscle. Recession of the lateral rectus in type I Duane's syndrome does not significantly affect the position of the eye in the primary position. Although the upshoot and downshoot mimic inferior and superior oblique overaction in the same eye, operating on these muscles is contraindicated.

SURGERY FOR PSEUDOPTOSIS IN DUANE'S SYNDROME

Occasionally, this may be a significant cosmetic problem and improvement can be achieved by recessing both the antagonist medial rectus muscle and the affected lateral rectus muscle in type I Duane's syndrome. This tends to diminish the retraction on attempted adduction and therefore diminish the pseudoptosis.

Caution: Resections of the lateral recti in type I Duane's syndrome should be avoided. Resections will have little if any effect on the position of the eye in the primary position, but the likelihood of retraction of the globe will be increased, as will the likelihood of pseudoptosis, and upshoots and downshoots on adduction.

Brown's Syndrome

Congenital Brown's Syndrome

This is caused by a short tight superior oblique tendon or sheath that prevents the eye from moving up in the adducted position. It can only be differentiated from an inferior oblique palsy by a forced duction test.[6] In children this is rarely indicated because it would require a general anesthetic.

Characteristics

The majority of patients are orthophoric in the primary position, on down gaze, and for reading. Their main problem is that, when they look up, the affected eye fails to go up properly (Fig. 14–2A). In the adducted position it does not go up at all and, indeed, usually goes down on adduction (Fig. 14–2B). The eye can be ele-

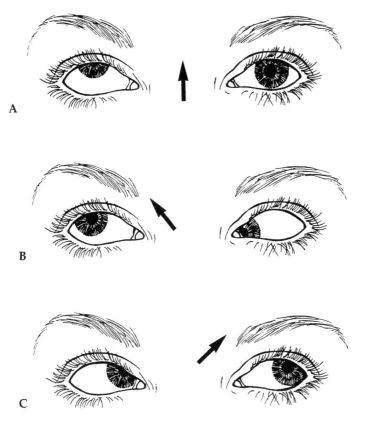

Figure 14–2. Left Brown's syndrome. (*A*) Looking up. (*B*) Looking up to the right. (*C*) Looking up to the left.

vated in the abducted position, although this may not be normal (Fig. 14–2C). Parents rarely detect any problem with the affected eye but want to know why one eye (the normal eye) rolls up under the upper lid much of the time (see the right eye in Fig. 14–2A). If the patient fixes with the affected eye, Hering's law causes the normal eye to overshoot in upgaze because the affected eye does not go up properly. The affected eye is held down and triggers excessive innervation of the elevators of the normal eye.

If the eyes are orthophoric in the primary position and on down gaze, treatment is not advised. The cosmetic defect is worse in children when they are small and everyone who is important to them, such as their parents, is much taller than they are so they look up a lot of the time. But, when the child is fully grown, the deviation can easily be disguised. Occasionally, the condition may spontaneously disappear.[1,7,25,33]

Congenital Brown's Syndromes that Require Treatment

Some patients have a hypotropia of the affected eye in the primary position and preserve their fusion and vision by tilting their chin up. If there is a hypotropia of approximately 10 to 15 prism diopters in the primary position with the head straight, a tenotomy of the involved superior oblique tendon and sheath should be performed between the trochlea and the superior rectus muscle. This will usually improve the vertical deviation and the secondary chin elevation. It also may help the inferior oblique muscle elevate the eye in the adducted position.

Tenotomy of the Superior Oblique: Important Surgical Details

1. The conjunctiva should be incised about 8 mm from the limbus between the medial and superior recti.

2. The surgical assistant should then place a strabismus hook under the superior rectus muscle and turn the eye down. If a lot of excyclotorsion results, the assistant can remedy it by placing a strabismus hook under the medial rectus as well.

3. The surgeon should now remove the conventional eyelid speculum and insert a Desmarres type of hand-held upper lid retractor in the conjunctival wound so that the distal conjunctival edge, as well as the upper lid, is held up (Fig. 14–3A). Adequate exposure is not possible using the conventional lid speculum, which holds both upper and lower lids open.

4. Good overhead light is focused on the exposed area, or a surgeon's headlight is used, to identify the superior oblique tendon in its sheath under direct vision (Fig. 14–3A). Its whitish color differs little from that of the surrounding tissue, so it can be difficult to spot. Patience is necessary so that the superior oblique tendon can be isolated with minimal dissection and trauma (Fig. 14–3B). The conventional eyelid speculum is then reinserted.

5. Two strabismus hooks should be placed under the superior oblique tendon, being careful to include all of the tendon (Fig. 14–3C).

6. The tendon and its sheath are then cut by scissors or cautery with minimal dissection of the sheath or surrounding fascia and check ligaments (Fig. 14–3C). This seems to allow recovery of superior oblique function a few weeks after the tenotomy. Presumably, the cut ends do not retract too far apart.

COMPLICATIONS OF TENOTOMY OF THE SUPERIOR OBLIQUE FOR BROWN'S SYNDROME

Tenotomy of the superior oblique may result in an overaction of the ipsilateral inferior oblique, which may then require a myectomy to restore the muscle balance. We have seen a more serious complication of diplopia in down gaze due to an incomitant vertical deviation. This patient had undergone surgery at another center for a Brown's syndrome that was orthophoric in the primary position. There was diplopia preoperatively only in up gaze in adduction on the affected side. This was exchanged for diplopia in down gaze with all the inherent problems, which were not alleviated by two surgical attempts. Similar cases of postoperative cyclovertical deviation that is worse in the functional positions of gaze with a significant torsional component resistant to therapy have been described.[37] We have not encountered these complications in our own cases, where surgical treatment is reserved for those patients with a head tilt and a hypertropia of approximately 10 prism diopters in the primary position.

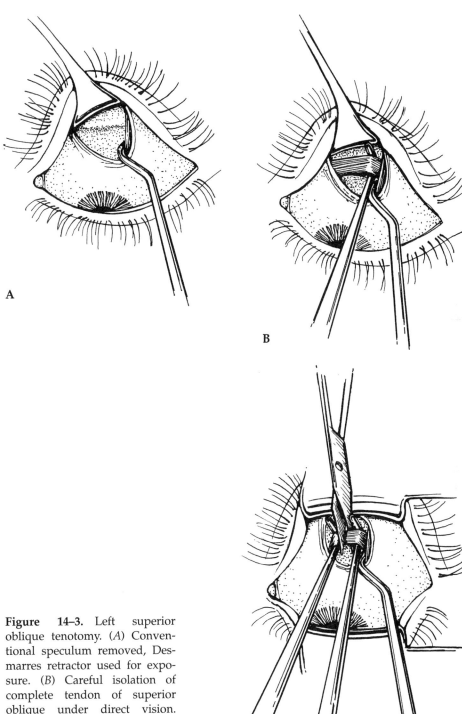

A

B

Figure 14–3. Left superior oblique tenotomy. (A) Conventional speculum removed, Desmarres retractor used for exposure. (B) Careful isolation of complete tendon of superior oblique under direct vision. (C) Conventional speculum reinserted, tendon divided.

C

WRIGHT'S SILICONE EXPANDER

Dr. Kenneth Wright described the insertion of a no. 240 silicone retinal band 6 to 10 mm in length, which was placed in the tenotomized superior oblique tendon 3 to 5 mm nasal to the nasal border of the superior rectus muscle to treat Brown's syndrome.[45] Stager et al. subsequently suggested using a no. 40 silicone band, which conforms more closely to the width of the superior oblique tendon,[42] elongating the tight tendon.

Acquired Brown's Syndrome

Acquired Brown's superior oblique tendon syndrome may be due to an abnormal nodule on the superior oblique tendon sheath, preventing it from gliding smoothly through the trochlea. This syndrome may result from trauma, or it may be due to an inflammatory disease or some collagen diseases.[3,22] The unusual movement of the eyes up and down, such as a musician playing the drums in a band, looking from one drum to the other and then up at the leader and back and forth, presumably caused a mild intermittent Brown's syndrome in one patient in our practice. In our experience, it may just come on for no apparent reason at any age. A tight superior oblique tendon from a surgical tuck also may cause the syndrome.

This syndrome may result in the eye getting "stuck" because the nodule has come through the trochlea and will not go back or vice versa. Commonly, such patients notice that their eye gets stuck after looking up or down for long periods of time. When it becomes free again they often notice a click and actually feel pain in the region of the trochlea.

TREATMENT

1. Conservative management with antiinflammatory medication should be tried.

2. Injection of steroid in the region of the trochlea should be tried. If these two measures fail to bring relief and the patient is having a lot of discomfort and functional problems and has a history indicative of a nodule, surgical exploration with attempted removal of any nodule on the sheath could be performed.

Inferior Oblique Palsy and Treatment

Inferior oblique palsy presents with the same clinical features as Brown's syndrome, except for a normal forced duction test up and in, the affected eye. If a negative forced duction test in the field of action of the inferior oblique is found in the presence of a hypotropia of 10 to 15 prism diopters, the diagnosis of an inferior oblique paresis is made. Tenotomy of the ipsilateral superior oblique tendon (the direct antagonist of the paretic inferior oblique muscle) is indicated. This should eliminate the vertical in the primary position and the chin elevation. It will not result in any elevation of the eye in the adducted position because the inferior oblique muscle is paralyzed.

Blow-Out Fractures of the Orbit

Blow-out fractures of the orbit usually involve the floor or the medial wall, or both. The incarceration of the inferior rectus muscle, inferior oblique, and surrounding tissue in the blow-out fracture often causes most of the problem. In such a situation, the eye may fail to go up, and downward movement also may be impeded. A less frequent hazard encountered is a paralysis of the nerve to the inferior rectus muscle from the trauma. This results in a complete inability to move the eye down in the field of action of the inferior rectus muscle, a hypertropia of about 15 prism diopters in the primary position and in the absence of any incarceration a normal forced duction test in the field of action of the inferior rectus muscle. Sometimes this paralysis may occur with an incarceration of the muscle as well, the diagnosis becoming clear only after surgery to free the muscle.

Management of Acute Cases

ADULT CASES (OVER AGE 20 YEARS)

Conservative management is advised for 1 week with active vertical duction exercises to allow the swelling to subside and to allow proper evaluation of the eye movements. If there is restriction of movement and if the patient is old enough, a forced duction test should be administered under topical anesthesia. If the eye movements and the forced duction tests demonstrate mechanical restriction, and if there is strabismus with diplopia in the primary position and down gaze without improvement by the end of a week, surgical exploration should be undertaken without further delay. The fractured floor may need to be supported, ideally by an artificial thin (0.4 mm) porous biocompatible sheet of material such as polythethylene that imparts sufficient support of the contents of the orbit but does not raise the eyeball.

CHILDREN AND TEENAGERS

In this patient group, a type of fracture may occur that may be more like a "greenstick fracture" in which the floor springs back after fracture and is particularly likely to entrap a rectus muscle, usually the inferior. This can occur in the absence of severe trauma and without much lid swelling, but with obvious restriction of eye movement in the field of the rectus muscle involved. Children may experience nausea and vomiting as a prominent symptom. Surgery is indicated without waiting for a week in such children, in whom marked restriction is present in the absence of much swelling or inflammation, sometimes referred to as "the white-eyed blow-out fracture."[21] The thin (0.44 mm) sheet of porous biocompatible polyethelyne material is recommended to repair the orbit, as in adults.

Old Blow-Out Fractures

Once healing has taken place, after only a few weeks, the restriction from the incarceration of the muscles is usually permanent. Attempts to replace the floor of the orbit and free the inferior muscle from the incarceration are difficult. It is safer to tackle the motility problems by moving the appropriate vertical rectus muscles involved.

Fixed Eyeball

Occasionally, one will see a patient who is orthophoric in the primary position and in side gaze to the right and left with good fusion but in whom the affected eye does not elevate or depress more than a few degrees either actively or with the forced duction test (Fig. 14–4). The treatment must involve recession of the inferior rectus muscle, which should improve both upward and downward movement but will create a hypertropia in the primary position. The superior rectus is recessed an equal amount to neutralize this. Therefore, a 5-mm recession of the inferior and superior rectus muscles of the same eye is indicated. This usually results in a marked improvement of motility in up and down gaze and does not usually disturb fusion in the primary position. If the patient is old enough for the adjustable suture technique, it is safer to perform these recessions on adjustable sutures. The guiding principle, in all motility surgery, where complete normalization is unlikely, is to achieve fusion in the practical positions of gaze, namely straight ahead and looking down, so that vision is single for driving, reading, and going up and down stairs, as well as for recreational pursuits such as hiking and skiing. Consequently, the reading and down position is checked and the inferior

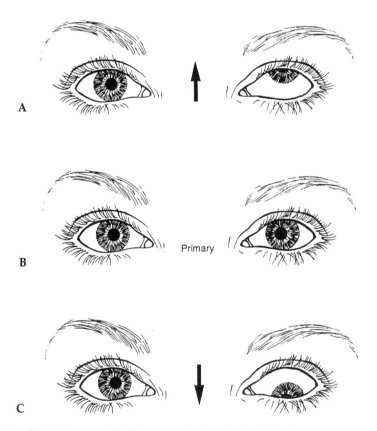

Figure 14–4.   Righ blow-out obital fracture, fixed eyeball. (*A*) Looking up. (*B*) Primary position. (*C*) Looking down.

rectus adjusted and tied off first, leaving the adjustment on the superior rectus to restore alignment first in the primary position and, secondly, in up gaze.

Thyroid Ophthalmopathy

Thyroid ophthalmopathy is a difficult and complicated subject.[34] This discussion only relates to the ocular motility side effects.

Features

One may see a patient with what appears to be an isolated acquired hypotropia with a positive forced duction test in the affected eye that cannot be moved upward from the hypotropic position. The patient may deny having had any hyperthyroid symptoms or treatment of any thyroid abnormality at any time. All the test results for thyroid dysfunction also may be normal. Sometimes such patients are thought to have an ocular tumor or some strange fibrotic condition of the orbit. However, in such a case, thyroid ophthalmopathy with fibrosis of the inferior rectus muscle is the diagnosis until proved otherwise. We have not seen any other acquired condition that results in the tethering of the inferior rectus muscle causing the marked mechanical restriction in the absence of trauma or any other obvious abnormality.

Some patients are unaware of the painless insidious fibrosis of the inferior rectus muscle and, in unilateral cases, may complain only about the "normal" eye being too high and that this eye tends to shoot up under the upper lid in response to Hering's law (Fig. 14–5) when they fix with the affected eye.

Presumably the patient has had some sort of thyroid problem that has resulted in the fibrosis of the inferior rectus described. Computed tomography (CT) scan may reveal thickening of the affected muscle, particularly in the posterior half of the muscle, seen primarily behind the posterior margin of the globe.[34]

Muscles Affected

Any muscle or muscles may be affected in one or both eyes, but the inferior and medial recti are most frequently involved.

Advice and Generalizations

1. Surgery should not be performed in the active phase of thyroid disease or when the ocular motor muscle imbalance is obviously changing. Six months of stable findings should be recorded before planning surgical treatment.

2. Prisms may occasionally be useful in alleviating diplopia in these circumstances, but the patient usually prefers to adopt a compensatory head position to obtain single vision unless the deviation is very marked, such as 40 prism diopters, when only surgery is feasible.

3. Adjustable strabismus surgery is the procedure of choice in an attempt to achieve a field of single binocular vision in the practical fields of gaze straight ahead and down once the condition has become stable.

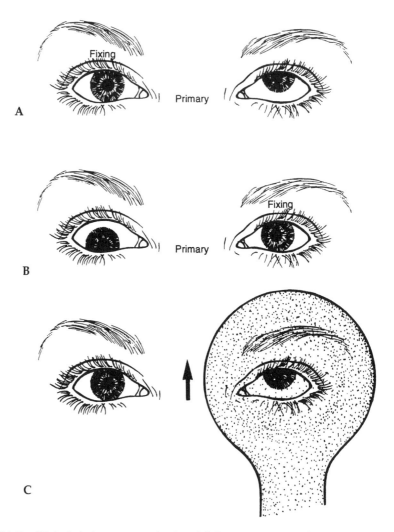

Figure 14–5. Right inferior rectus tethering. (*A*) Primary position fixing right eye. (*B*) Primary position fixing normal left eye. (*C*) Looking up, testing upward movement of right eye with opaque occluder over left eye.

Principles of Surgical Treatment for Thyroid Patients to Reduce the Restriction

Recession of the tethered affected muscle is necessary to reduce the mechanical limitation of eye movement. Adjustable sutures are used wherever possible.

Example: If the inferior rectus is tethered and is holding the eye down in a hypotropic position, the muscle should be dissected free and reinserted to the original insertion with an adjustable suture. The assistant should then rotate the eye upward approximately 10 to 15° above the horizontal straight ahead meridian being careful not to push the eye back into the orbit-if anything, pulling it out slightly. With the eye held in this position, the adjustable suture is then pulled up snugly and a bow tied to secure the suture placed in that position. This should allow minimum weakening and sufficient release of the restriction to restore good practical movement and single binocular vision in the straight ahead and down positions of gaze. The same principles can be exploited when addressing tethering of any of the other rectus muscles.

Caution: If possible any resection of any muscle to restore alignment should be avoided because this may cause further restriction and limitation of eye movement in addition to that caused by the disease process.

Potential Problems Associated with Recession of the Inferior Rectus

If at all possible, excessive recession of the inferior rectus muscle also should be avoided and, if necessary, the patient should be left with a very slight chin-up position in the primary position and the ability to maintain fusion in down gaze. This is important for going down stairs, walking, and reading. Making the patient orthophoric in the straight ahead position by too large a recession of the inferior rectus muscle causes an overcorrection in down gaze. However, there is no solution to the problem of trying to restore single vision in the primary or near primary position and down gaze when the eye is tethered 50 prism diopters hypotropically. An adjustable recession of the inferior rectus muscle of that eye (probably 10 mm or more) is needed to achieve an area of single vision slightly below the horizontal distance gaze position which is the most practical compromise.

Recession of the Lower Lid

Recession of the lower lid invariably occurs if the inferior rectus muscle has been recessed more than 3.0. mm, even though meticulous attention has been directed to separating all check ligaments, particularly all connections to the lower lid retractors. This is cosmetically noticeable, especially if any proptosis or upper lid retraction is present. The lower lid position is best assessed 2 months after the inferior rectus recession. Surgery, using eye bank sclera as a spacer at the lower end of the tarsal plate, allows the appropriate repositioning of the lower lid.

Contracture of Both the Superior and the Inferior Rectus Muscles

Sometimes, there is some contracture of the superior rectus muscle in the same eye as the tethered inferior rectus muscle, although this may not be noticed preoperatively. Surgery to release and recess the inferior rectus may result in an overcorrection, with hypertropia in the eye that was previously hypotropic. This develops within a few days of the surgery but, unfortunately, after the adjustable sutures have been tied off. It is important, however, to exclude overrecession of the inferior rectus as the cause for the hypertropia. CT scan showing involvement of the superior rectus and a positive forced duction test on downward movement in the field of action of the vertical recti implicates the superior rectus muscle. The affected superior rectus may then need adjustable recession surgery to optimize the area of single binocular vision and fusion.

Mechanical Restriction Following Retinal Detachment Surgery

The repair of a retinal detachment may involve an explant with an encircling tape that passes under the insertion of the rectus muscles. This may result in strabismus with or without mechanical restriction. Forced duction tests should be used to evaluate this. It is also important to test the patient's fusion ability to make sure that metamorphopsia is no barrier to fusion. Metamorphopsia may result from the retinal receptors falling back into place in a disturbed fashion, causing distortion of the image seen by that eye.

The surgical exploration of the appropriate muscles of an eye with an encircling tape should be cautiously performed, preferably exposing the tape and at least one muscle insertion before putting the strabismus hook round the muscle. The muscle is frequently scarred down, making passage of the hook more difficult. The muscle involved can be dissected off the tape, which is left intact. If a hang-back technique to suspend the muscle behind the tape is used, the possibility of using a nonabsorbable suture such as Dacron should be considered because the tape explant may interfere with the recessed or resected muscle growing back onto the sclera properly.

General Fibrosis Syndrome

This is a dominantly inherited condition characterized by a general fibrosis of the muscles around the eye and orbit.[13] It results in ptosis and various strabismus abnormalities. Commonly, the eyes are pulled down by severe involvement of the inferior recti and sometimes with an inability to elevate the eye even to the straight ahead midline. The patient is forced to adopt a marked chin-up position to function. In such cases it is difficult to evaluate the function of the levator muscle because the patient is unable to look up. It is therefore difficult to know how much of the ptosis is due to pseudoptosis and how much is due to real weakness of the levator. Improvement of the patient's function can usually be achieved by recessing both inferior rectus muscles on an adjustable suture an appropriate amount to give the patient the most practical area of single binocular vision. This is achieved usually with a slight chin-up position, which allows the patient to look down as well as function straight ahead. Unfortunately, recurrence of the hypotropia and esotropia is common, and a permanent improvement is not easy to achieve.

Progressive External Ophthalmoplegia

This is a rare condition associated with an abnormality in the mitochondria of the muscles. It is usually limited to the eye and orbit, resulting in bilateral ptosis and strabismus associated with a weak muscle. Many of these patients can be improved with ptosis and strabismus surgery, although care must be exercised to avoid raising the eyelids too much. These patients frequently have a poor or absent Bell's phenomenon due to the inability of the eyes to move upward properly. Although the condition is called progressive external ophthalmoplegia, progress varies from one patient to another and many years can go by with little noticeable deterioration in the patient's eye movement. Some of these patients have cardiac conduction abnormalities. An electrocardiogram should be performed before considering surgery. An electroretinogram should also be performed because pigmentary and other forms of retinal degeneration have been reported with this condition.

Moebius' Syndrome

This syndrome is associated with combined congenital sixth and seventh nerve palsies in both eyes.[27] Aplasia of the involved brain stem nuclei has been suggested as the etiology, and this may sometimes also affect the third nerve (oculomotor). Characteristically, the patient has restricted horizontal eye movements with better vertical movements. Improved alignment is often difficult to obtain. Recession of the medial recti muscles may give some improved cosmesis, although frequently it does not provide noticeably improved function.

Strabismus Fixus

We have seen three cases of this rare, presumed congenital, condition, two bilateral and all esotropic. It usually involves fibrous contracture of both medial rectus muscles, often with fibrotic bands and check ligaments mechanically anchoring the eyes in extreme esotropia.

Treatment

The surgical release of the involved muscle and fibrous bands should be performed until results of the forced duction test are normal. The affected muscle should then be recessed using the adjustable suture hang-back technique. The affected eye should be held forward "out of the orbit" and pushed over into maximum abduction in the case of esotropia before the suture is temporarily secured without tension or slack, allowing the medial rectus to hang back the appropriate amount. This must be combined with a 10-mm resection of the antagonist lateral rectus muscle in esotropic strabismus fixus. Considerable cosmetic improvement can be achieved.

Superior Oblique Myokymia

The patient with this condition presents with a typical history. It is usually easier to document than to actually see the myokymia. The patient describes torsional and slight vertical diplopia in the form of oscillopsia usually lasting a minute or two. The frequency of the attacks may vary from one or two a week to several times a day. If the patient is examined during an attack, the intorsional fine nystagmus may be seen with the naked eye, but it will be easier to see using the slit-lamp microscope. The etiology of this condition is not known, but it is generally thought to be benign. Medical treatment using such agents as carbamazepine (Tegretol) has been tried and reported as successful,[16,35] but we have never seen any benefit from this. We have not seen patients who were sufficiently bothered by the symptoms to want surgery. Tenotomy of the involved superior oblique combined with a myectomy of the antagonist inferior oblique is reported to relieve all the signs and symptoms.[16,24,31,36]

Myasthenia Gravis

Intermittent acquired ptosis, diplopia, or strabismus should make one think of the possibility of myasthenia gravis at any age, including young babies. Acquired strabismus, the etiology of which is difficult to explain, such as isolated medial, superior, or inferior rectus weakness or paralysis, may be due to myasthenia.

Such acquired cases warrant a neurologic investigation.

References

1. Adler, F.H.: Superior oblique tendon sheath syndrome of Brown. Arch Ophthalmol 48:264, 1959.
2. Arimoto, H.: Ocular findings of thalidomide embryopathy. Jap J Chin Ophthalmol 33:501, 1979.
3. Beck, M., Hickling, P.: Treatment of bilateral superior oblique tendon sheath syndrome complicating rheumatoid arthritis. Br J Ophthalmol 64:358, 1980.
4. Breinin, G.M.: Electromyography: A tool in ocular and neurological diagnosis. 11 muscle palsies. Arch Ophthalmol 57:165, 1957.
5. Brodsky, M.C., Pullock, S.C., Buckley, E.G.: Neural misdirection in congenital ocular fibrosis syndrome: implications and pathogenesis. J Pediatr Ophthalmol Strabismus 26:159–161, 1989.
6. Brown, H.W.: Congenital structural muscle anomalies. In: Allen, J.H., ed. Strabismus Ophthalmic Symposium 1. St. Louis: Mosby, 1950:205.
7 Brown, H.W.: Strabismus in the adult. In: Strabismus, Symposium of the New Orleans Academy of Ophthalmology. St. Louis: Mosby, 1962:248.
8. Burian, H.M., Cahill, J.E.: Congenital paralysis of medial rectus muscle with unusual synergism of the horizontal muscles. Trans Am Ophthalmol Soc 50:87–102, 1952.
9. Cruysberg, J.R.M., Mtanda, A.T., Duinkerke-Eerola, K.U., Huygen, P.L.M.: Congenital adduction palsy and synergistic divergence: A clinical and electro-oculographic study. Br J Ophthalmol 78:68–75, 1989.
10. Duane, A.: Congenital deficiency of abduction associated with impairment of adduction, retraction movements, contraction of the palpebral fissures and oblique movements of the eye. Arch Ophthalmol 34:133, 1905.
11. Hamed, L.M, Dennshy, P.J.,Lingua, R.W.: Synergistic divergence and jaw-winking phenomenon. J Pediatr Ophthalmol Strabismus 27:88–90, 1990.
12. Hamed, L.M., Lingua, R.W., Fanous M.M., Saunders, T.G., Lusby, F.W.: Synergistic divergence: Saccadic velocity analysis and surgical results. J Pediatr Ophthalmol Strabismus 29:30, 1992.
13. Hansen, E.: Congenital general fibrosis of the extraocular muscles. Acta Ophthalmol 46:469, 1968.
14. Helveston, E.M., Ellis, F.D.: Pediatric Ophthalmology Practice. St. Louis: Mosby, 1980:54–55.
15. Hotchkiss, M.G., Miller, N.R., Clark, A.W., Green, W.M.: Bilateral Duane's retraction syndrome. A clinico-pathological case report. Arch Ophthalmol 98:870, 1980.
16. Hoyt, W.F., Keane, J.R.: Superior oblique myokymia. Report and discussion on five cases of benign intermittent uniocular microtremor. Arch Ophthalmol 84:461, 1970.
17. Huber, A.: Electrophysiology of the retraction syndrome. Br J Ophthalmol 58:293, 1974.
18. Huber, A., Esselen, E., Kloti, R., Martenet, A.C.: Zum problem des Duane's syndromes. Graefes Arch Ophthalmol 167:169, 1964.
19. Isenberg, S., Urist, M.J.: Clinical observations in 101 consecutive patients with Duane's retraction syndrome. Am J Ophthalmol 84:419, 1977.

20. Jimura, T., Tagami, Y., Isayama, Y., Yamamoto, M.: A case of synergistic divergence associated with Horner's syndrome. Folia Ophthalmol Jpn 34:477–480, 1988.
21. Jordan, D.R., Allen, L.H., White, J., Harvey, J., Pashby, R., Esmaeli, B.: Intervention within days for some orbital floor fractures: The white-eyed blowout. Ophthalmol Plast Reconstr Surg 15:301–302, 1999.
22. Killam, P.J., McLain, B., Lawless, O.J.: Browns syndrome. An unusual manifestation of rheumatoid arthritis. Arthritis Rheum 20:1080, 1977.
23. Kirkham, T.H.: Duane's syndrome and familial perceptive deafness. Br J Ophthalmol 53:335, 1969.
24. Kommerell, G., Schaubele, G.: Superior oblique myokymia: An electromyographical analysis. Trans Ophthalmol Soc UK 100:504, 1980.
25. Lowe, R.F.: Bilateral superior oblique tendon sheath syndrome. Occurrence and spontaneous recovery in one of uniovular twins. Br J Ophthalmol 53:466, 1969.
26. Maruo, T., Kusota, N., Arimoto, H., Kikuchi, T.P.: Duane's syndrome. Jpn J Ophthalmol 23:453, 1979.
27. Miller, M.T., Owens, P., Chen, F.: Moebius and Moebius like syndromes. J Pediatr Ophthalmol Strabismus 26:176, 1989.
28. Miller, M.T., Stromland, K.: Ocular motility in thalidomide embryotapy. J Pediatr Ophthalmol Strabismus 28:47, 1991.
29. Nawratzki, I.: A typical retraction syndrome: A case report. J Pediatr Ophthalmol 4:32, 1967.
30. Noorden, G.K. von: Binocular vision and ocular motility. St. Louis: Mosby, 1990:399.
31. Noorden, G.K. von: Binocular vision and ocular motility. St. Louis: Mosby, 1990:418.
32. Pfaffenbach, D.D., Cross, H.H., Kearns, T.P.: Congenital anomalies in Duane's retraction syndrome. Arch Ophthalmol 88:635, 1972.
33. Pratt-Johnson, J.A.: Personal experience.
34. Rootman, J.: Diseases of the Orbit. Chapter 11. Philadelphia: J.B. Lippincott, 1988:241.
35. Roper-Hall, G., Burde, R.M.: Superior oblique myokymia. Am Orthopt J 28:58, 1978.
36. Sa, L.C. de, Good, W.V., Hoyt, C.S.: Surgical management of myokymia of the superior oblique muscle. Am J Ophthalmol 114:693, 1992.
37. Santiago, A.P., Rosenbaum, A.L.: Grave complications after superior oblique tenotomy or tenectomy for Brown's syndrome. J AAPOS 1:8–15,1997.
38. Scott, A.B.: Upshoot and downshoot. In: Souza Dias, C., ed. Smith Kettlewell Symposium on Basic Sciences in Strabismus. Guaruja, Brasil, October 16–17, 1976.
39. Scott, A.B., Wong, G.Y.: Duane's syndrome: An electromyographic study. Arch Ophthalmol 87:140, 1972.
40. Souza-Dias, C.: Considerascoes otiopatogenicas sobre a assim chamada divergencia sinergica. Rev Latinoam Estrabismo 3:42, 1979.
41. Spaeth, E.B.: Surgical aspects of defective abduction. Arch Ophthalmol 49:49, 1953.
42. Stager, D.R. Jr., Parks, M.M., Stager, D.R. Sr., Pesheva, M.: Long term results of silicone expander for moderate and severe Brown syndrome (Brown syndrome plus). J AAPOS 3:328–332, 1999.
43. Velez, G.: Duane's retraction syndrome associated with Goldenhar's syndrome. Am J Ophthalmol 70:945, 1970.
44. Wagner, R.S., Caputo, A.R., Frohman, L.P.: Congenital adduction deficit with simultaneous abduction, a variant of Duane's retraction syndrome. Ophthalmology 94:1049-1053, 1987.
45. Wright, K.W.: Superior oblique expander for Brown's syndrome and superior oblique overaction. J PediatrOphthalmol Strabismus 28:101–107, 1991.
46. Znajda, J.P., Krill, A.E.: Congenital medial rectus muscle palsy with simultaneous abduction of the two eyes. Am J Ophthalmol 68:1050–1052, 1969.

15

Strabismus in the Adult

General Remarks about Adults with Strabismus

Compared with children, adults make very demanding patients. They perceive even the tiniest cosmetic defect. They are acutely aware of any sensory change such as diplopia that may be precipitated by altering the alignment of their eyes. Many adults expect miracles from modern surgery. Some even expect to acquire fusion in adult life despite having the congenital strabismus syndrome and no fusion. Failure to recognize this will soon convince ophthalmologists that they do not wish to do any more strabismus surgery on adults.

Special Points in the History Taking

It is important to ask the patient, "What are you hoping to achieve with treatment?" This usually clarifies the patient's expectations: cosmetic improvement, relief of diplopia, or binocular vision with fusion and stereopsis.

Asthenopia

If the patient reports symptoms of asthenopia, it is important to ask how long the symptoms have been present. If they have only been present a few months in a patient with childhood-onset strabismus, it is unlikely that the asthenopic problems have anything to do with the strabismus. It is generally safe to assume that asthenopic symptoms are unrelated to strabismus if the patient has no fusion. Occasionally, the patient may be aware of a pulling sensation when their eye wanders. It is unlikely that this can be changed; therefore, it is better to avoid surgery for these symptoms.

Most patients with intermittent exotropia are unaware of when their eye diverges. However, they are often aware of closing one eye in bright sunshine. Occasionally, they may say they are aware of trying to control the position of the eye and that this annoys and tires them. Despite these claims, because the eye drifts out without the patient being aware of it most of the time, it is unlikely that surgery will make any difference to their symptoms.

Suppression Facts that Must Be Known

A patient with esotropia from infancy to visual adulthood who has not obtained any fusion will suppress the area of the visual field of the deviating eye that overlaps that of the fixing eye as long as the deviation remains esotropic.[6,8,10] However, if the deviating eye becomes exotropic, causing the image to cross the retinal midline from nasal to temporal retina by even as little as 1 prism diopter, diplopia will be triggered (Fig. 15–1). Similarly, a patient who has been exotropic from infancy through visual adulthood who either has not obtained fusion and has constant suppression or who intermittently fuses and suppresses (as happens in intermittent exotropia) will have suppression while exotropic but will have diplopia if any esotropia results from treatment. These patients immediately experience diplopia once the deviation becomes overcorrected and the image of the fixation target crosses even 1 prism diopter over the retinal midline. This is an exact and extremely sensitive rule (under section on Suppression in Chapter 2, see discussion on the hemiretinal trigger mechanism).

This hemiretinal trigger of diplopia should be exploited in confirming measurements in adult strabismus[10] (Fig. 15–1). Once the strabismus has been measured with the cross-cover test, the accuracy of the measurement should be checked by using a prism bar or rotary prism until the patient first sees double. This will confirm the exact amount of strabismus present in that gaze position. Occasionally, one will see an exception to this rule with the congenital strabismus syndrome with dissociated vertical divergence in which the patient appears to be

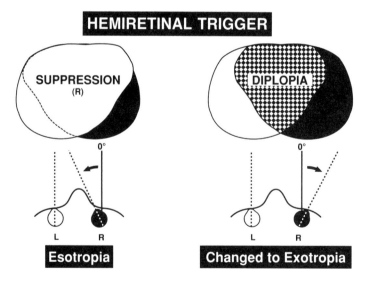

Figure 15–1. The crossing of the hemiretinal vertical line from nasal to temporal retina or vice versa determines whether suppression or diplopia occurs.

immune to diplopia. This scenario is unusual, but should be checked in congenital strabismus. Patients with intermittent exotropia have suppression when the eye is exotropic, but 100% of them experience diplopia if the eye is esotropic after surgery or if esotropia is simulated by the use of overcorrecting base in prisms by even as little as 1 prism diopter.

Caution: Any overcorrection is likely to give rise to diplopia.

Adjustable Suture Surgery

This should be used in all cases of adult strabismus unless specifically contraindicated (see Chapter 16).

Special Points in Assessing Adults with Strabismus

1. Every patient must be refracted.

2. Detailed measurements of the strabismus in all positions of gaze are needed at distance fixation with and without the full optical correction in place. The deviation also should be measured at near fixation with and without the full optical correction in place. It is important to make a note in the chart of whether the postoperative adjustment can be made without the patient's glasses or whether glasses make a difference to the deviation and must be worn for the adjustment. A patient who has no fusion and wears contact lenses need only wear the contact lens on the dominant eye to control the accommodative effects at the time of adjustment. This is useful if surgery is confined to the nonfixing eye. Surgery resulting in overcorrection in any gaze position will give rise to noticeable diplopia (see Chapter 19).

3. In patients who have strabismus with suppression and no fusion potential the visual field of the nonfixing strabismic eye is suppressed where it overlaps that of the fixing eye. However, that part of the visual field of the nonfixing eye (monocular temporal crescent) that does not overlap that of the fixing eye is not suppressed. Indeed, it complements the visual field of the fixing eye. A larger than normal binocular visual field is present in exotropia, and a smaller binocular visual field in esotropia.[8] The reduction in the binocular field of vision associated with the straightening of a large angle exotropia may be noticeable to the patient and should be explained before surgery. A bonus of straightening a marked esotropia without fusion is an expansion of the binocular visual field.

4. Symptomatic alternation may occur in nonfusers. Some patients who spontaneously alternate fixation and have no fusion will complain of symptoms associated with alternation.[2] The patient notes an apparent jump in position of the object of regard, in the process of changing conscious fixation from one to the other eye. Because there is an angle of deviation separating the eyes, fixation must be transferred in these patients before the previously strabismic eye is turned straight, causing an apparent jump in the visual environment. Occasionally, this may cause problems in driving, reading, or playing ball games. This seems more likely to cause problems in large-angle strabismus without fusion and may therefore be a consideration in advising surgery in addition to the cosmetic correction.[2]

5. Assessment of the angle kappa in each eye is needed to see what effect this has on the appearance of the visual alignment in patients undergoing cosmetic surgery (see also Chapters 3–5). Occasionally, the patient has a pseudostrabismus and has normal fusion and stereopsis. Surgery is obviously not indicated in these patients.

Acquired Loss of Fusion without Suppression: Central Fusion Disruption

Contrary to most accepted teaching, adults can lose their ability to fuse.[3,7,9] This causes intractable diplopia. Loss of the motor ability to maintain sensory fusion occurs occasionally following severe head trauma, the lesion probably being located in the mid-brain. A similar type of fusion defect may occur following improvement of vision in cases of unilateral sensory deprivation, such as a traumatic cataract, uncorrected unilateral aphakia, or severe corneal scarring reducing vision to less than 6/60 for many years. The longer the duration of the deprivation, the more likely this is to occur.[9]

Diagnosis of Central Fusion Disruption

The patient is able to obtain momentary superimposition of the diplopic images. However, there is a complete inability to maintain fusion; the images typically bob up and down as if the eyes are trying to avoid fusion. This can be appreciated subjectively when prisms are used to try to superimpose the diplopic images. Occasionally one eye may be observed bobbing up and down slightly when fusion is attempted. This fusion problem is easier to detect on the synoptophore. In a patient who has had a severe head injury, an inability to fuse may be caused by central fusion disruption or by excyclotorsion from a bilateral superior oblique palsy.

An orthoptist using a synoptophore is essential to distinguish between the two conditions (see also Chapter 12). It is possible for these conditions to coexist in the same patient.

Improving the vision in a previously sensorially deprived eye may make the patient aware of intractable diplopia, even if the vision is restored to the same level as that of the unaffected eye. In unilateral aphakia, approximate correction of the refractive error with a spectacle or contact lens is valid for testing fusion. Aniseikonia is not a barrier to fusion in the primary position.[1]

Treatment of Central Fusion Disruption

Unfortunately, recovery is rare. Some recovery may occur in cases resulting from a head injury if the images from each eye are superimposed by surgery or prisms or both combined. It is also very difficult but not impossible to regain fusion in cases resulting from unilateral sensory deprivation.[4] In both situations, treatment involves providing the best possible visual acuity in each eye and then superimposing the images from each eye by adjustable strabismus surgery and prisms. However, patients in this situation are still limited functionally because they have diplopia with images close to one another. One image is constantly moving. Driving, working, and reading with both eyes open becomes unrealistic. Occlusion of one eye with an occluding cosmetic contact lens or by a patch may be necessary to enable the patient to function normally. It is hoped that new methods of retraining fusion may become available in the future.

Uncorrected Refractive Errors and Strabismus Surgery

If a patient has no fusion and an amblyopic eye, only an uncorrected refractive error (especially hypermetropia) of the fixing eye may affect alignment. No matter what the uncorrected error is in the deviating nonfixing eye, it is irrelevant to the alignment of the eyes.

Strabismus Surgery Instead of Glasses

It should always be remembered that patients will eventually become presbyopic and need reading glasses. Hypermetropes tend to do so earlier than others. At that stage, exotropia may be induced by wearing glasses if surgery had made an esotropia without glasses cosmetically acceptable at a younger age.

Accommodative Esotropia

Patients with central fusion and fusional amplitude in excess of 30 prism diopters can often stop wearing their glasses after the age of 8 years and remain comfortable and aligned with good control until presbyopia occurs, if their refractive error is under +3.0 diopters. Some patients, however, may need their glasses to prevent asthenopia for close work or diplopia when tired. Patients who are uncomfortable or who cannot maintain alignment with clear vision without glasses are not helped by surgery for the strabismus. Their refractive error is usually greater than +3.0 diopters.

Partially Accommodative Esotropia

In these cases the deviation is reduced but not eliminated by the correction of their refractive error. If the patient has peripheral fusion and a small residual esotropia of under 10 prism diopters (monofixation syndrome), it is worthwhile trying just removing glasses. If these patients, and patients without fusion, look cosmetically good with glasses but noticeably esotropic without them, strabismus surgery may help to reduce the deviation and achieve satisfactory cosmesis without glasses if the refractive error is under +3.0 diopters. Many of these patients do not need the correction for comfortable vision and are rarely asthenopic as they suppress the fovea of the deviating eye and have plenty of accommodative reserve to cope with the refractive error in the dominant eye. In such a case the eye should be made as straight as possible, without diplopia, by adjustable strabismus surgery; postoperatively, the angle should be adjusted without glasses on. Results are variable.

Stability of Strabismus Surgery in Adults without Fusion

Although the alignment obtained by surgery in adults without fusion tends to be more stable than in childhood, it is important to inform the patient that although the adjustable suture technique should align the eyes so that they appear to be approximately straight immediately after surgery, the deviation may sometimes recur in as little as a few days to a few months. Conversely, the eyes may remain well aligned for the rest of the patient's life. There are no indications that help predict which result will occur. Recurrence is particularly common after surgery for exotropia in patients without fusion.

Consecutive Exotropia Following Congenital Esotropia without Fusion

Patients with a congenital esotropia syndrome who do not obtain fusion often present with a consecutive exotropia in adulthood. If the patient's eye has drifted out much before the age of 8 years, the patient may have developed suppression for exotropia. It is essential that all patients have their awareness of diplopia examined in detail. Are they aware of diplopia? If not do they experience diplopia when overcorrecting prisms are used? Patients with consecutive exotropia who are aware of diplopia if the deviation is overcorrected by prisms should be informed that although a slight surgical overcorrection of the deviation usually produces a better long-term result diplopia will be experienced while the overcorrection persists. They must understand that it may be necessary to operate again to eliminate the overcorrection if it does not wane in a few weeks. Despite the fact that some recurrence of the exotropia is likely most patients choose not to have the deviation overcorrected. They wish to avoid diplopia. In these circumstances adjustable suture surgery should be designed to cosmetically correct the strabismus in all fields of gaze without overcorrection.

Large-Angle Exotropia without Fusion Associated with Superior Oblique Overaction

If an exotropia in excess of 35 prism diopters in the primary position is found, the eyes should be examined specifically in down gaze. If there is a marked increase in the exotropia, it is almost always associated with overaction of the superior oblique muscles. If the eyes have been markedly exotropic for many years, it is thought that the superior oblique muscles take up the slack and are somewhat contracted, resulting in the increased exotropia in down gaze. In these cases a tenotomy of both superior oblique tendons between the trochlea and the medial aspect of the superior rectus should be performed. This should reduce the exotropia in the primary position by 5 to 10 prism diopters and markedly reduce the incomitance and increased exotropia in down gaze. The rest of the exodeviation should be eliminated with an adjustable suture on the horizontal rectus muscle. If attention is not directed to the overacting superior oblique muscles in such a situation, recurrence of the exotropia is common (see also Chapter 11).

Recurrent Congenital Exotropia

Almost all patients with recurrent congenital exotropia experience diplopia if they are made esotropic, by prisms or surgery, in any position of gaze. Surgery should therefore be designed to fully correct the deviation but not overcorrect it. The same general features apply to this condition as apply to consecutive exotropia from congenital esotropia without fusion.

Intermittent Exotropia

Problem of Surgical Overcorrection

It has been shown that adult patients with intermittent exotropia frequently experience recurrence of 10 to 15 prism diopters within a few months of surgery.[11] This has resulted in some surgeons advising a deliberate overcorrection in order to leave the patient with 10 prism diopters of esotropia immediately after surgery. However, it is essential to warn the patient, before surgery, of the inevitable occurrence of diplopia postoperatively if they become esotropic. If the esotropia does not resolve with the eye becoming slightly exotropic again, permanent diplopia that is only relieved by prisms or further surgery will result. Recommending a 10-prism diopter overcorrection is prudent if the patient wears glasses all the time. In this case if overcorrection persists the patient has the option of base-out stick-on Fresnel prisms while awaiting resolution. Spontaneous resolution is unlikely if the esotropia has persisted unchanged for at least 3 months.

Some exotropes may have a perfect postoperative result in all positions of gaze except one position, for example gaze to the right, where they are overcorrected and are esotropic. This will give rise to diplopia in this gaze position. If this is not recognized and acknowledged, these patients may be extremely upset if the importance of this symptom is dismissed and they are reassured that their eyes look much straighter and are not overcorrected in the primary position. These patients, who have never experienced diplopia before, may feel they are markedly incapacitated.

Caution: Always do a full postoperative examination in all fields of gaze to detect any incomitance.

Can an Intermittent Exotropia in an Adult Be Cured?

It is extremely unusual to obtain a sensory cure in a visual adult who has intermittent exotropia, but it is possible.[5] Surgery should cause a small permanent esophoria that prevents the eye from ever drifting out. These patients therefore never suppress, even though they have been doing so intermittently for their whole lives because the eye never becomes divergent now. They never experience diplopia from overcorrection because the deviation is phoric. Unfortunately, this is very difficult to achieve.

Winking in the Sunlight

Many adult patients with intermittent exotropia close one eye in sunshine or bright light and find this extremely annoying, particularly when they are driving. Surgery, in adults, which improves the alignment of the eyes but leaves them slightly exotropic, does not improve this symptom. Sunglasses, however, usually give the patient relief and avoid the necessity for closing one eye.

Refractive Surgery and Strabismus

Correcting a refractive error can change the nature of a strabismus, as discussed earlier in this chapter and in Chapter 21. The effect of refractive surgery on strabismus is no different from any other method of correcting the refractive error. Care must be taken not to disrupt the adult patient's sensory status. For example, inducing anisometropia may provoke fixation switch diplopia, as could correcting an anisometropia that has not been corrected previously. Any patient who is considering having refractive surgery, should be screened for strabismus first.

Strabismus and Monovision Contact Lens Correction for Presbyopia

Using contact lenses to correct one eye for near and the other for distance (monovision) can provoke diplopia in strabismic patients. A check for strabismus is important, before any patient is prescribed a monovision correction.

References

1. Lubkin, V., Linksz, A.: A ten year study of binocular fusion with spectacles in monocular aphakia. Am J Ophthalmol 84:700, 1977.
2. Lyons, C.J., Oystreck, D.T.: Presbyopia and strabismus: Old patients, new symptoms. In: Pritchard. C., et al., eds. Orthoptics in Focus-Visions for the New Millennium. Transactions of the IXth International Orthoptic Congress, Stockholm, Sweden, 1999. Nuremberg: Berufsverband der Orthoptistinnen Deutschland, 1999:119–122.
3. Pratt-Johnson, J.A.: Central disruption of fusional amplitude. Br J Ophthalmol 57:347, 1973.
4. Pratt-Johnson, J.A.: Fusion ability lost and regained in visual adults. Graefes Arch Clin Exp Ophthalmol 226:111, 1988.
5. Pratt-Johnson, J.A.: Intermittent exotropia: What constitutes a cure? Am Orthopt J 42:72, 1992.
6. Pratt-Johnson, J.A., Pop, A., Tillson, G.: The complexities of suppression in intermittent exotropia. In: Mein, J., Moore, S., eds. Orthoptics Research and Practice. London: Kimpton, 1979:172.
7. Pratt-Johnson, J.A., Tillson, G.: Acquired central disruption of fusional amplitude. Ophthalmology 86:2140, 1979.
8. Pratt-Johnson, J.A., Tillson, G.: Suppression in strabismus-An update. Br J Ophthalmol 68:174, 1984.
9. Pratt-Johnson, J.A., Tillson, G.: Intractable diplopia after vision restoration in unilateral cataract. Am J Ophthalmol 107:23, 1989.
10. Pratt-Johnson, J.A., Tillson, G., Pop, A. : Suppression in strabismus and the hemiretinal trigger mechanisms. Arch Ophthalmol 101:218, 1983.
11. Scott, W.E., Keech, R., Mash, A.J.: The post-operative results and stability of exodeviations. Arch Ophthalmol 99:1814, 1981.

16

General Comments on Extraocular Muscle Surgery

All the remarks in this chapter presuppose that a full strabismus examination has been performed as described in Chapter 3, and in Chapter 13 if a paretic element is present. It is also assumed that the aim of treatment has been logically deduced from the strabismus profile after summarizing the sensory and motor aspects of each case. Finally, these remarks apply to that part of the strabismus that remains after full correction of the refractive error.

Materials and Methods

Suture Material

Vicryl 6 × 0 (Polyglactin 910) or Dexon (polyglycolic acid) sutures are advised for all routine strabismus surgery, including all adjustable sutures. These sutures usually take months to absorb completely but rarely cause significant tissue reaction.

Allergy

Fortunately, allergic reaction to these sutures is rare. If it occurs, 5 × 0 plain or 6 × 0 chromic catgut can be substituted. For adjustable sutures, 5 × 0 plain or 5 × 0 chrome catgut can be substituted. Allergy to catgut sutures also may occur, and in such cases a nonabsorbable suture, such as white silk 6 × 0 or white Dacron 5 × 0, may be used, if necessary.

Nonabsorbable Suture

Occasionally a permanent suture is indicated, e.g., if a hang-back recession technique allows the muscle or sutures to pass over an encircling band or explant from a previous repair of a retinal detachment. Another rare example is in a reoperation caused by a muscle secured by a Vicryl adjustable or fixed suture failing to attach to the sclera and presenting suddenly a month or two after surgery as a lost muscle, a harrowing experience shared by doctor and patient. We have experienced this in only three patients, one after an adjustable suture and two after fixed suture techniques. White nonabsorbable sutures should be used to make them less conspicuous.

Colored Sutures

Colored absorbable sutures should always be used for adjustable suture strabismus surgery. Different colors such as violet Vicryl and green Dexon S are used if an adjustable suture is placed on more than one muscle in the same eye. This facilitates identification at the time of the adjustment.

Needles

A spatula needle is one of the safest and easiest needles to use for surgery.

Safest Way to Perform a Recession of an Extraocular Muscle: The Hang-Back Technique

Personal experience with over a thousand adjustable recessions performed with the hang-back technique confirms our initial impressions of its effectiveness, reliability, and safety. Only one of our patients, among well over a thousand adjustable and hang-back operations performed, had the muscle come loose spontaneously. The patient was a 60-year-old white man with thyroid ophthalmopathy. The superior rectus was recessed on an adjustable suture because it was contracted and tight, resulting in a hypertropia. It was thought to have been recessed about 6 mm when it was tied off. One month after surgery, he reported that his double vision had come back suddenly the day before. There was no associated pain. At surgery, the superior rectus was loose about 8 to 10 mm from the original insertion over the tendon of the superior oblique.

This technique used for adjustable sutures has been adapted for use with nonadjustable sutures. There are two methods of performing this procedure. Figures 16–1A, B, and C illustrate the main points involved in the first method, and Figures 16–1D, E, F, and G demonstrate the second method. In both methods, the insertion of the muscle to be recessed is exposed and check ligaments are cut. A 6-0 Vicryl (polyglactin 910) suture with a spatula needle at each end is then threaded through the muscle adjacent to the insertion and locked at each border using precisely the same technique as for an adjustable recession (Fig. 16–1D). The muscle is then cut from the sclera using scissors while preserving the suture intact.

In the first method, the two needles are inserted approximately 4 mm apart in the central portion of the original insertion stump (Fig. 16–1A). The assistant, using suture forceps, pulls the muscle forward until the cut border is flush with the insertion (Fig. 16–1B). A second suture forceps then grips both sutures at the desired position measured by calipers, which equals the amount of recession required (Fig. 16–1B). Several knots tie the sutures together at this point held by the forceps. The suture ends are cut, leaving about 2-mm ends protruding from the knots. The muscle is allowed to slide back and will come to lie against the sclera with the muscle recessed the desired amount (Fig. 16–1C).

Our preferred method is that suggested by Dr. P Fells and illustrated in Figures 16–1D, E, F, and G, which demonstrate another method of the hang-back

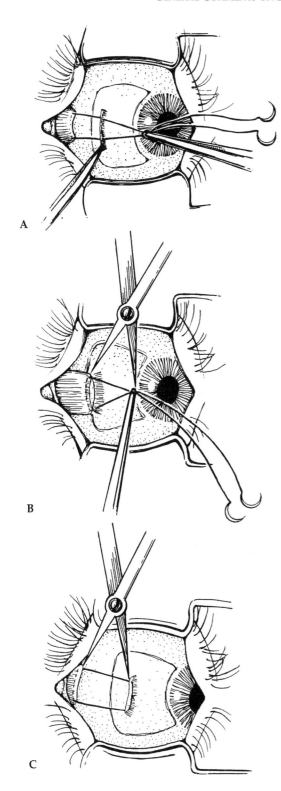

Figure 16–1. Nonadjustable recession of left medial rectus muscle. (*A*) Sutures placed into original insertion stump about 4 mm apart. (*B*) Forceps holds sutures to be knotted together securely at this measured point. (*C*) Muscle lies recessed the desired amount. (*Figure continued next page.*)

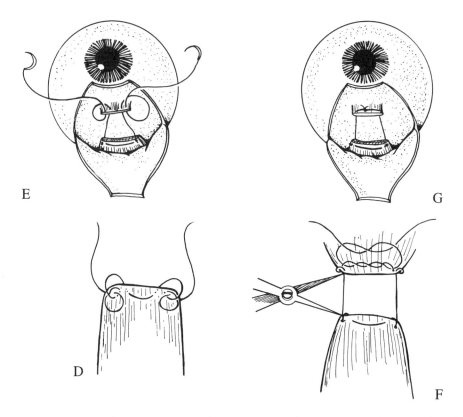

Figure 16–1. (*Continued*)   (*D*) Insertion of a 6-0 suture with a spatula needle on each end into the muscle adjacent to the insertion before cutting it from the scleral insertion. (*E*) The suture needle on each end is passed through the insertion stump twice, partially securing the muscle and preventing it from slipping back spontaneously. (*F*) The measurement of the amount of recession required with calipers. (*G*) The sutures are tied and secured with three knots and the ends cut.

technique. The needle on each end of the suture is passed twice through the insertion (Fig. 16-1E). This temporarily secures the muscle so that the amount of the recession can be adjusted to the desired amount and measurements checked without the help of an assistant (Fig. 16–1F). Adjustments are easily made. Once the surgeon is satisfied with the position of the recessed muscle, the sutures are tied and secured with three knots (Fig. 16–1G).

After either method, the muscle will attach to the sclera within 3 or 4 days as if it had been attached there with scleral sutures.

In recessions of more than 8 mm, a creeping forward of the muscle may occur by 1 or 2 mm. This does not occur with the medial rectus. If a recession of the superior, inferior, or lateral rectus muscle of more than 8 mm is mandatory for effective treatment, the muscle should be secured to the sclera directly at the measured amount of retroplacement. Insertion of the sutures, using the hang back technique, minimizes the danger from scleral perforation. In the unlikely event that the globe is inadvertently perforated, the forward location of the natural insertion of the rectus muscles makes subsequent retinal detachment or damage in the conscious visual field of the patient most unlikely.

Planning Strabismus Surgery

What Effect Can Be Expected?

Table 16–1 should act as a guideline for the effect of surgery on the previously unoperated extraocular muscles in an average patient. This gives the predicted effect in about 85% of our patients, meaning that reoperation with fixed suture surgery may be necessary in approximately 15% of patients.

Note how the effect on the horizontal muscles increases with the amount of surgery done, once this exceeds 5 mm. At 7 mm one tends to get at least 3 prism diopters of effect on the horizontal muscles, and at 10 mm the effect is as much as 5 prism diopters per millimeter. If a patient has a right angle exotropia of 90 prism diopters, it would be possible to correct this by surgery on the affected eye alone by approximately a 10-mm recession of the lateral rectus and a 10-mm resection of the medial rectus muscle. Surgery of this amount may give rise to weak ductions, especially in the immediate postoperative period before the muscles readjust and "take up the slack," after which surprisingly little weakness may be present, but this is unpredictable.

A recession or resection operation on the same eye tends to correct the same amount of deviation at distance and near measurements. Symmetrical surgery on the medial recti tends to produce a greater effect at near than at distance measurements. Symmetrical surgery on the lateral rectus muscles tends to produce more effect at distance as compared with near measurements.

Single muscle strabismus surgery may be used in deviations of small amount and is frequently exploited in vertical muscle surgery. However, recessions of one muscle larger than 7 mm may give rise to incomitance in the field of action of the muscle. Resection of one muscle has fewer disadvantages than a recession as far as incomitant results are concerned. Recession of one virgin medial rectus muscle may be used in patients who have an esotropia of under 20 prism diopters. However, careful assessment of the effects of this surgery on side gaze measurements are necessary preoperatively or at the time of adjustable strabismus surgery to assess if the patient will be overcorrected in gaze right or left with consequent diplopia. A similar sort of assessment is wise in all single muscle surgery, including the vertical recti.

Modification with Reoperations or Scarred Muscles

1.   Advancement, recession, or resection of a muscle, which has had several previous operations, yields more effect millimeter for millimeter as compared with surgery on previously unoperated muscles.

Table 16–1.   The Effect of Surgery, Recession or Resection, on Previously Unoperated Horizontal Muscles

Amount of Surgery (mm)	Probable Correction of Deviation
1–5	2.5Δ per mm
6–7	3Δ per mm
8–9	4Δ per mm
10	5Δ per mm

2.   Likewise, recession of the tight muscle that is associated with a positive forced duction test gives much more effect than surgery on a muscle without associated mechanical restriction. Adjustable sutures should be used whenever possible in unpredictable situations in similar cases.

Effect of Surgery on Virgin Vertical Rectus Muscles

The correction of the deviation to be expected from a recession or resection of the previously unoperated vertical rectus muscle is 3 prism diopters per millimeter up to 8 mm. A recession larger than 8 mm surprisingly does not produce further effect in the primary position, only some further weakening in the field of action of the muscle. This applies both to the superior and inferior rectus muscles from which the usual check ligaments have been cleaned and cut. This is because of the attachment to oblique muscles. The fascial connection running from the undersurface of the superior rectus to the superior oblique muscle, which is usually about 8 mm from the superior rectus insertion, is not cut in routine dissection. Careful dissection of all check ligaments and the lower lid retractors is routinely performed in surgery on the inferior rectus muscle, but attachment inferiorly further back involving Lockwood's ligament presumably prevents a complete weakening effect following recession of this muscle.

Special Values for Recession of a Virgin Inferior Rectus

There is usually more weakening effect in the field of action of the recessed vertical muscle if it is recessed more than 5 mm. However, this is more pronounced and of much greater practical significance in recessions of the inferior rectus. This effect is present in recessions of less than 5 mm. Therefore, it is suggested that the expected result from a recession of the inferior rectus muscle should be calculated on 3 prism diopters per millimeter in the primary position and 5 prism diopters per millimeter in the down gaze position, which is so vital for reading, navigating stairs, hiking, and skiing. Table 16–2 shows how to calculate the amount of surgery to do on the left inferior rectus in a case of a right superior oblique palsy.

Greater Effect from Muscle Surgery than Expected

When results appear to be grossly different from the expected effect in an infant, the possibility of the patient having some muscle tone abnormality, particularly cerebral palsy, should be considered.

Table 16–2.   Probable Effect of Left Inferior Rectus Recession 5 mm in Right Superior Oblique Palsy

	Vertical Deviation Preoperatively	*Probable Surgical Effect*	*Deviation Postoperatively*
Primary position	RHT* 15Δ	5 × 3 = 15Δ of correction	0Δ
Down position (reading, hiking, stairs, etc.)	RHT 30Δ	5 × 5 = 25Δ of correction	5Δ

* RHT: right hypertropia.

Maximum Effect from Recession of the Rectus Muscles: Hang-Loose Technique

Table 16–3 records the result of the hang-loose recession of the rectus muscles. These results were obtained on muscles that had not been treated surgically before and from which the check ligaments had been carefully dissected.[6] Most of all, careful dissections of the inferior rectus muscle, separating all connections between the lower lid retractors and the inferior rectus, were routinely performed. The connections between the levator and the superior rectus muscle were always carefully divided, but the check ligament between the inferior border of the superior rectus and the superior oblique was not divided. Adjustable sutures were inserted in the muscle end cut free from the sclera. The sutures were placed on the original insertion site, but the muscles were allowed to hang back with the sutures being completely limp and loose so the maximum recession effect on the muscle could be produced. At the time of the adjustment, a few hours after surgery, the appropriate saccades were induced to make sure that the muscle had not become adherent to the sclera. The results (Table 16–3) show that the average hang-loose recession effect on the vertical recti is only 20 prism diopters of vertical correction. The hang-loose recession effect on the virgin lateral rectus muscle is about 35 prism diopters of exotropic correction, and abduction is still possible to approximately 10° past the midline straight ahead position in many cases. However, rerecession of a lateral rectus muscle months or years after a previous recession now has much more effect as the muscle has taken up the slack. The hang-loose recession on the medial rectus muscle produces a complete inability to adduct the eye past the straight ahead midline position and converts a large esotropia to an exotropia of 70 prism diopters.

It is important to recognize that a vertical strabismus in excess of 20 prism diopters, with normal ductions, cannot be corrected by recessing one vertical rectus muscle. Likewise, it is important to recognize the limitation of correction that can be produced by a maximum recession of a virgin lateral rectus muscle with normal horizontal ductions.

Example: Cosmetic correction was required for an exotropia of 60 prism diopters in a patient with full ductions and normal versions. If a resection of the medial rectus of 5 mm was performed and an 8 mm adjustable suture recession was performed on the lateral rectus muscle, one would expect to correct $(8 + 5) \times 3 = 39$ prism diopters, so that a considerable exotropia remains. At the time of the adjustment, the lateral rectus muscle would be slackened off until the sutures are hanging loose, but approximately 10 prism diopters of exotropia still would remain because insufficient resection was performed on the medial rectus muscle. Maximum

Table 16–3. Maximum Effect from Hang-Loose Adjustable Recession in Previously Unoperated Rectus Muscles

	Rectus Muscle			
	Superior	Inferior	Lateral	Medial
Maximum correction	20Δ	20Δ	35Δ	140 + Δ

recession of the lateral rectus muscle will only correct 35 prism diopters. Therefore, at least 30 prism diopters must be corrected by resecting the medial rectus 9 mm to allow for some adjustment. It is possible to resect too much of the medial rectus, creating a mechanical restrictive type of esotropia with the inability to passively abduct the eye past the midline. This creates a new problem at the time of the adjustment of the induced esotropia, where the eye cannot be straightened by pulling up the lateral rectus muscle even right back to its original insertion site. This situation can be avoided by performing a forced duction test at the time of the resection. This is particularly important in the resection or advancement of a muscle on which much previous surgery has been performed. An alternative is to place an adjustable suture on the resected medial rectus as well as on the recessed lateral rectus.

Effect of Myectomy of One Inferior Oblique

If approximately 5 mm of muscle belly is excised midway between the inferior rectus and lateral rectus (see Fig. 12–3), correction of 5 to 20 prism diopters of hypertropia in the primary position can be expected. This operation is most forgiving, allowing the surgeon to perform exactly the same procedure for marked or for little overaction provided there is some clinical overaction of the inferior oblique and at least 5 prism diopters of hypertropia in the primary position. The muscle grows onto the sclera at just the right position to reduce the overaction in adduction and the hypertropia in the primary position to within the 5- to 20-prism diopter range. Although the action of the inferior oblique may be paralyzed for a few days to a few weeks, near normal action is usually restored 1 month after surgery.

Effect of Tenotomy of One Superior Oblique

If the tendon and sheath are cut through between the trochlea and nasal border of the superior rectus muscle with minimal dissection of check ligaments and fascial connections, the effect is correction of 10 to 15 prism diopters of hypotropia in the primary position increasing in adduction and down gaze, without paresis.

Effect of Tucking One Superior Oblique Tendon

If the superior oblique tendon is tucked until the slack is just taken up (usually about 8 mm) and if the tuck is performed temporal to the superior rectus muscle (see Fig. 12–4), correction of 10 to 15 prism diopters of hypertropia in primary position is usually obtained. A variable restriction may occur especially in attempted elevation in adduction (Brown's syndrome), but provided only 8 mm is tucked, this should not be a problem.

Effect of Vertical Transposition of Both Horizontal Rectus Muscles in the Same Eye

In our experience a variable correction of approximately 1 prism diopter of vertical deviation per millimeter of vertical displacement is achieved if both horizontal recti are moved in the same direction as the vertical correction is required, i.e., raising them for hypotropia or lowering them for hypertropia.[1,3–5]

Special Indication

This method is recommended if two horizontal muscles are already being treated surgically in the same eye and the vertical correction required is concomitant and less than 8 prism diopters.

Unforgiving Inferior Rectus Muscle

This muscle is prone to cause problems, including:

1.   Overcorrection of the deviation in down gaze. This may result from failing to observe the special allocation of 5 prism diopters per millimeter of correction in down gaze.

2.   Late overcorrection after adjustable recession of the inferior rectus. Slippage of the muscle seems to be the logical explanation of why a recession adjusted to slight undercorrection in the primary as well as down gaze spontaneously develops into an overcorrection a week or more after surgery. In our experience, this has not occurred with any of the other rectus muscles, but alignment is not usually so critical in the gaze directions that involve the other muscles. It is for this reason that in our practice a fixed type anchoring suture for surgery on the inferior rectus is advised when the vertical deviation is under 10 prism diopters and the outcome of surgery therefore reasonably predictable.

3.   Unpredictable results with reoperations. Original surgery on the inferior rectus should include careful and complete dissection of the anterior lid retractors and check ligaments. This seems to heal over with variable but sometimes severe scar tissue formation, which may make reoperation more difficult with considerable bleeding and the outcome less predictable.

Abnormal Appearance of Eye Muscles

It is rare to have noticeable variations in the rectus or oblique muscles, but it is not uncommon to pick up the wrong muscle or become disorientated with regard to the anatomy. If the muscle undergoing surgery seems to be too big or too small or in an unusual position, surgery should be stopped to allow time for reorientation with regard to the anatomy of the eye and orbit, and to make sure the wrong muscle is not being treated.

Complicated Reoperation

A patient who is a candidate for reoperation should be assessed as follows:

1.   The patient should be investigated like a fresh case with a repeat refraction and measurements of the deviation in all positions of gaze even if surgery has been performed only 3 or 4 months previously.

2. Forced duction tests should be conducted either using a local anesthetic, if the patient is old enough, or when the patient is under general anesthetic at the time of surgery to detect and evaluate significant mechanical factors.

3. The decision on what procedure to do should be based on the facts and not influenced by what was done before.

Example: A bimedial recession of 5 mm for an infantile esotropia of 35 prism diopters was performed, and a year later the patient has a consecutive exotropia of 20 prism diopters in the distance and 10 prism diopters at near. There is no significant refractive error. The fact that bimedial recessions were performed and that approximately 50 prism diopters of effect were produced should be disregarded. A decision should be based on the patient's present measurements.

The procedure indicated for such a strabismus would be a 4-mm recession of both lateral rectus muscles. It would not be better to advance one medial rectus in the hope that this would produce half the effect produced by previously recessing the medial rectus muscles. This approach does not work.

Repeat Muscle Surgery

The following precautions are necessary when trying to achieve satisfactory alignment in eyes on which many previous muscle operations have been performed:

1. The forced duction test should be performed before, during, and at the conclusion of surgery to evaluate any obvious mechanical restriction associated with the muscles, conjunctiva, or scar tissue.

2. All muscles on which surgery is planned should be exposed before deciding the plan of surgery. This is particularly important when performing adjustable strabismus surgery.

3. Adjustable sutures should be used on the recessions. In some instances adjustable sutures should be placed on all muscles, including those on which a resection is performed.

4. The distance at which the muscles are attached from the limbus should be measured using a caliper. In addition, the position on the sclera from which the muscle is being cut should be marked with a microcautery. If this precaution is not taken, the site from which one has cut the muscle may not be obvious in reoperations in contrast to a virgin muscle.

5. If a muscle is tight and scarred from multiple previous surgeries or from a disease process such as dysthyroid ophthalmopathy, the exact insertion to sclera may be difficult to identify. The insertion of the needles for recession is sometimes facilitated by the use of two strabismus hooks placed under the muscle adjacent to the insertion so that the needles can be placed between the two hooks, ensuring a secure bite of the muscle without perforating the sclera (Fig. 16–2).

6. In reoperations on the lateral rectus, always look for the inferior oblique muscle that may have been accidentally sewn into where the lateral rectus was reattached. Free the inferior oblique by blunt dissection in these cases. This will minimize any effect on the vertical alignment.

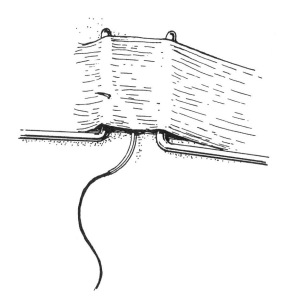

Figure 16–2. Insertion of needle using two hooks in scarred tight muscle reoperation.

Adjustable Sutures

Some Tips for Adjustable Suture Surgery

1. Use colored sutures, because they are easier to identify.

2. Always try to put the adjustable suture on the recessed muscle. Ophthalmologists who are inexperienced with the adjustable suture technique, should start with an adjustable recession of a virgin lateral rectus in the appropriate case, because this is the easiest to adjust. The conjunctiva should be opened with a limbal incision. A 6-0 Vicryl (polyglactin 910) suture with a spatula needle on each end should be threaded through the muscle adjacent to the insertion, locking the suture at each edge (Fig. 16–3A). Sufficient space must be left to safely cut the muscle from the sclera with scissors without cutting the sutures. The two needles are then inserted approximately 4 mm apart in the central position of the insertion stump (Fig. 16–3B). The muscle is allowed to hang back the desired amount and is secured temporarily in this position by a double throw knot and a single bow (Fig. 16–3C). The conjunctival flap should be left open to be sutured under topical anesthesia after tying off the adjustable suture in the final desired position at the time of the postoperative adjustment.

3. In adjustable surgery on the superior rectus muscle, it is important to ensure that the knot and bow temporarily securing the muscle are within 3 mm of the superior limbus to facilitate adjustment (Fig. 16–4). The needles of the double-armed suture can be passed intrasclerally, from the normal insertion forward to emerge about 3 mm from the limbus, or, if easier, the needles can reattach the muscle anterior to the normal insertion. At the time of the adjustment, the patient may find it uncomfortable to open the eye and look down. Indeed, Bell's phenomenon may encourage upward drift of the eye, making visualization difficult. A Desmarres-

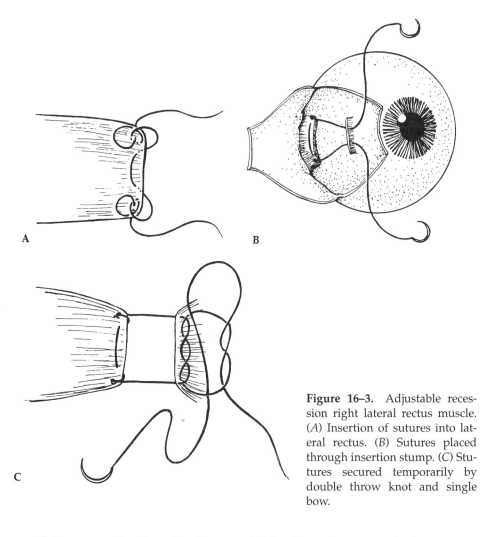

Figure 16–3. Adjustable recession right lateral rectus muscle. (*A*) Insertion of sutures into lateral rectus. (*B*) Sutures placed through insertion stump. (*C*) Sutures secured temporarily by double throw knot and single bow.

type lid retractor placed under the upper lid by the assistant may facilitate exposure (Fig. 16–4).

4.   In complicated reoperations all muscles on which it is intended to operate should always be exposed prior to putting on the adjustable suture so the relative amounts of surgery can be planned. This is particularly applicable in those cases where details of previous surgery are not available.

5.   If the optical correction makes a difference to the deviation, the patient should wear the correction at the time of adjustment. In purely cosmetic cases without fusion, correction is only necessary for the dominant eye.

6.   At the time of adjustment, attention should always be directed to which eye is fixing. In patients without fusion, fixation with the dominant eye must be ensured.

7.   It is important always to inform the anesthetist that an adjustable suture technique is planned so that nonreversible and long-term sedative acting drugs can be avoided.

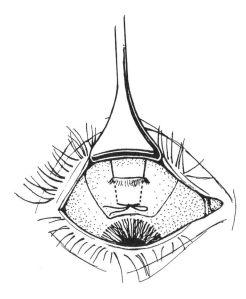

Figure 16–4. Adjustable recession of right superior rectus muscle (see text).

8. If surgery is being performed on muscles that have previously been surgically treated and the result is unpredictable, adjustable sutures may be placed on all the muscles involved. When an adjustable suture type resection is performed, the amount of resection is calculated and an additional 3 mm added so that the muscle can be slackened off 3 mm from the insertion to enable adjustment after surgery to be made.

9. The anesthetist should be asked to avoid the use of droperidol as an antiemetic. Some patients have great difficulty opening their eyes and coordinating their eye movements after this drug has been used even when they are otherwise fully awake.

10. Postoperative preadjustment pain: Intramuscular codeine should be used routinely, provided the patient is not allergic. Intravenous morphine can be used for severe pain in difficult reoperations with pain-sensitive patients. This is most effective in controlling pain and seldom interferes with the patient's ability to cooperate.

11. Eye ointment should be avoided and only eye drops, or nothing, used at the time of surgery to avoid blurring the cornea.

12. Patients may have their suture adjusted any time from immediately upon awakening from the anesthetic to 24 hours later. Preferably, it should be done a few hours postoperatively.

13. Patients should always be placed on appropriate parenteral and topical antibiotics when they have had an adjustable suture type surgery.

14. Adjustable sutures are indispensable in the treatment of adults and most children over the age of 10 years. The following modified technique can be used in difficult cases with young children. (a) The child should be booked twice on the operating room slate, i.e., at the beginning of the slate and a couple of hours later on the same slate, after other cases. (b) The anesthetist should put in and leave in an intravenous drip. The patient is kept in the postoperative recovery room. (c) Tetracaine ½% eye drops or another topical anesthetic should be instilled just as the patient is becoming conscious and the patches are removed. (d) If the alignment is as desired at the examination in the recovery room, the patient is sent out to the daycare area or the hospital ward, if admitted, and discharged when fully recovered from the anesthesia. (e) If the alignment is unsatisfactory, when the patient is examined in the recovery room, he or she is taken back to the operating room, easily reanesthetized through the intravenous drip, intubated again, and the position of one muscle adjusted with sutures.

This is preferable to the ordinary technique of adjustable sutures, where the adjustable suture is left tied only by a bow and the conjunctiva left open, which would commit the patient to a second anesthetic, even if the eyes are aligned perfectly, so that the suture can be tied off and the conjunctiva repaired.

15.   If there is a very marked overcorrection at the time of adjusting a recessed muscle, two possibilities should be considered: (a) Has the muscle slipped? (b) Is there a topical anesthetic paralysis? This anesthetic paralysis has happened twice in over 1000 cases in our practice. It spontaneously passed off 3 hours later.

16.   Adjustable recession may be done on both vertical recti in one eye. Occasionally, one is confronted with a problem of a patient with a hypertropia that is present predominately in down gaze below the horizontal meridian with good up and down movements of both eyes. Most of these patients have a superior oblique palsy that has been treated previously by surgery in an effort to restore comitance and a better muscle balance.

Example: If the deviation is mainly concomitant in side gaze and on head tilting and the main discrepancy is in down gaze, one should consider operating on both vertical recti in the same eye. This means recessing the yoke inferior rectus to reduce the vertical deviation in down gaze and then recessing the superior rectus of the same eye to neutralize the overcorrection caused in the primary position. These should be done at the same time.

Calculate:

a.   3 prism diopters per millimeter of recession for both superior and inferior recti in the primary position.

b.   5 prism diopters per millimeter of recession of the inferior rectus in down gaze.

c.   1 prism diopter per millimeter in down gaze following a recession of the superior rectus muscle.

Example: The amount of surgery required is described in Table 16–4. The table shows the expected result on the vertical deviation by recessing the left inferior rectus muscle 5 mm for a right superior oblique palsy and the planned effect of recessing the left superior rectus muscle 4 mm to remedy the overcorrection in the primary position from recessing the left inferior rectus muscle 5 mm.

Table 16–4. Adjustable Recession on Both Vertical Recti of the Left Eye to Improve Residual Vertical Imbalance in an RSO Palsy*

Position of Gaze	Preoperative Measurement	Planned Surgical Effect	Result Expected
		5 mm LIR Recess*	
Up	3Δ RHT*	2Δ per mm = 5 × 2 = 10Δ	7Δ LHT*
Primary	3Δ RHT	3Δ per mm = 5 × 3 = 15Δ	12Δ LHT
Down	30Δ RHT	5Δ per mm = 5 × 5 = 25Δ	5Δ RHT
	After LIR Recess	**4 mm LSR Recess***	
Up	7Δ LHT	3Δ per mm = 4 × 3 = 12Δ	5Δ RHT
Primary	12Δ LHT	3Δ per mm = 4 × 3 = 12Δ	0
Down	5Δ RHT	1Δ per mm = 4 × 1 = 4Δ	5–10Δ RHT

* RSO Palsy: right superior oblique palsy; LIR recess: left inferior rectus recession; LSR recession: left superior rectus recession; LHT: left hypertropia; RHT: right hypertropia.

Therefore, at surgery:

a. Recess left inferior rectus 5.0 mm on an adjustable suture.

b. Recess left superior rectus 4.0 mm on an adjustable suture.

c. The inferior rectus adjustment should be done first, aiming to leave the preoperative vertical deviation in down gaze slightly undercorrected. The patient will have developed some fusional amplitude for this and will have none available if the hyperdeviation is reversed in down gaze.

d. When satisfied with the down gaze position obtained by adjusting the inferior rectus, the superior rectus should be adjusted to neutralize the overcorrection in the primary position caused by recessing the inferior rectus muscle.

e. There will probably be residual diplopia in up gaze and in far down gaze, but this is the trade-off for securing single binocular vision straight ahead and hopefully some in down gaze.

Contraindications to Adjustable Sutures

1. Surgery involving angulation or displacement of the tendon at the new insertion, for example, in the management of some cases of the A/V syndrome (see Chapter 12).

2. The Harada-Ito type of partial superior oblique displacement to correct torsion (see Fig. 12–8). Errors in torsion assessment can be induced by tilting the trial frame in which the double Maddox rods or Bagolini lenses are placed or if the patient fails to hold the head straight. In addition, the appreciation of torsion disappears if the patient fuses. For these reasons, using the patient's responses for guidance during the adjustment is unreliable. It is more expedient to transpose the anterior two thirds of the superior oblique tendon temporally until it is tight and anteriorly until it is close to the normal superior rectus insertion and then to tie it off permanently. This will produce the desired overcorrection, which will disappear within a month or two.

3. Variable horizontal deviations due to the patient constantly trying to control the deviation. This may make accurate adjustment very difficult.

4. In reoperation on the occasional case where a muscle has become detached from the sclera several weeks postoperatively using the hang-back technique of adjustable sutures.

5. Small-angle vertical deviations of less than 10 prism diopters in which surgery on the inferior rectus muscle is involved. Precise anchoring of this muscle is preferred in this type of case (see special problems of inferior rectus).

Posterior Fixation Suture (Faden Operation)

This operation involves placing a mattress 6-0 Vicryl suture or several sutures to bind the muscle belly to the sclera as far back as is surgically possible.[2] Theoretically, this retroplaces the effective insertion, thereby decreasing the muscle power in the field of action of the muscle without affecting the position of the eye in the primary position (Fig. 16–5A and B). It can be combined with a recession of appropriate amount if some correction is required in the primary position.

Theoretical Indications for the Posterior Fixation Suture (Faden Operation)

1. High AC:A ratio: suture on both medial recti.

2. Dissociated vertical divergence: suture on the superior rectus.

3. Vertical strabismus present only in down gaze: suture on inferior rectus of hypotropic eye.

4. Incomitant strabismus: suture on the appropriate rectus muscle for the desired weakening effect.

Problems Associated with the Posterior Fixation Suture

1. The results, in our experience, are disappointing and vary from 0 to 10 prism diopters of weakening effect in the field of action of the muscle sutured.

2. It is a difficult procedure to safely suture the muscle to the sclera 15 mm or more from the limbus.

3. Possible hazards include inadequate exposure resulting in tearing a vortex vein or perforating the eyeball in a noticeable part of the visual field.

Practical Value of the Posterior Fixation Suture

1. The operation is best reserved for vertical strabismus with diplopia only in down gaze, particularly if there is no significant deviation in the other gaze positions and the vertical in down gaze is under 10 prism diopters.

2. Placement of the posterior fixation suture on the inferior rectus belonging to the eye that is lowest in down gaze sometimes produces a noticeable improvement (Fig. 16–5A and B).

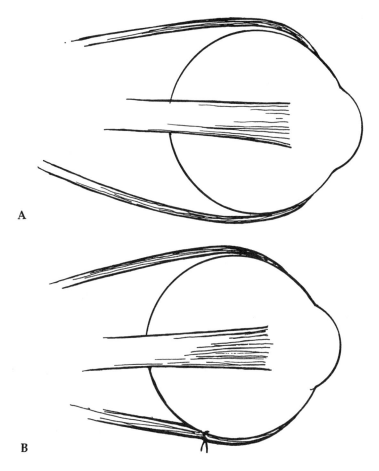

Figure 16–5. Posterior fixation suture, right inferior rectus muscle. (*A*) Normal inferior rectus muscle. (*B*) Posterior fixation suture in place.

Example: Constant diplopia remains in down gaze following surgical treatment for left superior oblique palsy.

The "Lost" Medial Rectus Muscle

The only cure for this condition is to find the muscle even if the muscle has been lost for many years.

Example: A 43-year-old man presented with a large left exotropia of approximately 60 prism diopters with absent adduction, although the eye could be adducted passively during the forced duction test. He was unable to move the left eye to the right past the midline position (Fig. 16–6A). The diagnosis was a lost left medial rectus muscle. The patient had been told by his parents that he had been like this ever since surgery was performed on both eyes when he was a 1-year-old child with congenital esotropia. Several surgical attempts elsewhere to improve the alignment were unsuccessful. A computed tomography (CT) scan clearly showed the muscle (Fig. 16–6B). The muscle was reattached, and a recession of the left lateral rectus muscle on an adjustable suture was performed. Figure 16–6C show the satisfactory alignment 2 days after surgery, and Figures 16–6D and E show good horizontal ductions despite the medial rectus being unattached for more than 40 years. We have seen several other patients in our practice who have had a lost medial rectus for over 20 years with restoration of good alignment and eye movement after the muscle has been recovered. The muscle is surprisingly normal in appearance and functions well, giving the patient good horizontal ductions except for limitation in the extremes of side gaze.

The following measures are helpful in locating a lost muscle:

1.   A CT scan to visualize the muscle.

2.   The case should be booked for 2½ hours to allow plenty of time to look for the muscle without being pressured.

3.   The anesthetist should be asked to avoid using atropine preoperatively so that the vasovagal oculocardiac reflex may be observed if a structure that might be the muscle is pulled. If the heart then slows considerably, it is likely to be the muscle that is being pulled.

4.   A large incision just in the limbal side of the plica should be made.

5.   The operating microscope should be used.

6.   Once the medial rectus muscle has been secured, it should be sewn back onto the eye with the eye held in full abduction so that the muscle is firmly stretched to prevent a mechanical limitation to abduction. If this is difficult, i.e., in the case of a previously resected medial rectus that has been lost or one on which several previous operations have been performed, it is advisable to put the muscle on an adjustable suture.

7.   The lateral rectus muscle and conjunctiva are probably contracted in response to the eye being markedly exotropic ever since the medial rectus muscle was lost. If a forced duction test result is positive, a limbal incision of conjunctiva to expose the lateral rectus muscle should be performed, followed by a repeat passive duction test, pushing the eye over into maximum adduction to see if the conjunctiva was the cause of the restricted movement. If it was not, the lateral rectus muscle should be recessed on an adjustable suture and the passive duction test repeated when the muscle has been cut from the sclera to make sure that the eye can be fully adducted.

8.   Many of these patients show marked postoperative reaction because of the hunting for the muscle as well as the fact that there have probably been many previous operations. It is therefore important to do the adjustment within a few hours of the patient awakening from the general anesthetic, before undue swelling takes place.

9.   Some experienced ophthalmologists have located a lost muscle in a cooperative patient under topical anaesthesia. The location of the lost muscle may be indicated when the patient attempts to look in the field of action of the lost muscle. This is only possible if minimal swelling is present. We have had no success with this method.

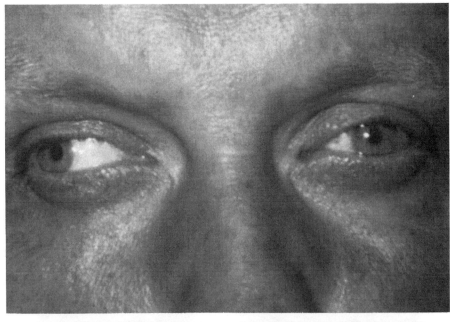

A

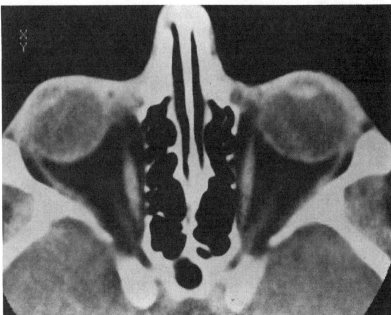

B

Figure 16–6.   Left medial rectus muscle, "lost" for 41 years, was found and reinserted. (*A*) Absent left adduction as patient looks in right gaze preoperatively. (*B*) CT scan shows "lost" left medial rectus muscle. (*Figure continued next page.*)

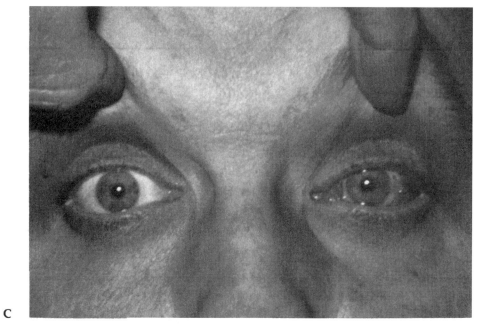

C

D

Figure 16–6. (*Continued*)   (*C*) Good alignment 2 days postoperatively. (*D*) Good abduction 2 days postoperatively.

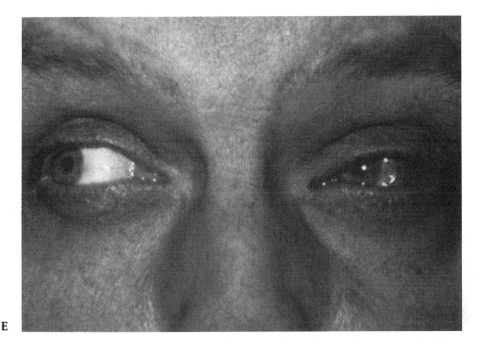

E

Figure 16–6. (*Continued*)   (*E*) Good adduction 2 days postoperatively.

References

1. Alvaro, M.E.: Simultaneous surgical correction of vertical and horizontal deviations. Ophthalmologica 120:191, 1950.
2. Cüppers, C.: The so called "Fadenoperation." 11 Kong. I.S.A. Marseille. 1974, S 395. Paris-
   Marseille: Diff Gen Libr, 1976.
3. Foster, J., Pemberton, E.C.: The effect of operative alterations in height of the lateral rectus in-
   sertia. Br J Ophthalmol 30:88, 1946.
4. Jones, S.T.: Treatment of hypertropia by vertical displacement of horizontal recti. Am Orthopt J 27:107, 1977.
5. Paque, J.T., Mumma, J.V.: Vertical offsets of the horizontal recti. J Pediatr Ophthalmol Strabismus 15:205, 1978.
6. Pratt-Johnson, J.A.: Adjustable-suture strabismus surgery: A review of 255 consecutive cases.
   Can J Ophthalmol 20:105–109, 1985.
7. Pratt-Johnson, J.A.: Complicated strabismus and adjustable sutures. Aust N Z J Ophthalmol
   16:87–92, 1988.

17

Complications of Strabismus Surgery

Ocular Alignment Problems

Our experience using fixed suture techniques is that a postoperative position of the eyes consistent with what had been planned preoperatively is obtained in about 85% of simple cases. Fifteen percent, therefore, are under- or overcorrected. Using the adjustable suture technique, the reliability of ocular alignment is much better than the fixed suture technique, particularly in more complex cases. It is important for the patient to recognize, however, that although the immediate postoperative alignment is invariably satisfactory, if no fusion is present the eyes may wander again after just a few weeks.

Muscle Shock: Fusion Resetting the Muscle Balance?

We have occasionally seen adult patients with normal fusion ability who had an unexpected marked overcorrection after surgery with consequent diplopia. A sudden and unexplained recovery of the muscle balance and fusion 5 to 6 weeks after the surgery was just as startling to the patients as it was to us. Was this a recovery from muscle shock? Did the recovery of fusion reset the muscle balance so virtually no phoria remained?

Case Histories

1. A 28-year-old female surgical resident presented with intermittent diplopia. She was wearing −8.0 diopter sphere (DS) right and (−10.0 DS left with prisms to correct 20 prism diopters of esophoria. She wanted to wear contact lenses, and because she had normal fusion with good fusional amplitudes and 40 seconds of arc stereopsis with the Titmus test at near, adjustable strabismus surgery on her left eye was advised. An adjustable recession of the left medial rectus muscle of 5.0 mm was combined with a 5.0-mm resection of the left lateral rectus. There was an exophoric flick of less than 5 prism diopters with her myopic correction without prisms at the time of the adjustment 4 hours after surgery, and no adjustment was made. She returned 10 days later with constant diplopia in all fields of gaze, as well as an exotropia of 25 prism diopters at distance and near and in all fields of gaze except in gaze right, where it measured 30 to 35 prism diopters of exotropia. Versions appeared to be normal. The patient was, understandably, upset and demanded more surgery. However, being aware of this strange muscle shock phenomenon, we advised a review in 6 weeks. Six weeks after surgery she returned with a broad smile as the diplopia had resolved over a 2-day period and was now only present in extreme right gaze where she had an exotropia of 10 prism diopters. She was orthophoric with correction in all other positions. Versions showed a slight limitation of the left eye looking in extreme right gaze. The marked overcorrection and the dramatic recovery 6 weeks later were documented on the Lees screen and synoptophore.

2.   A 31-year-old man presented with a bilateral superior oblique palsy. He had undergone a myectomy of the inferior oblique muscles. He could only obtain fusion in up gaze by depressing his chin, and in this position he was orthophoric with 40 seconds of arc stereopsis at near with the Titmus test. In the primary position he had an esotropia of 2 prism diopters and a right hypertropia of 1 prism diopter. The esotropia increased to 12 prism diopters in down gaze. Twelve degrees of excyclotorsion in down gaze was not a barrier to fusion when the esotropia and minimal hypertropia were neutralized on the synoptophore. He was assessed 1 week following a recession of both medial recti of 3.5 mm with a half tendon width downward displacement. Twenty-five prism diopters of exotropia were present in all fields of gaze with normal horizontal versions. Diplopia was present everywhere. The patient was not impressed. He was offered prisms but preferred to close one eye to relieve the diplopia. He was reviewed 4 weeks later. He happily reported how the diplopia was noticeably better when he awoke one morning, and it had virtually disappeared over the next 2 days. He had an exophoria of only 2 prism diopters in the primary position. He had a right hypertropia of 10 prism diopters in gaze left, which gave him diplopia if he looked more than 25° to the left. He had a large area of single binocular vision. His remarkable experience was documented preoperatively, 1 week postoperatively, and after recovery 5 weeks postoperatively on the synoptophore and Lees screen, as well as with the prism cover test.

Diplopia

Postoperative diplopia may be due to a number of causes (see Chapter 19).

Conjunctival Complications

Prolapse of Tenon's Capsule

A small piece of Tenon's capsule may prolapse through the conjunctival wound, although difficult to see at the time of surgery. Postoperatively it appears much more obviously white in contrast to the conjunctiva and is usually cosmetically obvious.

   Prophylaxis: Careful cleaning of Tenon's capsule from the operative site combined with good wound closure of the conjunctiva will make this a rare occurrence.

Treatment options: (1) Wait a few days. Tenon's capsule may shrink back inside the conjunctiva. (2) Excise it under topical drops if the patient is old enough. A general anesthetic is not necessary for treating this complication.

Suture Granuloma

Occasionally an inflammatory slightly tender lump over the suture site may develop within 1 or 2 weeks of surgery. It is a foreign body reaction either to the suture itself or some other foreign matter such as cotton wool fibers.

Treatment: Corticosteroid drops. If this does not bring resolution, removing the suture and excising the small lump should be considered provided more than 10 days have elapsed since surgery, at which time the muscle should be firmly adherent to the sclera.

Suture Abscess

An abscess localized to the suture knot may occur within a few days of surgery.

Treatment: (1) A smear and culture should be taken before starting appropriate topical and parenteral antibiotics. If the abscess is not resolving within 2 days, consideration should be given to removal of the suture provided it is not in the medial rectus. In the latter case, drainage should be encouraged, but do not remove the suture until 10 days after operation. (2) The ends of any protruding suture should be trimmed. (3) Topical corticosteroid drops four times a day should be used. Treatment usually results in slow resolution over 10 days.

Allergic Reaction to Sutures

This is rare but occurs occasionally with polyglycolic acid sutures. It used to be more common, occuring in as much as 10% of cases when catgut was used.

Cysts

Epithelial inclusion cysts may arise at the site of the conjunctival incision. These may be small, insignificant, and nonprogressive, or they may enlarge to be cosmetically and mechanically disturbing, reaching a size larger than the average pea.

Treatment: Careful excision, using the operating microscope, is necessary to ensure that the cyst does not return.

Dellen Formation

Dry spots on the cornea, near the limbus, may be produced by folds of conjunctiva preventing adequate distribution of the tear film with blinking in the postoperative period.

Treatment: Artificial sterile tears and forced frequent complete closure of the lids with a blink may bring relief. It is sometimes necessary to refashion the conjunctiva if a Dellen formation persists.

Mobile Conjunctiva

The conjunctiva normally falls back flush with Tenon's capsule and the sclera without taking any particular measures to attach it to the underlying tissues. Occasionally, the conjunctiva will not adhere properly to the underlying tissues, and a mobile conjunctiva that moves around with the eye movement may be seen mimicking the appearance of chemosis. If this is in the lower part of the conjunctiva, when the patient looks down the conjunctiva will overlap the limbus inferiorly. When the patient looks up it will be stretched right against the underlying tissue, and the protrusion of the conjunctiva will disappear.

Treatment: In such a situation where the mobility of the conjunctiva postoperatively is symptomatic, a small elipse may be excised and the conjunctiva actually sutured to the underlying sclera in addition to closing the conjunctival wound. Care should be taken to excise only as much conjunctiva as is necessary to eliminate the apparent excess and to avoid any restriction.

Conjunctival Scarring and the Plica

A permanent scar always remains following conjunctival incision. However, in most patients it is not particularly noticeable and produces no symptoms. In patients who have had multiple procedures, increased conjunctival vascularization may result in more obvious scarring. This tends to be particularly troublesome on the medial aspect of the conjunctiva, and if it is associated with some contracture of the conjunctiva between the limbus and the plica, the plica is drawn out of the medial canthal area toward the limbus, giving rise to an obvious reddish lump, and is symptomatic (Fig. 17–1). In such patients, when the patient looks medially in adduction, the plica overlaps the medial limbus, is uncomfortable, and looks very red and unpleasant cosmetically (Fig. 17–1). The patients have burning and irritable tearing eyes when they go out in the sun or after prolonged periods of driving or reading.

Treatment: Excise the lumpy tissue of the plica that has been displaced (Figs. 17–2 and 17–3). This can be cut and excised right down flush to the level of the conjunctiva. If there is marked shortage of conjunctiva between the plica and the limbus and the conjunctiva is freely mobile above and below between the vertical recti and the medial rectus, slips of conjunctiva can be brought down and joined

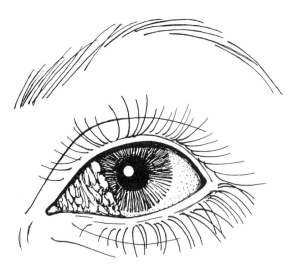

Figure 17–1. Plica pulled by scarring to overlap the limbus in primary position left eye.

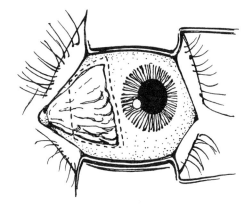

Figure 17–2. Line of excision of plica.

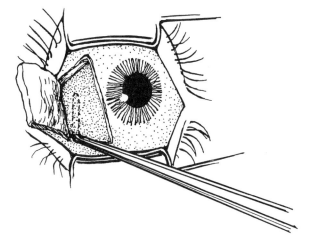

Figure 17–3. Excising plica, preserving the medial rectus muscle.

together in the interpalpebral fissure. The conjunctiva, from which the plica has been excised, can then be sutured down to the sclera in the internal canthal area. It is important, when operating in this area over the medial rectus muscle, that this muscle be isolated on a strabismus hook so that it is not accidentally damaged or cut from the sclera (Fig. 17–3).

There seems to be a reluctance shared by most strabismus surgeons to touch the plica, but in our experience the best method of treating a plica, which is pulled toward the limbus, is to excise most of it. After excising the plica, the conjunctiva is sutured above and below (Fig. 17–4). The medial rectus is covered, but bare sclera is left between the medial rectus insertion and the cut edge of the conjunctiva on the medial side. There are several millimeters of flat unvascularized conjunctiva extending from the limbus nasally, which was hidden by the plica being drawn over it toward the limbus. This is left undisturbed (Fig. 17–4). The bare area of sclera is soon epithelialized. The conjunctiva in the medial canthal area is firm and tight but does not cause any significant limitation of abduction because it exerts its effect too far back on the medial side. This procedure improves cosmesis noticeably and relieves symptoms of irritation and watering (Fig. 17–5).

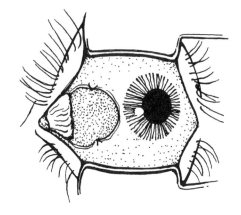

Figure 17–4. Conjunctiva sutured above and below.

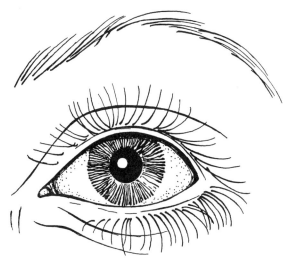

Figure 17–5. Two months postoperative appearance.

Case History: A 45-year-old woman presented with a large-angle right exotropia. She had already undergone several surgical procedures for strabismus as a child in New Zealand. Following as adjustable strabismus surgery, she was pleased with her alignment but annoyed by the red conjunctiva and plica that overlapped the medial edge of the cornea when she looked straight ahead or to the left (Fig. 17–6A). She had the plica excised (see Figs. 17–1 through 17–5). Figure 17–6B shows her appearance 2 months after the surgery, which gave her markedly improved cosmesis and relieved all her symptoms.

Red Lumpy Subconjunctival Appearance from Fat Pad Disturbance

It is important in strabismus surgery to avoid damaging the fat pad that is present in the orbit. If Tenon's layer, which keeps the fat back 10 mm or so from the limbus, is broken, the fat may prolapse forward subconjunctivally, causing ugly subconjunctival lumps and a conjunctiva that is chronically red, inflamed, and uncomfortable. If surgery has inadvertently caused much bleeding and disturbance

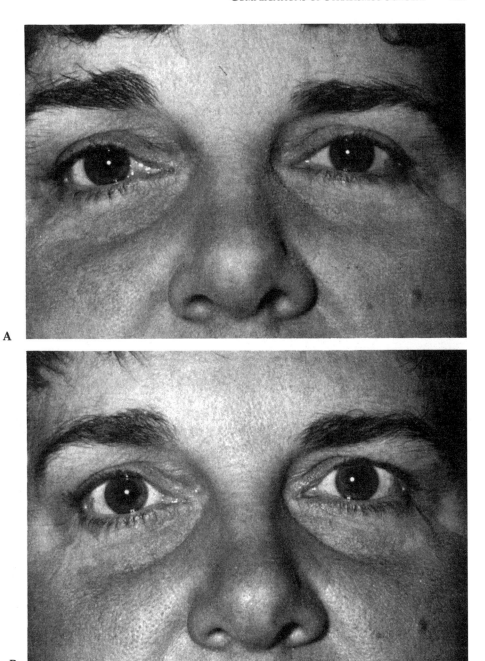

Figure 17–6.   (*A*) Plica pulled and scarred toward limbus right eye. (*B*) Marked cosmetic improvement 2 months after surgery.

of the fat, some mechanical restriction may result in as little as a week postoperatively. This is particularly a problem on the medial aspect of the eye if the fat pad is disturbed. This results in a red lumpy conjunctiva up to the medial aspect of the limbus and is very obvious and cosmetically disturbing, and causes a prickly foreign body sensation.

Treatment: Prophylaxis is the most important thing to remember because it is difficult to obtain a satisfactory resolution of this problem. The conjunctiva should be opened along the previous scar and the subconjunctival fat excised by clamping and cauterizing the fat as one would do in a blepharoplasty. Careful attention to prevent bleeding is important. Peel as much fat from the conjunctiva, leaving the conjunctiva as thin as possible, if necessary using the operating microscope.

Mechanical Restriction as a Complication of Strabismus Surgery

Multiple Surgery

The more operations that are performed on the same eye muscles, the more likely it is that fibrous and some mechanical restriction will result, particularly if the fat pad has been disturbed.

Postoperative Restriction of Up Gaze after Surgery on the Inferior Oblique Muscle

This is a rare complication in our experience after inferior oblique myectomy surgery. It has been referred to as the adherence syndrome.[7] We have seen only three cases in 30 years during which time many hundreds of inferior oblique myectomies between the inferior and lateral rectus muscles have been performed in our practice. If the fat has been grossly disturbed and much bleeding has occurred, postoperative scarring may occasionally result in mechanical restriction of the eye moving upward as soon as a few days after surgery. This may be associated with a positive forced duction test result, but this is often difficult to demonstrate. The restriction is the reason for the increased hypotropia in up gaze. Further surgery is almost always necessary, and because there is an increasing hypotropia of the affected eye in up gaze, the most effective treatment is a recession of the inferior rectus muscle in the affected eye, calculating 3 prism diopters per millimeter of effect for the hypotropia in the primary position. This usually improves the situation but rarely normalizes the eye movements and muscle balance. This is therefore a serious complication, but fortunately it is rare if attention is focused on a careful and gentle technique in performing the myectomy between the inferior and lateral rectus muscles, cauterizing the cut ends thoroughly in addition to using a cautery to stop any other bleeding.

"Lost" Muscle

Lost Muscle at the Time of Surgery

The medial rectus muscle is the only muscle that creates a potential major problem if it slips back inadvertently into the orbit either at the time of surgery or subsequently. We have seen a medial rectus lose its attachment completely 1 month after surgery, presumably when the 6-0 Vicryl sutures began to disintegrate. The other muscles are usually easy to recover due to the many fascial connections between the inferior rectus and inferior oblique, the lateral rectus and inferior oblique, and the superior rectus, levator, and superior oblique.

It is advisable to lock all sutures placed in the medial rectus muscle for recession or resection with at least two knots. If the scleral sutures should spontaneously come out during another phase of the surgery, such as during lateral rectus resection on the same eye, the muscle can usually be distinguished from surrounding Tenon's capsule and soft tissue by using magnification provided by operating loupes or an operating microscope and by identifying the suture knots. Care must be taken to avoid disturbing the fat pad lying approximately 10 mm from the limbus between the medial wall of the orbit and the muscle while looking for and securing the muscle (see also Chapter 16).

Lost Medial Rectus Muscle Recognized after the Patient Has Recovered from General Anesthesia

This presents as a large exotropia of 60 to 70 prism diopters with absent adduction past the midline primary position. The medial rectus will have retracted into the orbit. Occasionally a rectus muscle may come loose from the sclera weeks after surgery and occur as an acute sudden deviation. Presumably, the sutures have absorbed and the muscle has failed to grow onto the sclera, resulting in its immediate retraction into the orbit. Fortunately, this is rare but it has involved the medial rectus twice and superior rectus once in our practice.

The medial rectus may be caught at the Tenon's capsule exit approximately 10 mm from the limbus or may sometimes remain attached to the sclera by only a flimsy piece of Tenon's capsule. However, clinically, if there is any attachment of the muscle, slight but definite adduction past the midline will be present. Extreme care should be exercised in exposing the area involved, tracing back all strands of Tenon's capsule that may lead to the muscle (see also Chapter 16).

Postoperative Infection

Prophylaxis

Povidone-iodine (Betadine) solution as a preoperative preparation of the skin of the eyelids and eyebrows as well as instillation of a drop of the half strength solution into the conjunctival sac of each eye is advised in an attempt to reduce or eliminate bacteria just before surgery.[1,2] This must not be used if the patient is allergic to iodine.

Conjunctivitis

Topical antibiotic drops may be instilled in both eyes after anesthesia and before starting the surgery. Topical broad spectrum antibiotic drops or ointment are used at the conclusion of the surgery.

The use of topical antibiotic medication four times per day for 4 days after surgery is advised if the patient is compliant enough to allow their use. If this is resisted, more harm than good may result, so observation only for any signs of infection is recommended. If an infection is starting, the use of appropriate systemic antibiotics, guided by a smear and culture, is advised.

Orbital Cellulitis

If there is any postoperative infection of the conjunctiva, infection may spread to the orbit along the paths that were opened up in performing the muscle surgery. A warning sign is undue swelling of the upper and lower lids, pyrexia, and pain. Orbital cellulitis in a young child may be life threatening, and immediate treatment is mandatory. In a young child admission to the hospital for intravenous broad-spectrum antibiotics preferably chosen based on the results of a smear or culture examination should be arranged without delay. In older patients, if any of these early signs or symptoms are present within a few days of surgery, swabs and culture of any discharge should be performed. The patient should be given appropriate systemic antibiotics in addition to hourly instillation of appropriate broad-spectrum antibiotic drops and kept under close observation (seen at least daily). Any progress of the symptoms necessitates an intravenous antibiotic appropriately chosen on the basis of smear and culture technique.

Endophthalmitis

This is the one nightmare complication, and fortunately it is rarely seen following strabismus surgery. It can result in the total loss of all vision and even loss of the eye itself. Presumably, this only follows perforation of the globe. Fortunately, we have never experienced this complication.

Treatment: Treatment is urgent and involves the intravitreal injection of appropriate broad-spectrum antibiotics after obtaining a small amount of vitreous, so that a smear and culture can be done for organisms. After 24 to 48 hours of observation, if there is no improvement, an emergency vitrectomy may be indicated. These drastic measures are urgently needed after early diagnosis if the sight is to be saved.

Perforation of the Globe

The sclera alone may be perforated by the passage of the needle or all layers of the eye perforated. If perforation of the globe with leakage of vitreous occurs, a small ring of cryotherapy surrounding the perforation should be performed. If possible, this should be visualized through the dilated pupil. A culture should then be taken from the lashes and conjunctiva. Appropriate broad-spectrum antibiotic should be liberally lavaged around the perforation site. Postoperatively, the patient should be seen on a daily basis for a thorough eye examination in case signs of endophthalmitis should start, in which case reference could be made to the previous culture and a smear taken at the time of surgery for some guidance as to which intravitreal antibiotic to use. If possible, an ophthalmologist experienced in retinal surgery should be consulted immediately after surgery. It is rare to encounter any complications following a needle perforation of the globe in strabismus surgery.

Anterior Segment Ischemia

Anterior segment ischemia[3,6] is most likely to occur in persons over 60 years of age. Anterior segment ischemia is rare in children. It is more likely to occur in patients with vascular problems and arteriosclerosis and in those patients who are undergoing muscle surgery for a strabismus that has followed retinal detachment surgery with an encircling band.

Prophylaxis

1. Operating on three rectus muscles at the same sitting in one eye should be avoided. If more than two muscles need to be treated surgically in one eye, do this at two separate operations, treating two muscles initially and the other muscle or muscles at a subsequent operation after an interval of at least 4 months.

2. Muscle surgery sparing the anterior ciliary vessels (see Figs. 13–1 and 13–2). It is possible to operate on a rectus muscle and yet dissect out and preserve the anterior ciliary vessels.[3–5] This is particularly easy on the vertical recti, where two distinct arteries are usually present, allowing easy dissection of the vessel out of and away from the muscle. It is usually possible to preserve at least one of the two vessels in the vertical recti using this technique.

Signs

The patient presents within 24 hours of surgery with corneal edema and a mild anterior uveitis.

Treatment

Use corticosteroids topically and, if there are no contraindications, systemically as well.

Malignant Hyperthermia*

Malignant hyperthermia is a rare but potentially lethal hereditary disorder characterized by a fulminant hypermetabolic state of skeletal muscle. It may be precipitated by general anesthesia and, perhaps, by stress or exercise. In particular, the volatile anesthetics such as halothane and the muscle relaxant succinylcholine are known triggering agents. The diagnosis is confirmed by a positive halothane-caffeine contracture test on a biopsy of skeletal muscle.

The syndrome should be suspected when otherwise unexplained tachycardia, tachypnea, muscle rigidity, cardiac dysrhythmias, and pyrexia are observed while the patient is under anesthesia and a coincident metabolic and respiratory acidosis is identified. The diagnosis may not always be obvious—mild presentations have been described.

---

*Michael F. Smith, M.D., F.R.C.P.(C). Pediatric Anesthetist, British Columbia's Children's Hospital, University of British Columbia, Canada.

The treatment of the acute malignant hyperthermia episode must be initiated promptly. It requires the immediate elimination of all triggering agents and hyperventilation of the patient with 100% oxygen. Reversal of the crisis can be achieved by intravenous dantrolene sodium in an initial dose of 2.5 mg/kg body weight. Subsequent doses up to 10 to 20 mg/kg may be required to normalize the clinical signs. The metabolic acidosis should be corrected and active cooling measures begun. Cardiac dysrhythmias, if persistent, are best treated by intravenous procainamide 3 mg/kg body weight. The patient must be transferred to an intensive care unit for further treatment and monitoring until stable.

For patients known to be at risk for malignant hyperthermia who require general anesthesia, all triggering agents must be avoided. Safe drugs include local anesthetics, barbiturates, narcotics, nondepolarizing muscle relaxants, atropine, the anticholinesterases, and ketamine.

References

1. Apt, L., Isenberg, S., Yoshimori, R., Paez, J.H.: Chemical perforation of the eye in ophthalmic surgery: 111. Effect of poviodine-iodine on the conjunctiva. Arch Ophthalmol 102:728, 1984.
2. Apt, L., Isenberg, S.J., Yoshimori, R., Spierer, A.: Outpatient topical use of poviodine-iodine in preparing the eye for surgery. Ophthalmology. 96:289, 1989.
3. France T.D., Simon J.W.: Anterior segment ischemic syndrome following muscle surgery: The A.A.P.O.S experience. J Pediatr Ophthalmol 23:87, 1986.
4. Freedman, H.L., Waltmann, D.D., Patterson, J.H.: Preservation of anterior ciliary vessels during strabismus surgery: A non-microscopic technique. J Pediatr Ophthalmol Strabismus 29:38, 1992.
5. McKeown, C.A., Lambert, M., Shore, J.W.: Preservation of anterior ciliary vessels during extraocular muscle surgery. Ophthalmology 96:498, 1989.
6. Noorden, G.K. von: Binocular Vision and Ocular Motility. St. Louis: Mosby, 1990:529
7. Parks, M.M.: The weakening surgical procedures for eliminating overaction of the inferior oblique muscle. Am J Ophthalmol 73:107, 1972.

18

Why Does the Patient
Have a Head Tilt or Turn?

There is nearly always a significant reason for an abnormal head position. The patient may adopt an abnormal head position unconsciously. It is therefore important to look specifically for it at the beginning of the examination. If a heterotropia in excess of 10 prism diopters persists with the abnormal head position, the head position was not adopted in order to permit fusion.

Head Tilt or Turn to Fuse and Avoid Diplopia

A patient may adopt a constant compensatory head position to avoid diplopia. In order to prove that this is the reason for the patient's abnormal head position, it is necessary to show that the eyes are straight or within a few prism diopters of being straight with the adopted head position so that central or peripheral fusion can be obtained. Further proof is obtained by turning the patient's face or head in the opposite direction and seeing if this provokes diplopia and a larger heterotropia.

Example: A patient with a right superior oblique palsy adopts a head tilt to the left. With the head tilted toward the left shoulder, the eyes are perfectly straight and the patient obtains fusion. When the head is tilted toward the right shoulder, there is a right hypertropia (see Fig. 12–1) and the patient appreciates diplopia.

Occlusion Test

If an abnormal head position is assumed to maintain fusion and avoid diplopia, occluding one eye prevents diplopia or fusion; therefore, the need for the head tilt will disappear and the head will straighten. This is a useful test where other tests are not possible, particularly in a young child.

Head Tilt or Turn to Improve Vision: Nystagmus Null Zone

The most common cause of a head tilt or turn, in our experience, is nystagmus. Patients with nystagmus may adopt a compensatory head position in order to improve their visual acuity. The head is positioned so that the eyes are within the null zone of the nystagmus where the foveation time is greatest. If a patient has an unexplained head tilt and a congenital strabismus, micronystagmus is almost certainly the cause, particularly if no fusion is present (see also Chapters 8 and 20). In these cases there is a manifest strabismus even with the abnormal head position. The nystagmus may be difficult to detect (micronystagmus). Sometimes it can only be confirmed by covering one of the patient's eyes, which usually increases the amplitude of the nystagmus, and then turning the patient's head away from the preferred position. The fovea of the unoccluded eye should then be examined with a visuscope or a direct ophthalmoscope with a fixation target that is projected on the fovea. By this method, tiny oscillations of previously undiagnosed nystagmus may become apparent. These patients do not adopt the abnormal head position when they are walking or running around. Usually, they only assume it for detailed visual observation, such as watching television, watching a movie, or reading the Snellen chart.

The abnormal head position is often not as noticeable at near because the convergence associated with near vision tends to block the nystagmus. Nystagmus is usually worse when the patients are under physical or emotional stress. Patients may then adopt a head tilt or turn to improve visual acuity in circumstances in which they would not normally do so.

Occlusion Test and Micronystagmus

The abnormal head position is not usually altered by occlusion of one eye, particularly if it is the nondominant deviating eye that is occluded. Sometimes a different null zone is adopted under uniocular conditions, the most common being a face turn so that the unoccluded eye is adducted.

Mechanical Restrictions

Mechanical restrictions of movement of one or both eyes may be the reason for the patient adopting an abnormal face or head position to preserve fusion or, sometimes, to facilitate vision in the fixing eye when there is no fusion. For example, type I Duane's retraction syndrome usually has a small esotropia in the primary position with the head straight. In order to maintain fusion, the patient adopts a face turn toward the side of the affected lateral rectus muscle. Patients with the general fibrosis syndrome usually adopt a chin-up head position due to severe fibrosis and contraction of the inferior rectus muscles. Any of the extraocular muscles may be involved with mechanical restriction, causing a compensatory head posture. Fibrosis in thyroid ophthalmopathy also may result in a compensatory head position. Mechanical restrictions may cause a compensatory abnormal face or head position, even in the absence of fusion, if the dominant eye is involved. The patient tries to position this eye in the most useful direction.

Ptosis

Children with severe unilateral or bilateral ptosis may adopt a chin-up position to preserve fusion by looking below the lids. If a child who has been doing this ceases to do so, this should be taken as a warning of amblyopia or loss of fusion.

Optical Causes

Oblique astigmatism may be the reason for a patient adopting an abnormal face or head position, although this is most unusual. Once the refractive error is properly corrected, the abnormal position disappears.

Wider Separation of Diplopic Images

Occasionally patients with incomitant strabismus may adopt a face turn or head tilt in order to increase the separation of the images if they have constant diplopia and cannot fuse. This makes the diplopia less disturbing.

Congenital Fibrosis of the Sternomastoid Muscle on One Side

Although this may be the most common cause of an abnormal head position in an orthopedic practice, it is most unusual for these patients to present first in an ophthalmologic practice.

Unilateral Deafness

Occasionally, a young child may turn the face to the side away from the normal ear if they have unilateral deafness.

Habit and Idiopathy

Occasionally a patient may adopt either a face turn or head tilt, for no demonstrable cause. These patients see just as well with the head straight and the preferred head position and even with the head turned in the opposite direction. The patients do not appreciate diplopia in any direction of gaze and are unable to offer any reason why they assume the abnormal head position. The abnormal head position may persist into adult life in these patients.

19

Why Does the Patient Have Double Vision?

Many patients who complain of double vision (diplopia) do not have a strabismus or even binocular diplopia. In order to determine the cause of the complaint, and therefore its management, a steplike process of elimination should be followed.

Is the Diplopia Monocular or Binocular?

Establish whether the diplopia is present only when both eyes are open (binocular diplopia) or if it persists when only one eye is open (monocular diplopia), and if so, which eye. The causes of monocular diplopia can usually be seen in the offending eye and are mainly refractive or optical, such as an uncorrected refractive error or a dislocated intraocular lens. If double vision is present only when both eyes are open, proceed to the next step.

Is the Diplopia Functional or Real?

1. Ask the patient to look at a fixation light at the end of the examining room. Ask how many lights there are and how they are separated—horizontally, vertically, tilted or any combination of these. Then ask the patient to look first at one light and then at the other light while you observe the patient's eyes. All patients with true binocular diplopia will have a movement of their eyes when they look from one light to the other. If there is no movement of the eyes, the diplopia is functional in origin.

2. Check that the diplopia described by the patient is correct for the objective signs (crossed in exotropia, uncrossed in esotropia, lower in hypertropia). Rarely a patient with abnormal retinal correspondence may be seen who has incongruous or even paradoxical diplopia.

3. Check that the images move correctly when prisms are used.

When it has been established that there is true binocular diplopia, the patient's binocular status must be evaluated further.

Does the Patient Have the Ability to Fuse?

1. Can the patient bring the images together anywhere by a change of eye or head position? Can the images then be kept together?

2. Can the patient fuse if the images are superimposed with the aid of prisms (in free space)?

3. Can the patient be made to fuse using a haploscopic device such as a synoptophore? In particular, is torsion preventing fusion? Bilateral superior oblique palsies may have little to show for the palsy other than an esotropia in down gaze and marked bilateral excyclotorsion in excess of 10° in the primary position, which increases in down gaze. This can be missed unless specifically sought. Cyclotorsion cannot be neutralized with prisms. It is essential to use a haploscopic device such as a synoptophore to neutralize the cyclotorsion and determine whether or not the patient is able to fuse when this has been done.

If fusion is present under any of the conditions just described, treatment involves mechanically realigning the eyes so that the patient can regain single binocular vision.

If the Patient Is Unable to Fuse, There Are Several Possibilities: Changes in Suppression

Is the Diplopia Caused by a Disruption of Suppression?

If the patient's eyes were convergent during visual immaturity and have become divergent now that the patient is a visual adult, the patient will be unable to suppress.[8,10] This is because suppression was developed in response to a convergent deviation. As a visual adult the patient is unable to develop suppression in response to the new eye position (see section on Suppression in Chapter 2). This problem may be tested by overcorrecting the deviation by prisms to see if the double vision then disappears. A similar situation occurs in divergent strabismus that has become convergent. It is important to check for this phenomenon in all fields of gaze in case the strabismus is incomitant. Dense amblyopia does not prevent a patient from becoming aware of diplopia in these circumstances, even if the vision is as low as counting fingers in the deviating eye (see also Chapter 21).

Treatment is adjustable suture strabismus surgery to realign the eyes to where suppression will again eliminate the diplopia.

Has Suppression Been Weakened by Antisuppression Exercises or by the Patient Making a Deliberate Attempt to Use the Deviating Eye on a Regular Basis?

Many patients who have had a strabismus since visual immaturity believe that they must keep using both eyes, or attempting to use both eyes all their life, otherwise they will become severely amblyopic in one eye.

In such a case, explanation and reassurance of the patient is all that is required. An adult patient should be told about suppression and that ignoring the image from the deviating eye will not cause amblyopia as it would do in childhood. The patient should be encouraged to concentrate on using the dominant eye and to ignore the second image to encourage the normal process of suppression.

Changes in Fixation

Is Diplopia Caused by the Patient Switching Fixation with the Habitually Nonfixing Eye Now Being Used for Fixation?

Such a situation may arise in a previously nonalternating strabismus in which the nonfixing eye is relatively amblyopic (e.g., 6/9 vision). If the originally fixing eye becomes myopic so that the vision drops below that of the amblyopic eye, fixation may change for distance and the patient may then experience diplopia because of an inability to suppress the image from the previously dominant eye.[2]

Correction of the refractive error so that the patient is able to fix once again with the usually dominant eye will eliminate the diplopia.

Rapid Alternation of Fixation

In a case of strabismus present from childhood, rapid alternation is occasionally mistakenly described as diplopia because the patient notices the shift in the apparent position of the fixation target when fixation changes from one eye to the other.

The patient should be encouraged to develop a dominant eye, as outlined in a previous paragraph.

Central Fusion Disruption

This is due to central disruption of fusional vergences without the development of suppression. The lesion is thought to be in the mid-brain.[7] It results in a distressing situation where the patient is unable to fuse and unable to suppress. The result is constant double vision, often without the patient being aware of which is the true image.

The term *horror fusionis* was used many years ago in the literature to describe cases of binocular diplopia without the ability to fuse or suppress, but case details are scarce and confusing.[1,3,4] For this reason, we prefer the term central fusion disruption.

The etiology of this condition is usually severe head trauma, but it can be due to other causes.[9] It is characterized by momentary fusion or superimposition of the images and a total inability, from a motor standpoint, to keep the images superimposed and fused. The condition is most easily confirmed with the aid of a haploscopic device, such as a synoptophore, and fusion targets. Prisms in free space also may be used to indicate the presence of this condition, provided there is no cyclotorsion in the primary position. Serious head injury also may cause a bilateral superior oblique palsy with marked excyclotorsion. In such a case, diplopia may be due to the excyclotorsion itself or to central fusion disruption. If cyclotorsion is present in the primary position, a synoptophore or similar haploscopic device, not prisms, must be used to establish which entity is responsible for the diplopia.

Some patients with a unilateral traumatic cataract appear to lose their fusion ability if there has been a long interval, usually of several years, between the loss of vision and the restoration of good (6/6) vision by cataract extraction and the correction of the resulting refractive error by a contact lens or an intraocular lens.[11] In the interval a strabismus has developed. This strabismus is usually exotropic and hypotropic with excyclotropia.

Other causes of long-standing visual deprivation also may result in the motor loss of fusion in a visual adult; examples include corneal scarring from keratitis and corneal distortion caused by keratoconus, which reduces vision to the 6/60 range. These patients behave similarly to those in whom there has been a traumatic central disruption of fusional vergences.[6] It appears to be mainly a motor vergence loss in that the patient is able to momentarily superimpose the images but is unable to maintain fusion. In both the traumatic and this variety of central disruption of fusional vergences, the patient notices a strange vertical bobbing movement of the image seen by the nonfixing eye when an attempt is made to superimpose the images either by prisms or on the synoptophore. At times it is possible to observe a similar movement of that eye as the patient attempts to superimpose the images.

The occasional patient with central fusion disruption responds to surgical or prismatic elimination of the strabismus by recapturing fusion. However, the prognosis is poor.[6]

Other Causes of Diplopia

Could It Be Metamorphopsia?

The major cause of this is retinal detachment surgery in which the retina has become reattached in such a way that the retinal elements are more crowded or less crowded together or are distorted. Thus, the image seen by one eye is a different shape from that seen by the other eye. The best way of diagnosing this is to ask the patient to look at a square box at the end of the examining room to see whether or not it appears to be any different seen through one eye compared with the other. These patients can superimpose the images but they cannot hold them together. Sometimes it is easier to show these differences by using a haploscopic device such as a synoptophore.

Unfortunately these patients are incurable.

Patients with Abnormal Retinal Correspondence

Patients with abnormal retinal correspondence (ARC) may occasionally appreciate paradoxical diplopia in the immediate postoperative period, but usually this disappears with time. Paradoxical diplopia also may be demonstrated or elicited in patients with ARC when the angle of deviation is altered by prisms. The diplopia described by the patient is opposite to that which would be expected for the type of deviation found by the cover test. If a patient with an esotropia has diplopia, it will be uncrossed provided the patient has normal retinal correspondence, but it will be crossed if the patient has ARC.

Aniseikonia

Aniseikonia itself, i.e., the actual difference in the image size presented to each retina, is rarely the cause of the diplopia. Patients can tolerate the image size difference of unilateral aphakia corrected with glasses.[5] However, diplopia is provoked by the prism induced if the patient fails to look through the optical center of the glasses. The second image varies in direction of displacement depending on whether the patient is looking up or down or in side gaze. This dancing around of the virtual image is particularly disturbing. Spectacle-corrected unilateral aphakia is an example of marked anisometropic amblyopia. This same mechanism operates in the correction of any anisometropia with spectacles.

Physiologic Diplopia

Sometimes, an observant patient may complain of double vision that has a normal physiologic explanation. Objects in front of or behind the fixation point do not fall on corresponding retinal points and therefore are seen double. The fixation point itself is single.

Example: A patient complained that recently he was seeing double. Further history revealed that he frequently noticed it when he was looking out of his office window at the flag fluttering on a nearby building. The blind cord hanging down in the middle of his window was double. He was disturbed by this and his worries were not allayed by an explanation of physiologic diplopia.

Treatment: The blind cord hanging in his window was excised.

Visual Confusion

Each fovea of a patient with a strabismus receives an image of a different object. Because the foveas are corresponding points, the patient will see the two different images as superimposed and may describe it as double vision. This problem is rare because retinal rivalry and suppression usually eliminate it quickly.

Inexplicable Diplopia

Unfortunately there are occasional cases of diplopia that do not seem to have any explanation. Fortunately these are rare.

References

1. Bielschowsky, A.: Congenital and acquired deficiencies of fusion. Am J Ophthalmol 18:925–937, 1935.
2. Boyd, T.A.S., Karas, Y., Budd, G.E., Wyatt H.T.: Fixation switch diplopia. Can J Ophthalmol 9:310, 1974.
3. Duke-Elder, Sir S., Wybar, K.: System of Ophthalmology. Vol VI. Ocular Motility and Strabismus. London: Henry Kimpton, 1973:243, 510.
4. Grant, H.W.: Some observations on divergent strabismus with anomalous retinal correspondence. Am J Ophthalmol 28:472–485, 1945.
5. Lubkin,V., Linksz, A.: A ten year study of binocular fusion with spectacles in monocular aphakia. Am J Ophthalmol 84:700, 1977.

6. Pratt-Johnson, J.A.: Fusion ability lost and regained in visual adults. Graefes Arch Clin Exp Ophthalmol 226:111–112, 1988.
7. Pratt-Johnson, J.A.: Fusion and suppression: Development and loss. 18th Annual Frank Costenbader Lecture. J Pediatr Ophthalmol Strabismus 29:4–9, 1992.
8. Pratt-Johnson, J.A., Pop, A., Tillson, G.: Suppression in strabismus and the hemiretinal trigger mechanism. Arch Ophthalmol 101:218–224, 1983.
9. Pratt-Johnson, J.A., Tillson, G.: Acquired central disruption of fusional amplitude. Ophthalmology 86:2140–2142, 1979.
10. Pratt-Johnson, J.A., Tillson, G.: Suppression in strabismus-An update. Br J Ophthalmol 68:174–178, 1984.
11. Pratt-Johnson, J.A., Tillson, G.: Intractable diplopia after vision restoration in unilateral cataract. Am J Ophthalmol 107:23–26, 1989.

20

The Patient with Nystagmus

The whole field of congenital nystagmus is a changing and growing area of knowledge. The term congenital is controversial because only children with motor nystagmus are born with or develop the nystagmus within a few days of birth. Congenital sensory nystagmus does not develop until about 2 months after birth. In this book the term *congenital nystagmus* will be applied to sensory or motor nystagmus present from the first few months of life.

Classification of Congenital Nystagmus

Congenital nystagmus can be divided into sensory and motor types.[8]

Sensory Nystagmus

The cause of sensory nystagmus is loss of foveal fixation due to an organic abnormality of the media, macula, retina, or optic nerve. Etiologies include foveal hypoplasia associated with albinism, congenital cataracts, aniridia, macula defects, Leber's congenital amaurosis, congenital stationary night blindness, and achromatopsia.[5,6]

The importance of recognizing the sensory etiology is for giving a prognosis and for genetic counseling and, in some cases, such as congenital cataracts, for treatment. For instance, oculocutaneous albinism usually has associated autosomal-recessive inheritance, whereas ocular albinism tends to be X linked. Aniridia, on the other hand, usually follows an autosomal-dominant pattern.[6]

Patients with sensory nystagmus tend to have poor vision from organic causes in addition to the limited foveation time resulting from the nystagmus.

Motor Nystagmus

This term is used when a sensory cause for nystagmus cannot be found. Because the fovea is usually not affected by any obvious organic pathology, the vision tends to be better than in sensory nystagmus. Some patients with motor nystagmus may see 6/6.

Diagnostic Importance of the Null Zone

The null zone is a position of gaze in which the nystagmus is dampened and the patient sees better. Commonly, the patient adopts a face turn or possibly a head tilt or chin-up or -down position in order to bring the eyes into the null zone. A null zone is often present in motor nystagmus, but it is not so characteristic of sensory nystagmus. A null zone is rarely present in nystagmus from an acquired central lesion. Convergence tends to dampen all types of congenital nystagmus. The patient may not assume the null zone position under ordinary visual circumstances but may seek it out only when looking at fine material or fine print in the distance or, particularly, when interested in seeing small detail. The null zone position frequently is present with only one eye open, but there may be a different null zone position for each eye separately.

General Features of Congenital Motor Nystagmus

This type of nystagmus is associated with much better vision than that in sensory nystagmus. It is usually in the range between 6/24 and 6/6 vision with both eyes open. There is often a null zone where the nystagmus is less marked and the patient sees better. If a null zone is present, the patient assumes a head position, either a head tilt or face turn, to maximize the null zone.

Convergence Blocked Nystagmus

The characteristic feature of motor nystagmus is the dampening of the nystagmus by convergence. This feature is particularly noticeable in some patients with the congenital strabismus syndrome and seems to play a part in the size of the esotropia (see also Chapter 5).

Exaggeration of Nystagmus with Stress

The amplitude and frequency of congenital motor nystagmus increase with stress, particularly emotional stress. As a result, the visual acuity decreases due to decreased foveation time, and the patient commonly uses the null zone if one is available. This is why the visual acuity, tested in the distance, is sometimes variable in motor nystagmus in the same patient tested at different times. This feature must be considered when interpreting the alleged benefit of any treatment.

Latent Nystagmus

Characteristically, congenital motor nystagmus is made worse in the fixing eye by closing or by cutting down the light entering the other eye. Latent nystagmus is often described as being present only when one eye is occluded and absent when both eyes are open. Although the nystagmus may be difficult to detect when both eyes are open, the patient with so-called latent nystagmus can be shown to have nystagmus of small amplitude with both eyes open. Many of these patients will assume a head tilt position to use the null zone, suggesting that nystagmus must still be present. This is commonly seen in the micronystagmus associated with the congenital strabismus syndrome. In some of these cases the nystagmus may not be obvious in casual observation of the patient when both of the patient's eyes are open. Because nystagmus is exaggerated by occluding or cutting down the light entering one eye, it is important to test the visual acuity by blurring the vision in the non-fixing eye with a +10.00 lens rather than an occluder.

Spasmus Nutans or Head Nodding and Nystagmus

This syndrome consists of patients with congenital motor nystagmus who have a nodding of the head in addition to an abnormal head posture. The nodding may be an attempt to increase foveation. It varies and, like nystagmus, is increased when the patient is under stress, particularly emotional. It may persist into adulthood. There is considerable confusion, in the literature, concerning the terms *spasmus nutans* and *head nodding*, but in this book these terms are used synonymously to describe the syndrome discussed in the following paragraph.

In the vast majority of cases the head nodding appears to be a part of motor nystagmus and does not appear to be associated with any other particular abnormality. Occasionally, the nystagmus is more prominent in one eye and may be called dissociative nystagmus. However, there is the occasional case of head nodding that is caused by intracranial neoplasm such as optic glioma.[4] Typically, this is associated with nystagmus acquired after 4 months of age. Congenital motor nystagmus, present from or within a few days of birth, may not be noticed by the parents until the child is over 4 months old. This is the reason why it is essential to have all preverbal children with nystagmus and head nodding (spasmus nutans) assessed by a neurologist. The term *spasmus nutans* is used in different centers with different interpretations and therefore needs to be clearly defined if it is used.

Types of Oscillations Found in Congenital Motor Nystagmus

The frequency may vary from slow to fast. The amplitude may vary from small to large. The direction of the nystagmus may be horizontal, vertical, rotatory, or a combination. Characteristic wave motion may be a jerk pattern with a fast and a slow component, or pendular. It is common to have different patterns present in the same patient at different times, jerk features being replaced by pendular. In describing the clinical features, comments on the frequency, amplitude, and direction should be included.

Investigations in the Preverbal Age Group

1. History: Is there a family history of strabismus, nystagmus, or conditions such as albinism that may be associated with sensory nystagmus?

2. Complete eye examination: This should eliminate obvious causes of sensory nystagmus. Transillumination of the iris indicates albinism.

3. Electroretinogram: This may help diagnose some causes of sensory nystagmus.

4. Neurologic examination: This is necessary if head bobbing (spasmus nutans) is present. It is also necessary if the nystagmus is an acquired one presenting after the first 4 months of age.

Clinical Associations of Motor Nystagmus

Motor Nystagmus without Strabismus

The nystagmus is usually present from birth. Many of these patients have a family history of nystagmus, and the hereditary patterns may vary. These patients usually have good fusion and stereopsis, although higher degrees of stereopsis may only be present in patients with good visual acuity.

Motor Nystagmus Associated with the Congenital Strabismus Syndrome

Motor nystagmus is common in this syndrome no matter whether there is an esotropia or an exotropia. In one study, approximately 50% of patients with the congenital esotropia syndrome had detectable nystagmus.[16] It may manifest itself as the nystagmus block syndrome in congenital esotropia. In these patients both eyes may be simultaneously markedly esotropic, making a total combined angle of approximately 90 prism diopters. Any attempt to abduct either eye provokes obvious nystagmus. Sometimes the strabismus is variable and the eyes only become markedly esotropic when the child is really trying to look carefully at something. The diagnosis in these children may be confused with bilateral sixth nerve palsies because both eyes are turned in. Bilateral congenital sixth nerve palsy is rare in children, whereas this syndrome is common. If nystagmus is present on attempted abduction, the diagnosis is almost certainly nystagmus block syndrome associated with congenital esotropia (see also Chapter 8).

An additional feature is the persistence of the convergent position of the fixing eye if one eye is occluded, forcing the child to adopt a face turn in the direction of the fixing eye, for example, turning the face to the right if the patient is fixing with the right eye, the left eye being occluded. One is often unable to get the child to abduct either eye even by using the doll's head phenomenon or holding the child up and spinning to the right or left rapidly. Sometimes shining a bright light, like the indirect ophthalmoscope, into the dilated pupil can cause the eye to abduct as the child tries to avoid the misery of looking at the light. However, even if it cannot be confirmed that the eye goes past the straight ahead midline position, the chances are that this is a cross-fixating congenital esotropia with or without the nystagmus block syndrome and not a bilateral sixth nerve palsy. Occlusion of one eye for several hours may encourage movement of the other eye past the midline.

In the absence of any other neurologic signs, the diagnosis is almost always congenital strabismus syndrome. The nystagmus and other features of the congenital esotropia syndrome are sometimes referred to as Ciancia's syndrome.[7]

Head Tilt or Face Turn Acquired in Later Life

Some patients with motor nystagmus associated with a congenital strabismus syndrome may not have had the convergent blocking feature of the nystagmus block syndrome or it may not have been recorded or noticed in the infancy period before surgery. However, some of the children who had the nystagmus block syndrome as well as others who were not noticed to have it may later develop a face position or head tilt after they have had their eyes straightened and they have reached the age where they demand the clearest visual acuity. The most common cause of a head tilt or face turn seen in our practice is congenital motor nystagmus associated with the congenital strabismus syndrome. To differentiate nystagmus as a cause for the head tilt or turn from a paretic strabismus, such as a superior oblique palsy, see Chapter 18.

Sometimes the nystagmus is difficult to diagnose because it is of small amplitude and slow frequency. The best way to see it is by dilating the patient's pupils and then occluding one of the patient's eyes to bring out the latent element of the nystagmus. It is helpful to tilt or turn the patient's face in the opposite direction to the preferred head position during this part of the examination. A simple visuscope target such as the circle in the Welch-Allyn ophthalmoscope is then used. The patient is asked to look at the circle target with the ophthalmoscope turned down to about half its normal intensity so that the patient can use the fovea to look at it without discomfort. The examiner is then able to observe the small movements of the fovea. In addition, it is usual for a head position or face turn because of nystagmus to persist when one eye is occluded, although it may not always be in the same direction. Conversely, if the patient is assuming the abnormal head position to avoid diplopia (as in a superior oblique palsy with fusion) the head becomes straight when one eye is occluded.

Periodic Alternating Nystagmus

This nystagmus is caused by posterior fossa lesions and should not be confused with the occasional case of congenital nystagmus in which a null zone is chosen looking in right gaze as well as sometimes in left gaze.[15] Periodic alternating nystagmus is characterized by repetitive cycles of directional change of the nystagmus separated by brief periods of apparent cessation of the nystagmus. Congenital hydrocephalus, myelomeningocele, Arnold-Chiari malformation, and acquired posterior fossa lesions may cause periodic alternating nystagmus.[3,10]

Acquired Nystagmus and Other Types

Seesaw nystagmus, downbeat nystagmus, and all cases of acquired nystagmus must be referred to a neurologist for investigation. The presence of a well-established single null zone, seen so often in congenital motor nystagmus, almost never occurs in acquired nystagmus.

Treatment of Congenital Nystagmus

Refractive Errors

1.   In young patients in whom a visual acuity cannot be obtained, refractive errors should be corrected in the hope that this may improve the foveal visual acuity and stabilize the nystagmus. If the patient is old enough to reliably record distance and near visual acuity, it is possible to evaluate whether the correction of the

refractive error could make any difference to the visual acuity. Unless correcting the refractive error improves the visual acuity in a patient with nystagmus, corrective lenses are seldom helpful. Glasses should therefore only be prescribed in the unlikely event that the patient's eyes are more comfortable with the refractive error corrected.

2.   Contact lenses are often an advantage over glasses for patients who assume a null zone that causes them to look away from the optical center of their glasses.

3.   Near vision is usually adequate when the reading matter is held close to the eyes. This helps to dampen the nystagmus by using convergence and also magnifies the retinal image. Hence, visual aids for near are rarely required in congenital nystagmus unless an organic lesion of the fovea is present.

4.   Monocular telescopic aids for distance are useful in nystagmus, but frequently the patients do not have the motivation to use these aids until they are approaching adolescence. They would rather manage just by sitting in the front of the class and walking up to the blackboard if necessary than be teased about the use of a monocular telescope.

Surgery to Move the Null Zone Nearer to the Primary Position

Kestenbaum Procedure

Special points to consider when evaluating patients for null zone surgery[11]are described as follows:

1.   It is important for the patient to maximize visual acuity by using the null zone position. Frequently patients will not turn their face maximally until they are attempting to read the small letters on the Snellen chart, which causes them to struggle. The visual acuity of each eye as well as the visual acuity with both eyes open should be tested using this technique. Record the best corrected visual acuity with both eyes open and the head straight in the primary position to compare with the best corrected visual acuity with both eyes open using the null zone position.

2.   The near visual acuity of each eye individually as well as with both eyes together should be tested. It is important to record the distance at which the patient is holding the reading chart. This will assess whether there is convergence block improving the visual acuity at near compared with at distance. If this is significant, there is frequently less or no face turn at near. If a face turn at near is present, the visual acuity should be recorded, with both eyes open, at near with the preferred face turn and with the head straight.

3.   The patient should be asked directly what the limitations are with everyday functioning such as reading, writing, playing sports, enjoying recreational pursuits, riding a bicycle, driving a car, etc.

Explaining Informed Consent

It is important for the patient to recognize that null zone surgery is a trade-off—surgery is rarely advised except for a marked face turn. In order to improve the face turn position in such cases, extensive surgery is necessary, producing significant gaze restriction. For instance, if the eyes are moved maximally to the right for a marked right face turn position, by performing 10-mm surgery on all four horizontal muscles, the patient will not be able to move the eyes significantly to the left of the midline position after surgery. This will mean that the patient's head rather than the patient's eyes would have to turn whenever the patient wished to look to the left.

Surgery is not advised for the null zone position unless there is an improvement of distance visual acuity of several lines with the face turn. Because a sophisticated assessment by the patient of his or her needs is necessary, surgery for this condition is seldom performed until the patient is old enough to make such a judgment. This may vary from 8 years to teens. It is important to recognize that unless sufficient surgery is performed to produce a gaze restriction, the surgery is of limited benefit. The gaze restriction gradually reduces postoperatively, so that the face turn returns, much to the disappointment of both surgeon and patient.

Indications for Surgery in Patients with Nystagmus and a Face Turn

1. Improved corrected visual acuity of at least two Snellen lines with the head turn.

2. Adopted face position causes significant problems in work, driving, recreation, and cosmesis. In order to satisfactorily assess this question, a certain maturity of the patient is necessary.

3. Patient always turns the face to the same side. (Confirm this by asking patient and parents.)

4. Patient understands and accepts the permanent side effect of markedly restricted gaze to one side after surgery.

Caution: Some improvement in the head posture may occur as the patient matures; therefore, surgery should be delayed until the patient is over 8 years old.

Surgery

The surgical technique involves turning the eyes in the same direction as the patient turns the face to reach the null zone.[14,15] For instance, if a patient's face is habitually turned maximally to the right, both eyes would be moved maximally to the right. Occasionally, a patient seeks a null zone, turning the face in one direction 95% of the time. Rarely, the patient may turn the face in the opposite direction to obtain a null zone. Surgery on such a patient is contraindicated because it will result in a constant marked face turn to the opposite side. Patients who use a face turn both to the right and left are untreatable. For over 15 years if treatment was indicated, we have used a 10-mm recession/resection operation on all four horizontal muscles to move the eyes maximally in the direction of the preferred face turn. Fusion has never been lost in a patient who had fusion preoperatively. However, the success of the operation is directly proportional to the gaze restriction in the opposite direction to the way the eyes were turned. The best results are frequently seen within a month after surgery. One year after surgery, some recurrence of the head turn may occur. Overcorrection with a face turn past the midline primary position to the opposite side is rare unless the patient has two null zones—one in gaze to the left and one in gaze to the right. Surgery would be contraindicated for a patient who has two null zones as already described.

Surgery for the Nystagmus Block Syndrome

Surgery is no different for patients with congenital esotropia who have, as an additional feature, the nystagmus block. These patients, characteristically, have a large-angle strabismus and therefore require a lot of surgery. The general principles explained in Chapter 16 should be followed. In most patients surgery would involve a recession of both medial rectus muscles of 6 to 7 mm. For a patient with a 90-prism diopter esotropia with each eye turned in about 45 prism diopters, this would be combined with a 10-mm resection of one lateral rectus muscle.

Surgery for the Null Zone in Older Children or Adults

Approximately half the patients with the congenital strabismus syndrome have nystagmus.[16] It is not unusual to see older patients who adopt a face turn or head tilt position on this basis. Many of these patients may not have a turn that is sufficiently severe to warrant surgery.

Surgery for the Null Zone in Patients with Horizontal Strabismus without Fusion

When nystagmus coexists with strabismus without fusion, the fixing eye is turned maximally with a 10-mm recession/resection operation on the horizontal recti.[15] The amount of surgery in the strabismic nonfixing eye is designed to straighten the strabismus relative to the new position of the fixing eye.

Example 1: A patient has a left esotropia of 20 prism diopters without fusion potential. There is a maximum face turn to the right and best corrected vision of 6/6 in the right eye and 6/12 in the left eye. Surgery would be designed to straighten the eye as well as improve the face turn. Both eyes would therefore need to be moved to the right, but less surgery would be done on the left eye to reduce the esotropia to a smaller angle esotropia for cosmesis. The following surgery would be suggested: right medial rectus recession of 10 mm, right lateral rectus resection of 10 mm, left medial rectus resection of 8 mm, and left lateral rectus recession of 8 mm.

Example 2: A patient presents with a left esotropia of 50 prism diopters without fusion potential. The best corrected vision is 6/6 in the right eye and 6/60 in the left eye. The patient also has a marked face turn position to the right. Naturally the patient is expecting surgery on the left eye with the poor vision, and this would be the best course to follow for cosmetic improvement of the strabismus alone.

However, if the patient is interested in attempting to improve the face turn position as well as the strabismus, it will be necessary to perform surgery on the right fixing eye, turning it to the right. Surgery could be confined to the right eye alone, performing 7-mm recession of the right medial rectus and 7-mm resection of the right lateral rectus. This would probably reduce the strabismus to a small cosmetically unnoticeable esotropia, calculating approximately 3 prism diopters per millimeter effect (see Chapter 16 and Table 16–1). This may also improve the head position. However, if the head position is disturbing to the patient but results in a marked increase in visual acuity over the primary position, it may be better to perform the standard 10-mm recession/resection procedure on the right eye. This will overcorrect the strabismus, producing an exotropia. To avoid this, an adjustable recession of the left lateral rectus of 3 to 4 mm and a resection of the left medial rectus muscle of 3 to 4 mm at the same operation would be indicated. Frequently, however, when there is a markedly amblyopic eye opposite a normal eye, the patient will not give consent to operate on the fixing eye. In this case the patient would not get rid of the face turn position but only have a better alignment of the eyes.

Chin-Up or Chin-Down Abnormal Head Position and Nystagmus

In predominantly vertical congenital nystagmus, a chin-up or chin-down position may be implemented to utilize a null zone. In our practice, several of these patients have undergone recession/resection surgery on the vertical muscles of both eyes, moving the eyes in the same direction that the patient moves the chin. Surgery did not exceed 6 mm on each muscle because of anticipated side effects of doing the necessary "crippling" surgery to cure the chin position. For this reason, the results have been disappointing, the patients showing little permanent improvement.

Head Tilt and Nystagmus

Some patients with congenital motor nystagmus assume a head tilt rather than a face turn position or chin-up or chin-down position. Treatment of these patients involves a rotation of each eye in the direction of the head tilt.

Example 1: If a patient tilts the head to the right shoulder to obtain improved visual acuity, the right eye would have to be extorted and the left eye intorted to improve this situation. Because this involves surgery on the oblique muscles, it would be unlikely that this could be achieved without disrupting fusion in at least a vertical plane. For this reason, surgery is not advised if the patient has fusion.

However, in a situation where the patient has strabismus and no fusion, torsional correction of the dominant fixing eye may produce noticeable improvement and therefore is advised if the patient is disturbed by the head tilt position.[15]

Example 2: A patient has a head tilt to the right shoulder and has had previous horizontal muscle surgery for the congenital strabismus syndrome, resulting in cosmetically excellent horizontal and vertical alignment without fusion. If there is a significant improvement of visual acuity in the adopted right head tilt position, surgery to improve the head tilt position is advised. Surgery should be planned to turn the right eye into maximum excyclotorsion. This would involve a tenotomy of the anterior two thirds of the superior oblique insertion, leaving only the posterior fibers attached to minimize vertical effect. The right inferior oblique muscle would then be tucked to increase its excyclo torsion. If there was a hypotropia present in the right eye of approximately 10 prism diopters before surgery, it would be better to perform a complete tenotomy of the right superior oblique rather than a tenotomy of the anterior two thirds. However, one can anticipate producing a

10- to 15-prism diopter right hypertropia if a full tenotomy is performed, whereas preserving the posterior fibers should minimize this. Because no fusion is present it is not necessary to operate on the left eye.

Example 3: A patient has had previous horizontal muscle surgery for the congenital strabismus syndrome with good horizontal results. The patient now assumes a head tilt to the left shoulder but fixes with the right eye and has no fusion. If surgery is indicated because of significant visual acuity improvement with the tilt, it is designed to maximally intort the right fixing eye. The modified Harada-Ito transposition procedure should be performed on the anterior two thirds of the fibers of the right superior oblique (see Fig. 12–8) and combined with a myectomy of the right inferior oblique muscle. This surgery would not result in a significant vertical strabismus, and the change in position would not affect suppression or precipitate diplopia provided the patient's eyes are left in the same horizontal position. Diplopia would occur if an esotropic eye became exotropic as a result of the cyclovertical muscle surgery (see Chapter 19).

Driver's License and Nystagmus

The laws regarding the visual acuity necessary to drive an automobile vary in different parts of the world. Patients with borderline vision and nystagmus are often frustrated trying to meet the standard. Patients may fail the test once and yet pass the same test subsequently, the variability being due to the exaggeration of the nystagmus under stress. Occluding one eye to assess the visual acuity of the other eye usually increases the nystagmus while decreasing the visual acuity. It is important to inform the testing authorities about the unusual features of nystagmus, emphasizing repeated tests without duress and assessing the visual acuity with both eyes open. In our experience two procedures may improve visual acuity in order to pass the driver's test: (1) the prescription of contact lenses instead of glasses, particularly if any head position is assumed by the patient, and (2) surgery to center a null zone if the assumed position is awkward for driving and if the visual acuity in the null zone position improves to the level necessary.

In patients with fusion we have tried to encourage convergence, hoping to dampen the nystagmus by creating an exophoria with prisms in spectacles. This is unfortunately ineffective. The same idea has been tried by surgically inducing an exophoria.[1,9,12] Surgery involving large recessions of all the rectus muscles also has been tried.[1,2,13] It would appear that some improvement may result, but this is controversial. We have no experience with the latter two procedures.

References

1. Berard, P.V., Quere,, M.A., Roth, A., Spielmann, A., Woillez, M.: Chirugie des strabismes. Paris: Masson: 1984:430.
2. Bietti, G.B., Bagolini, B.: Traitement medicochirugical due nystagmus. Ann Ther Clin Ophthalmol 11:268, 1960.
3. Buncic, R.L., Lloyd, L.A.: In: Crawford, J.S., Morin, D.J., eds. The Eye in Childhood. New York: Grune & Stratton, 1983:416.

4. Buncic, R.L., Lloyd, L.A.: In: Crawford, J.S., Morin, D.J., eds. The Eye in Childhood. New York: Grune & Stratton, 1983:421.
5. Carruthers, J.D.A.: Human albinism: Recent advances in neurology and motility. Am Orthopt J 35:139, 1985.
6. Carruthers, J.D.A.: The practical assessment of nystagmus in infants. Am Orthopt J 36:77, 1986.
7. Ciancia, A.: La esotropia en al lactante, diagnostico y traitmento. Arch Chil Oftalmol 9:117, 1962.
8. Cogan, D.G.: Nystagmus. In: Haik, G.H., ed. Strabismus Symposium of the New Orleans Academy of Ophthalmology. St. Louis:Mosby, 1962:119.
9. Cüppers, C.: Probleme der operativen therapie des okularen nystagmus. Klin Monatsbl Augenheilkd. 159: 145, 1971.
10. Kestenbaum, A.: Periodisch umschlagender nystagmus. Klin Monatsbl Augenheilkd 84:552, 1930.
11. Kestenbaum, A.: Nouvelle operation du nystagmus. Bull Soc Ophthalmol Fr 6:599, 1953.
12. Kaufman, K., Kolling, G.: Operative therapie bei nystagmus patienten mit binokularfunktionen mit und ohne kopfzwangshaltung. Berl Deutsch Ophthalmol Ger 78:815, 1981.
13. Noorden, G.K. von, Sprunger, D.T.: Large rectus muscle recessions for the treatment of congenital nystagmus. Arch Ophthalmol 109:221, 1991.
14. Pratt-Johnson, J.A.: The surgery of congenital nystagmus. Can J Ophthalmol 6:268, 1971.
15. Pratt-Johnson, J.A.: Results of horizontal rectus muscle surgery to modify the null-zone position in congenital nystagmus. Can J Ophthalmol 26:219–223, 1991.
16. Pratt-Johnson, J.A.: Fusion and suppression: Development and loss. J Pediatr Ophthalmol Strabismus 29:14, 1992.

21

Common Mistakes in the Management of Strabismus

This chapter discusses the problems that may arise, particularly in adult patients, if both sensory and motor factors are not considered when correcting refractive errors, operating to alter the eye alignment, or when giving orthoptic exercises.

The most difficult problems in the management of strabismus are caused by the failure to consider the patient's current and potential sensory status. Visual acuity and the potential for fusion and stereopsis are vital parts of the assessment of a strabismic patient. Without this information the evaluation is incomplete. Unless the sensory status is taken into consideration, altering the motor status of a patient can cause or increase sensory problems.

Motor alignment of the eyes can be changed by optical (correction of refractive errors) and surgical means. The sensory status can be altered by changes in motor alignment as well as by prisms, occlusion, and orthoptic exercises. Each of these methods, alone or in combination with any or all of the others, can influence a patient's sensory status.

Prisms do not change the motor alignment of the eyes; they simply move the image received by the eye behind the prism to a different area of its retina. In a patient with strabismus and fusion ability, appropriate prisms should move the image nearer to the fovea to regain fusion while the prisms are being used. However, the patient may become more aware of diplopia that was easily ignored before if the images are moved closer together without fusing.

Sometimes prisms can help by moving the unwanted image onto an area of the retina where the patient has previously learned to suppress. Orthoptic exercises may help in establishing control of a strabismus in a very small group of patients who already have good fusion potential.

Failure to Recognize that Refractive Errors Influence Strabismus in Adults as well as Children

It is important to recognize that refractive errors, whether corrected or uncorrected, have a major impact on strabismus throughout life. Failure to take this into account often leads to unexpected results. Although correcting a refractive error may improve visual acuity, it also may change the strabismus, not necessarily for the better.

Many methods of correcting refractive errors are now available to patients. No matter how the refractive error is corrected, the effects are the same.

Before any refractive error is corrected, it is important to check the patient's extraocular muscle balance. A simple cover test for near and distance fixation is often all that is needed. This will help avoid inducing symptoms from a previously asymptomatic strabismus. Glasses and contact lenses can be used by patients of all ages. Intraocular lenses and refractive surgery are newer methods of treating refractive errors, and their indications and contraindications are still evolving. The age of patients who can be treated in these ways is changing with technology and experience.

Whatever the method used to correct refractive errors, in adults as well as children, the principles remain the same.

Effects of Refractive Errors on Muscle Balance

1. Esodeviations are frequently reduced by the correction of a hypermetropic (hyperopic) refractive error.

2. Esodeviations are often increased by the correction of a myopic refractive error.

3. Exodeviations are frequently increased by the correction of a hypermetropic (hyperopic) refractive error.

4. Exodeviations are often decreased by the correction of a myopic refractive error.

5. The fixing eye determines the amount of accommodation exerted. In patients who have a heterotropia and no potential for fusion, it is the refractive error of the normally fixing eye that influences the strabismus. Correcting the refractive error of the deviating eye in adult patients who suppress an eye and do not have fusion ability will not influence the deviation unless the correction causes them to switch fixation. Such patients should not have the vision improved in the deviating eye to a level that is equal to or better than that of the fixing eye because of the risk of precipitating fixation switch diplopia.

6. Accommodation and convergence are linked. The dominant or fixing eye determines the amount of accommodation and therefore the amount of convergence that is exerted. In strabismic patients who suppress an eye, correcting the refractive error of that eye will not change the deviation, but correcting the dominant eye may do so.

These six principles apply whether the deviation is latent or manifest (heterophoric or heterotropic).

Visually immature patients may gain better control of a strabismus simply by gaining optimal visual acuity in each eye when the refractive error is corrected and any amblyopia eliminated. However, it also may be necessary to modify the strength of the prescription slightly. It is important to keep in mind the points listed above.

Failure to Realize the Effect that Refractive Surgery, Intraocular Lenses, Contact Lenses, or Glasses Have on Adult Strabismus

Refractive surgery, intraocular lenses, contact lenses, or glasses may be used to correct refractive errors. There are many published descriptions of the symptoms—such as diplopia, visual confusion, and asthenopia—induced when contact lenses and intraocular lenses first became popular as ways of correcting refractive errors.[6,9,12,14,17,24,27,28] Presbyopes with strabismus who have the refractive error of one eye corrected for near and the other for distance, the so-called monovision correction, also may develop these symptoms. More recently reports have emerged of similar problems for strabismic patients who have had refractive surgery.[15,16,18,33]

The presence of a strabismus should be excluded by the use of a cover test before correcting a refractive error. The presence of a strabismus may mean that any correction planned for the refractive error has to be modified. No matter what method is used to modify the refractive error, it can affect the strabismus.

Precaution: Before refractive surgery or intraocular lenses are used for patients who have a strabismus, an initial trial with contact lenses or glasses is advisable to determine whether the patient is able to tolerate the proposed changes to their refractive error and their potential effect on the strabismus.

Changes in Refractive Error Precipitating Fixation Switch Diplopia

If a strabismic patient has a preferred eye for fixation, and always suppresses the deviating eye, even small changes in the refractive error in either eye can provoke a switch of fixation.[13,15] The development of as little as half a diopter of myopia in one eye can cause this problem, and it is more likely to happen if there was only a small difference in vision between the two eyes before the refraction changed. For example, myopia in the previously dominant (preferred) eye may reduce its distance visual acuity below that of the previously deviating eye, causing a switch of fixation and consequently diplopia for distance, such as when driving or for board work at school. Another example is the patient who develops half a diopter of myopia in the deviating eye. In this case the patient may switch fixation when reading, thus provoking diplopia at near. This is not unusual in teenagers and may easily be dismissed as an excuse to avoid studying unless a cover test is performed while the patient fixes a detailed target at both near and distance. In both examples the solution is explanation and the prescription of glasses to correct the refractive error and restore fixation to the previously dominant eye.

Refractive Error Correction Permitting Alternation

Adult patients with a history of a long-standing strabismus may be made symptomatic by the correction of their refractive error. This happens, for example, if a previously uncorrected strabismic eye is fully corrected and the visual acuity becomes almost equal in the two eyes. This may encourage spontaneous alternation of fixation, with the patient describing symptoms of "things jumping" or "moving over" from the periphery to straight ahead.[15]

Refractive Error Correction Precipitating Asthenopia and Diplopia

The wearing of a presbyopic correction for reading has the same effect as a hyperopic correction. Presbyopes who have an exophoria at near may develop a convergence insufficiency when they receive their correction for reading. A course of orthoptic exercises to improve their convergence is usually all that is needed to make them symptom free again.

Adult patients with anisometropia may develop problems of asthenopia and even diplopia when their refractive error is corrected, especially if it is for the first time. The varying prismatic effect of an anisometropic spectacle correction in different directions of gaze can induce diplopia.[19,20]

Anisophoria Induced by Correction of Anisometropia

Anisometropic corrections are usually well tolerated by children, but patients who either acquire anisometropia in adult life or receive their correction for the first time are often very unhappy. This is particularly so if there is sufficient difference in the prescription for each eye that a prismatic effect is induced in gaze directions other than straight ahead.[19,20] This is termed anisophoria. Many patients learn to address the horizontal problem by fusion or by turning the head to avoid side gaze and maintain fixation through the optical center of the lens. The vertical prismatic effect is more difficult to address because the vertical fusional range is small even in normal individuals.

Monocular Diplopia Induced by Uncorrected or Poorly Corrected Refractive Errors

This form of diplopia may be vertical, horizontal, or intermittent. Monocular diplopia may be appreciated by each eye. The use of a pinhole can usually quickly differentiate cases of monocular diplopia from true binocular diplopia.[6,10]

Monocular diplopia can be particularly confusing when the problem occurs for distance in persons with a small hyperopic refractive error. It is often first noticed for distant brightly illuminated objects such as the moon. It may be the first indication of presbyopia-the patient is able to "force" adequate accommodation for near and therefore deny any reading problems.

Failure to Recognize that Anisometropic Amblyopia and Bilateral Ametropic Amblyopia May Improve with Correction of the Refractive Error Alone

Patients who have anisometropia or high bilateral refractive errors but do not have an associated strabismus may only need a period of wearing their appropriate correction before achieving their best visual acuity.[29] A minimum of 1 month of wearing this correction full time should be allowed before visual acuity is reassessed and occlusion therapy instituted. If there is some improvement of visual acuity at the follow-up visit, the patient should continue with the glasses alone, even if some amblyopia persists. Occlusion is only needed if the visual acuity with correction does not continue to improve.

Problems Associated with Presbyopia

The onset of presbyopia is in itself a problem.[15] Patients who have worn glasses for many years suddenly notice a new problem and fear that their eyes are getting worse. Strabismic patients often feel that the problem is caused by overuse of their fixing eye and try to rest it by closing it and trying to read with the "bad" eye. This can disrupt their suppression mechanism and provoke diplopia or alternation of fixation with images "jumping." This presbyopic patient who happens to be anisometropic as well is often more comfortable with the same reading add for each eye without the refractive error of the deviating being corrected for distance. Presbyopic patients who have never worn glasses often seek to avoid them by alternative methods such as monovision correction.

Monovision Correction of Presbyopia

The term *monovision* has been accepted as the word to describe correction of one eye for distance and the other for near vision. For the past 20 to 30 years, monovision correction has been used in presbyopic patients. This technique is most successful in patients who do not have a strabismus. Some patients cannot tolerate the blurred vision, the aniseikonia from the induced anisometropia, and the reduction in their stereoacuity. Others can tolerate this in the early years of presbyopia when only a small reading add is needed, but not later as the strength of the add needed increases to more than +1.00 diopter sphere (DS). Monovision is achieved by the use of contact lenses, intraocular lenses, or refractive surgery, where one eye is corrected for near vision and one for distance vision. This induces a form of anisometropia. It is unpredictable as to how well a patient will tolerate this, particularly if fusion and stereopsis are weak or absent. Strabismic patients are particularly at risk for the precipitation of symptoms, as discussed in the next section.

   Caution: A trial with contact lenses is advisable initially to determine whether the patient is able to tolerate monovision and to test if ocular dominance is changed before refractive surgery or intraocular lenses are used.

Monovision Precipitating Fixation Switch Diplopia in Presbyopes

Monovision correction may make a previously asymptomatic patient with a strabismus symptomatic by disrupting the suppression mechanism and inducing fixation switch diplopia.[15] Patients are now forced to fix with one eye for distance and the other for near. This means that for a large part of every day they are fixing with the eye that they normally suppress. Because they do not have fusion, they will be aware of diplopia whenever they switch fixation. Teachers, trial lawyers, and judges are examples of persons who during the course of a normal day's work are constantly switching fixation from printed material at the reading distance to objects and persons at varying distances from them in the classroom or court. Monovision correction has the potential to severely interfere with their work if such a person is presbyopic and has a strabismus without fusion ability. The need to constantly switch fixation during a lecture or a trial causes an annoying diplopic image that keeps "jumping" into view whenever they are forced to fix with their previously suppressed eye. Not all of these patients easily suppress again even if their correction is adjusted, so that they revert to fixing with the same eye at all distances. They may remain troubled by the diplopia for many years.

Failure to Recognize the Importance of Assessing the Patient's Sensory Status

Information about the patient's current and potential sensory status is as essential, as information about the motor alignment of the eyes when planning the management of a strabismus.

The patient's expectations of the outcome of treatment may be unrealistic. Many adult patients with strabismus and no fusion ability hope for improved visual acuity, normal fusion, and stereopsis. When they realize that this is not possible, they may decide against further treatment.

Only visually immature patients have any chance of developing fusion, even if there is no evidence of its existence at the initial visits. There is an ever-decreasing chance of a patient developing fusion the further the child is into the development period without any evidence of fusion potential.

Orthoptic exercises cannot teach a patient to fuse. Orthoptic exercises can only help those patients who already have the ability to fuse. They can enlarge already well-established fusional amplitudes. Orthoptic exercises are contraindicated in all patients who do not have proven potential for fusion. Only aligning the eyes of visually immature patients with the constant stimulation of similar images falling on corresponding retinal elements provides the opportunity for fusion to develop where it does not currently exist.

By the time a patient is old enough to cooperate with exercises, they are too old to develop fusion ability if they have not done so already. Suppression is then the patient's defense mechanism against intractable diplopia. Care needs to be taken not to disrupt this mechanism.

As the child ages, the goal of management gradually changes. The goal no longer is to give the child the chance of developing normal binocular single vision. It becomes one of providing the best possible visual acuity in each eye and a stable residual deviation that is small enough not to be noticed by other people. This often involves an operation to align the eyes. It is therefore important to check for the possibility of postoperative diplopia when planning the treatment of those patients who have no potential for fusion.

Failure to Check Strabismic Patients for the Risk of Postoperative Diplopia

A test for the possibility of postoperative diplopia should be performed in every visually adult patient with strabismus during the preoperative evaluation. This is especially important in patients that do not appear to have the potential for fusion or if there is any doubt about the patient's binocular status. The patient is asked to fix a distance target in the primary position. If the near angle of deviation is different from that in the distance, the test also should be given using a near fixation object. The target should be as detailed as possible, depending on the visual acuity of the deviating eye. Prisms of increasing strength are placed before the deviating eye to gradually correct the deviation. The patient is asked to report if one target or two targets are seen. The patient must be encouraged to maintain fixation with their dominant eye throughout the test. If the patient switches or repeatedly alternates fixation during the test the patient may mistakenly report diplopia, but close questioning will reveal that the patient is really noticing the image shifts position as fixation shifts. Strabismic patients will usually become aware of diplopia immediately if the deviation is overcorrected. This is an example of the hemiretinal trigger mechanism (see Chapter 15). This mechanism also can be used to confirm the objective measurement. It is useful in patients who have nystagmus or other fixation difficulies. If the patient has abnormal retinal correspondence, diplopia may be elicited before the deviation is fully corrected. In these unusual circumstances a prism can be prescribed to see if the patient can learn to suppress the second image. Using prisms usually allows an immediate assessment of the amount of change in the deviation that can be tolerated before the patient becomes aware of diplopia. This test can be performed and the results evaluated in a matter of minutes. It can be given anywhere that prisms are available and does not require any additional equipment. An operation to correct the strabismus can be planned using the information gained from this test. The adjustable surgery technique can be used to reduce further the risk of overcorrecting the deviation and provoking diplopia.

Failure to Recognize that Amblyopia Does Not Protect a Patient from Binocular Diplopia

It must not be assumed that a patient who has deep amblyopia will not suffer from binocular diplopia. Only patients with no perception of light in the deviating eye are safe from diplopia. Patients with strabismus and amblyopia with corrected vision of less than 20/400 in the strabismic eye are just as likely to suffer from diplopia, if their strabismus is overcorrected, as is a patient with an alternating strabismus without fusion and 20/20 vision in each eye. The mechanism of diplopia in esotropia and in exotropia is shown diagrammatically in Figures 21–1 and 21–2. In strabismus, diplopia is caused by the suppression, present from visual immaturity disappearing. If the strabismus is overcorrected, even by a few prism diopters, diplopia is triggered (the hemiretinal trigger mechanism) (see Fig. 15–1). The second image cannot be suppressed because it is the reduplication of the object of conscious attention seen by the fixing eye. For this reason, it also is

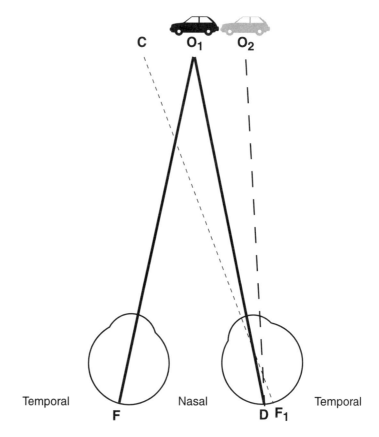

Figure 21–1.   Diplopia in right esotropia (convergent strabismus).

difficult to ignore, particularly if the diplopic images are close together, when there is only a few prism diopters of overcorrection. The nearer the diplopia point is to the fovea, the clearer and more disturbing the diplopic image. The bitter complaints from a patient whose strabismus has been overcorrected may appear to be unreasonable, ungrateful, and even hysterical to the ophthalmologist because the strabismus is now unnoticeable. These complaints, however, emphasize the shock of becoming diplopic for the first time in life.

Case Report

A 35-year-old taxi driver was finding it difficult to continue his work because of double vision. His best-corrected vision was right eye 6/4.5, left eye 6/120. His left eye had turned in from an early age. He had had two operations to align the eyes, but mentioned that he felt the second operation had ruined his eyes. His job and peace of mind were at stake. Examination showed a left exotropia of approximately 8 prism diopters in the primary position. He experienced crossed diplopia. The diplopia disappeared when base-in prisms of greater than 10 diopters were placed in front of the left eye. The strabismus was unnoticeable to

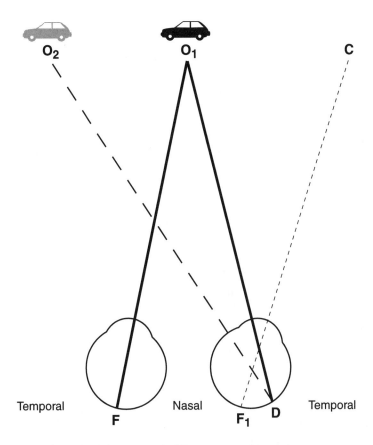

Figure 21–2. Diplopia in right exotropia (divergent strabismus).

a casual glance. An adjustable suture recession of the left lateral rectus eliminated the exotropia and diplopia in the practical positions of gaze, while preserving reasonable cosmesis. He was very grateful because it enabled him to return to work. Two other ophthalmologists whom he had consulted were reluctant to touch such a good cosmetic result because they would be unable to improve it. They discounted the patient's complaints because of the deep amblyopia. They felt that the possibility of worker's compensation might be the motivating factor for the complaints.

Failure to Check for Torsion and to Understand Its Significance

The brain is able to tolerate about 10° of torsion in the average person with fusion. The following facts are relevant to treating complaints of torsion:

1. Torsion is a symptom of acquired strabismus, usually a superior oblique palsy.

2. Prisms cannot neutralize torsion. Obliquely held prisms only have horizontal and vertical effects.

3. In our experience almost all cases in which torsion per se requires treatment are confined to patients with bilateral acquired superior oblique palsy, which usually follows severe trauma. Torsion usually exceeds 15° in these patients, particularly in down gaze.

4. Patients who complain of torsion usually have horizontal or vertical diplopia as well. If the clinician can get rid of the diplopia purely by neutralizing the horizontal and vertical deviation with prisms, the torsion can be totally ignored because it will obviously disappear once the patient can fuse after successful treatment of the vertical and horizontal strabismus.

5. Torsion should always be assessed.in down gaze as well as in the primary and the reading positions.[23]

6. In the unusual case where torsion does not disappear on neutralization of the vertical and horizontal strabismus, an evaluation by an orthoptist using a synoptophore is necessary to exclude central fusion disruption (see Chapter 12) and to confirm that fusion is likely to be present once all the elements of the strabismus and specifically the torsion are corrected surgically.

7. If torsion is a barrier to fusion, it must be corrected first, before the hypertropia and the esotropia in down gaze (see Chapter 12).[23]

Inappropriate Use of Orthoptic Exercises

Orthoptic exercises are a valuable adjunct to other methods of treating strabismus in suitable cases. Unfortunately, in the past there have been unrealistic expectations of orthoptic exercises. This is still the case today in some parts of the world, although fortunately to a much lesser extent. Elsewhere the value of orthoptic exercises in the management of some types of strabismus is overlooked because of the history of their inappropriate use, often over several years, in patients who had no hope of achieving binocular single vision. Orthoptic exercises can enhance the results already achieved. In some cases they are all that are necessary to reestablish comfortable binocular single vision for all distances.

Patients Can Be Taught to Maximize What Fusion Ability They Have but They Cannot Be Taught to Fuse

Antisuppression exercises should never be used unless there is evidence that the patient has a strong fusion potential that they will be able to use more efficiently. Orthoptic exercises cannot develop fusion or stereopsis ability if it is absent.

Some patients with a fully accommodative esotropia and a refractive error of less than +3.50 DS can be taught to control the esotropia that occurs when glasses are removed. Many are subsequently able to dispense with glasses, at least until presbyopia begins. The only other cases that respond to orthoptic exercises are convergence insufficiency, some heterophorias, and intermittent strabismus. The one thing that all these cases have in common is that by definition they already have fusion and stereopsis. Orthoptic exercises can teach them to use their fusion ability more efficiently. Some heterophorias and intermittent strabismus also may require that the angle of the deviation be reduced by surgery before orthoptic exercises can help establish comfortable control.

The use of convergence exercises in the management of convergence insufficiency is well known and is very effective, provided there is adequate supervision and follow-up. These orthoptic exercises are discussed in more detail in Chapter 6. It is important that the patient's progress be closely supervised.

Failure to Assess Preoperatively the Difficulties Involved in Postoperative Follow-Up

In large countries with remote areas and in many developing countries follow-up care after operation may be a problem.

Parents who witness a satisfactory cosmetic result from strabismus surgery or see the replacement of the abnormal white pupil of a cataract with a normal looking black pupil may feel that the result is good enough for them. They may choose not to come for the needed postoperative supervision and care if it involves a lot of travel and inconvenience, particularly if it involves walking and carrying the child 100 km to the doctor.

Failure to Recognize that a Small Residual or a Consecutive Esotropia Increases the Risk of Amblyopia in Children

The incidence of amblyopia in untreated congenital esotropia is much less than that found in young children who have had an operation to align their eyes before 2 years of age in the hope that they may be able to develop some fusion ability[1,2,7,22] (see Chapters 7 and 8). Postoperative follow-up is essential ideally about every 3 months until patients are over 8 years of age. If follow-up is unlikely, it is better to delay surgery and forego the 50% chance of developing some fusion for the increased chance of having a child with good vision in each eye. Unfortunately, the need for this approach is reinforced by the frequent incidence of traumatic blindness in one eye in many developing nations.

Similarly, it may be prudent to postpone surgical correction of intermittent exotropia in a young child if adequate follow-up is not possible. Surgical correction is ideally performed before 4 years of age for the best chance of cure.[21] However, if the child has a consecutive esotropia postoperatively, amblyopia may develop in an eye that otherwise would have had normal vision. The vision would be safeguarded and good appearance with a reduced chance of complete cure would be obtained at 8 years of age.

Failure to Recognize the Potential Advantage from Delaying Surgery to Correct an Abnormal Head Posture

The many causes of an abnormal head posture are discussed in detail in Chapter 18.

If the adopted head posture is compensatory, i.e., in the interest of preserving fusion such as in a patient with a superior oblique palsy or other complex strabismus (see Chapter 12) or to obtain better vision in a patient with nystagmus (see Chapter 20), it is frequently advantageous to delay surgical treatment until proper assessment of the problem is possible. This will include a prism cover test in the diagnostic positions of gaze and on head tilting to either side as well as Hess chart analysis in the case of strabismus, and detailed assessment of visual acuity in cases of nystagmus (see Chapter 20). By 6 years of age patients can usually perform these tests. Treatment will not be adversely affected by this delay, provided that the head posture is maintained because it indicates fusion in strabismus or optimum vision in nystagmus. The eventual outcome of treatment will not have been adversely affected by this delay but indeed may be enhanced.

Failure to Recognize the Role of Active Duction Exercises in the Prevention of Some Forms of Restrictive Strabismus

There are reports of postoperative diplopia following the injection of local anesthetic agents, when given as either a retrobulbar or peribulbar injection, before cataract surgery.[3–5,8,14,26,31] Possible causes mentioned include the direct neurotoxic effect of the injection of fluid agent on the ocular muscles fibers themselves, particularly if epinephrine is included.[32] The trauma of the needle piercing the belly of the muscle, or the injection of fluid itself are other possible causes.

The vertical recti are most commonly involved. Although the inferior rectus is the most common, injection in the inferolateral aspect of the orbit may directly involve the superior rectus as well.[4] The muscle fibers affected degenerate, and this may be followed by regeneration. Clinically the mechanism may involve an early mild contracture or a weakness, which may get better or may be followed by a more permanent scarring with restriction of movement. Clinical signs vary but may include an initial hypotropia, later followed by a hypertropia of the affected eye.

Diplopia also has been described following surgical treatment of pterygia.[11,25,30]

If postoperative diplopia occurs active duction exercises may help in the patient's recovery and may help to prevent adhesions and contractures that could cause restriction of movement and may require another operation for relief (see Chapter 13). These active duction exercises are only effective in the immediate postoperative period before adhesions develop. They may help also in new cases of blow-out fractures of the orbit and in preventing contracture of an extraocular muscle in recently acquired paretic strabismus.

Inappropriate Prolonged Occlusion of an Eye with a Recently Acquired Paresis of an Extraocular Muscle

The sudden onset of diplopia is distressing and incapacitating. It is natural for the patient to try to find the easiest way of eliminating the unwanted second image so that they can resume most of their daily activities. They therefore occlude the affected eye while waiting for spontaneous recovery or for treatment. The fixing (unoccluded) eye determines the amount of innervation received by each eye. This can lead to contracture of the unopposed direct (ipsilateral) antagonist muscle. This is another example of Hering's law. The most frequent occurrence of this is a case of a paresis of a lateral rectus muscle, which could lead to contracture of the ipsilateral medial rectus. To try to guard against the development of a contracture, the patient should be encouraged to occlude the unaffected eye for at least half the time. They should use a compensatory head posture to obtain single vision whenever practical instead of occluding an eye. Patients do not like occluding the unaffected eye because they feel that it upsets their balance even more, but if they occlude the eye at home it is often easier for them to tolerate. Following this regimen may help recovery, and treatment may be simplified by avoiding the need for surgery to deal with the contracture (see also Chapter 13).

References

1. Calcutt, C.: The natural history of infantile esotropia. A study of the untreated condition in the visual adult. In: Tillson, G., ed. Advances in Amblyopia and Strabismus. Transactions of the 7th International Orthoptic Congress. Nuremberg, Berufsverband der Orthoptistinnen Deutschland, 1991:3.
2. Calcutt, C., Murray, A.D.: Untreated essential infantile esotropia: Factors affecting the development of amblyopia. Eye 12(part 2):167, 1998.
3. Capo, H., Guyton, D.L.: Ipsilateral hypertropia after cataract surgery. Ophthalmology 103:721–730, 1996.
4. Capo, H., Roth, E., Johnson, T., Munoz, M., Siatkowski, R.M.: Vertical strabismus after cataract surgery [see comments]. Ophthalmology 103(6):918–921, 1996.
5. Carlson, B.M., Komorowski, T.E., Rainin, E.A., Shepard, B.M.: Extraocular muscle regeneration in primates. Local anesthetic-induced lesions. Ophthalmology 99:582–589, 1992.
6. Freeman, R.S.: Diplopia following cataract surgery. Am Orthoptic J 44:2–10, 1994.
7. Good, W.V., da Sa, L.C.F., Lyons, C.J., Hoyt, C.S.: Monocular visual outcome in untreated early onset esotropia. Br J Ophthalmol 77:492–494, 1993.
8. Grimmett, M.R., Lambert, S.R.: Superior rectus muscle overaction after cataract extraction [Comment]. Am J Ophthalmol 115:126–128, 1992.
9. Hamed, L.M., Helveston, E.M., Ellis, F.D.: Persistent binocular diplopia after cataract surgery. Am J Ophthalmol 103:741, 1987.
10. Hansen, V.C.: Evaluation and management of monocular diplopia. Am Orthoptic J 44:50–55, 1994.
11. Kenyon, K.R., Wagoner, M.D., Hettinger, M.E.: Conjunctival autograft transplantation for advanced and recurrent pterygium. Ophthalmology 92:1461–70, 1985.
12. Kushner, B.J.: Abnormal sensory findings secondary to monocular cataracts in children and strabismic adults. Am J Ophthalmol 102:349, 1986.
13. Kushner, B.J.: Fixation switch diplopia. Arch Ophthalmol 113:896–899, 1995.
14. Lyle, T.K.: The importance of orthoptic investigation before contact lens fitting in unilateral aphakia. A preliminary report. Trans Ophthalmol Soc UK 73:387, 1953.
15. Lyons, C.J., Oystreck, D.T.: Presbyopia and strabismus: Old patients, new symptoms. In Pritchard, C., eds. Orthoptics in Focus-Visions for the New Millennium. Transactions of the IXth International Orthoptic Congress, Stockholm, Sweden, 1999. Nuremberg: Berufsverband der Orthoptistinnen Deutschland, 1999:119–122.
16. Mandava, N., Donnenfeld, E.D., Owens, P.L., Kelly, S.E., Haight, D.H.: Ocular deviation following excimer laser photorefractive keratectomy. J Cataract Refract Surg 22:504–505, 1996.
17. Maurer, Y.: Survey of patients referred for orthoptic examination from the contact lens department with special reference to cases of unilateral aphakia. Br Orthoptic J 19:62, 1962.
18. McDonnell, P.J., Sadun, A.A.: Acquired accommodative esotropia following overcorrection by myopic epikeratophakia. Cornea 9:354–356, 1990.
19. Milder, B., Rubin, M.L.: The Fine Art of Prescribing Glasses without Making a Spectacle of Yourself, 2nd ed. Gainesville, FL: Triad Publishing, 1991:145–146.
20. Parkinson, J., McMain, K.: Diplopia in pseudophakes-Case presentation and review of anisometropic adaptation. Am Orthoptic J 47:172–180, 1997.
21. Pratt-Johnson, J.A., Barlow, J.M., Tillson, G.: Early surgery in intermittent exotropia. Am J Ophthalmol 84:689, 1977.

22. Pratt-Johnson, J.A., Tillson, G.: Sensory results following treatment of infantile esotropia. Can J Ophthalmol 18:175, 1983.
23. Pratt-Johnson, J.A., Tillson, G.: The investigation and management of torsion preventing fusion in bilateral superior oblique palsies. J Pediatr Ophthalmol Strabismus 24:145, 1987.
24. Pratt-Johnson, J.A., Tillson, G.: Intractable diplopia after vision restoration in unilateral cataract. Am J Ophthalmol 107:23–26, 1989.
25. Raab, E.L., Metz, H.S., Ellis, F.D.: Medial rectus injury after pterygium excision. Arch Ophthalmol 107:1428, 1989.
26. Rainin, E.A., Carlson, B.M.: Post-operative diplopia and ptosis. A clinical hypothesis based on the myotoxicity of local anesthetics. Arch Ophthalmol 103:1337–1339, 1985.
27. Ridley F: Contact lenses in unilateral aphakia. Trans Ophthalmol Soc UK 73:373, 1953.
28. Tillson, G., Pratt-Johnson, J.A. Fusion loss from longstanding unilateral cataracts in adults. In: Lenk-Schäfer, M., ed. Orthoptic Horizons: Transactions of the Sixth International Orthoptic Congress. British Orthoptic Society, London, England, 1987:327–331.
29. Verhoeff, K., Grootendorst, R.J., de Faber, J.T.H.N.: In: Lennerstrand G., ed. Ametropic Bilateral Amblyopia in Advances in Strabismology. Buren: The Netherlands, Æolus Press, 1999:26–28.
30. Vrabec, M.P., Weisenthal, R.W., Elsing, S.H., eds. Subconjunctival fibrosis after conjunctival autograft. Cornea 12:181–183, 1993.
31. Wakeman, B.J.: A review of the myotoxic effects of retrobulbar anesthetics. In: Pritchard, C., et al., eds. Orthoptics in Focus-Visions for the New Millennium. Transactions of the IXth International Orthoptic Congress, Stockholm, Sweden, 1999. Nuremberg: Berufsverband der Orthoptistinnen Deutschland, 1999:200–204.
32. Yagiela, J.A., Benoit, P.W., Buoncristiani, R.D., Peters, M.P., Fort, N.F.: Comparison of myotoxic effects of lidocaine with epinephrine in rats and humans. Anaesthesia Analgesia 60:471–480, 1981.
33. Zwaan, J.: Strabismus induced by radial keratotomy. Milit Med 161:630–631, 1996.

22

Vision 20/20: The Right to Sight and the Prevention of Amblyopia in Developing Countries

Vision 20/20: The Right to Sight

The Director General of the World Health Organization (WHO) announced in 1999 the launching of Vision 20/20, "The Right to Sight." This initiative is supported by a coalition of 18 international blindness prevention organizations from 11 countries, who, together with the International Association for the Prevention of Blindness, have endorsed the concept of ridding the world of the preventable and treatable causes of blindness by the year 2020.

It is estimated that one and a half million children are blind in the world and that 90% of them live in developing nations. If the aim of Vision 20/20 is to be achieved, all nations of the world must be involved, including the more industrialized and wealthy nations, who must lend their resources and expertise. Every health-care worker in ophthalmology should be aware of this huge project. Surveying the worldwide status of childhood blindness, it is estimated that 30% to 72% is avoidable, 9% to 58% is preventable, and 14% to 31% is treatable in different parts of the world.[6]

Prevention of Amblyopia in Developing Nations

It is essential that children with problems that are potentially amblyogenic, such as cataract, corneal opacities, strabismus, and very poor vision from uncorrected refractive errors, are treated as soon as the abnormality is noticed for any chance of restoring or preserving useful vision.

The most common cause of blindness in children is a combination of measles, vitamin A deficiency, and the use of traditional eye medicines[6] that result in corneal scarring and even loss of the eye. Corneal scarring in a child under 8 years of age results in amblyopia, which, if severe, will prevent the sight from returning. Even if a corneal graft can be successfully performed to remove the corneal scar, improvement in vision is rare. In many parts of the world, corneal scars that prevent children from seeing properly are often caused by a drying of the cornea and conjunctiva (xerophthalmia) associated with lack of vitamin A and then an infection by measles. This combination by itself is enough to rob the child of sight. An additional hazard is the treatment of the red eye with unclean concoctions from the traditional healer. This often causes a complicating infection that finally wipes out any chance for sight.

This scenario is totally preventable by:

1. Measles vaccination and a mass campaign to eradicate measles as smallpox was eradicated.

2. Adequate intake of vitamin A. Diet should include dark green leafy and yellow vegetables not only for children, but also for their mothers, who transmit the vitamin A via breast milk. Mothers should continue breast feeding as long as possible.

3. Administer capsules of vitamin A prophylactically on national immunization days.[4]

4. Administer capsules of vitamin A immediately if xerophthalmia is present, followed by a capsule on the next day and 4 weeks later.[4]

5. The universal distribution schedule of WHO for preschool children advises the administration of vitamin A capsules every 3 to 4 months from age 6 months to 6 years.[4]

6. Obtain the cooperation of traditional healers, witch doctors, and herbalists, who are the primary health-care contacts and treaters of patients in many developing nations. For instance, Nepal has a population of 22 million, but there are few medically qualified doctors, particularly in the rural and mountainous regions of the country. There are, however, 500,000 traditional healers; one for every 44 people in Nepal.[3] It was essential to devise some way of getting the cooperation of these traditional healers. Providing them with free topical antibiotics for use in "red eyes" has been effective in gaining their cooperation in Nepal. Additional education and providing the traditional healers with other useful remedies has resulted in children being referred to a hospital where there is an ophthalmologist as soon as possible when the healers realize they cannot cure their eye problems.[3]

Measures to Reduce Amblyopia from Cataracts, Microphthalmos, Glaucoma, and Strabismus

The use of rubella vaccine should follow the recommendations of WHO, which includes emphasizing the paramount importance of first protecting all females of child-bearing age, as well as the immunization of infants and children to prevent the congenital rubella syndrome. A combined measles-rubella vaccine is available.

Congenital rubella syndrome is associated with eye involvement in 72% of cases,[1] the most common of which is congenital cataract. There is a fourfold increase in the incidence of strabismus,[7] compared with the normal population. Sixty-six percent of involved eyes may be microphthalmic.[2] This is associated with high hypermetropia and, if it is unilateral, especially if it is combined with a congenital cataract, is a severe hindrance to the normal development of vision.

Congenital glaucoma occurs in about 10% of cases.[5] Even if the glaucoma is successfully treated, the cornea and anterior segment are often stretched out of shape by the high intraocular pressure before it is controlled. This produces high irregular astigmatic refractive errors, which are often overlooked in the preoccupation of controlling the intraocular pressure. Glasses may not give a clear enough definition to prevent amblyopia; consequently, contact lenses, if available, may be the only solution. Amblyopia lurks in the background, among these various ocular problems in this young age group. Its dangers may go unrecognized, but its toll on vision is relentless and ruthless.

Populations where consanguinity (spouse from the same family) is common should be counseled that this practice has the disastrous consequences of a marked increase in the incidence of inherited diseases, such as congenital cataracts, glaucoma, strabismus, and refractive errors.

Prevention of Amblyopia Due to Trauma in Children under 8 Years of Age

It is essential that the ophthalmologists who are used to treating patients of all ages are acutely aware of the dangers of amblyopia when they are treating children under 8 years of age. The covering of one eye for as little as 1 week in a child under the age of 3 years may induce amblyopia quite apart from other ocular problems that may be associated with the trauma. Amblyopia induced by patching of one eye following a corneal abrasion, or by occlusion resulting from bruising of the lids, where sight out of the eye is prevented by "the black eye," or poor vision resulting from a traumatic cataract is often the reason for failure for the vision to improve in the affected eye, rather than the injury itself, even if the injury is well cared for.

Tragically, traumatic injuries in children are common in developing nations. It is not only one of the common causes of unilateral blindness, but also contributes to blindness in both eyes when trauma involves the good eye in a patient with severe amblyopia in the other. Education of the whole community is necessary for the prevention of trauma in this age group.

Vital Role of Orthoptics and Optometry

Ophthalmologists are at a premium in most developing nations, the few that are available are preoccupied with the management of elderly adult patients blind from cataracts. The whole field of childhood blindness is therefore neglected in many countries. In this situation, a huge difference can be made by training personnel to understand and treat the nonsurgical aspects of strabismus and amblyopia. Such a person must be well trained and qualified in orthoptics, and must be able to refract and prescribe glasses. Many children become amblyopic because they have a significant refractive error that blurs the vision at all distances, and they have no opportunity of getting the correct glasses until they are visual adults (ametropic amblyopia). These trained professionals should also supervise all aspects of screening and prevention programs through public health nurses, teachers, and community workers, as well as volunteers. It is difficult to see how the aims of Vision 20/20 can be realized without training.and using many such individuals, ideally by the establishment of accredited training schools to produce the needed personnel.

Intractable Amblyopia and Congenital Cataracts

Cataracts present from birth or infancy may produce intractable amblyopia unless they are removed within the first 2 months of life. Dense cataracts in both eyes from birth will result in sensory nystagmus unless they are both removed and the aphakic refractive error corrected before 2 months of age. In microphthalmos, the refractive error may be as high as +25 diopters, which may be impractical to correct. There are strong arguments for preventing as many cases of congenital cataracts as possible: glasses of this magnitude and weight need support on the flat infant nose to keep the glasses in place. This can be aided by a head band. The unavailability and expense of contact lenses and the contraindication to the use of intraocular lenses, mentioned earlier, are more reasons. In many of the developing nations, these insuperable odds mean that most children born blind from cataracts remain blind for life despite treatment.

Unilateral Congenital Cataract

The odds that treatment of this condition in most developing countries will result in an improvement of vision are so poor that surgery to remove the cataract is not recommended. These cataracts can be removed at a later age for cosmetic reasons to get rid of the "white pupil." Surgery is the easiest part of the treatment—the real hurdle is the correction of the refractive error with a contact lens, and then the almost insuperable problem in most developing countries of supervised patching of the good eye. The child needs to be reassessed at least every 3 months until the child is over 8 years of age.

Bilateral Congenital Cataracts

Both cataracts need to be removed and the resulting large hyperopia corrected accurately by glasses or contact lenses before 2 months of age to prevent amblyopia and sensory nystagmus. Intraocular lenses are contraindicated at this age because they provoke too much inflammatory reaction. In most developing countries, particularly away from big centres, safe pediatric anesthesia is unavailable from both a lack of trained anesthetists and the lack of the necessary equipment.

In these situations, ketamine anesthesia offers the infant the only hope of getting cataracts removed by approximately 2 months of age. Because frequently the only medically qualified person in the operating room at the time of the administration of ketamine is the ophthalmologist who will perform the removal of the cataract, it seems appropriate to include information on the properties of the drug and on the optimum and safest method to administer this anesthetic agent in these circumstances.

Ketamine Anesthesia*

Mechanism of Action

Ketamine is thought to produce a dissociation between the thalamoneocortical and limbic systems, secondary to blockage of the N-methyl-d-aspartate receptor. This accounts for its anesthetic properties.

Advantages: It is inexpensive and easily stored, and no anesthetic machine is needed. The cardiac output, blood pressure, and pulse rate are increased. The functional residual capacity is maintained, and bronchodilation occurs.

Disadvantages: There is frequently an increase in the intraocular pressure, along with nystagmus, but the corneal and light reflexes remain intact. For these reasons, a retrobulbar block using injectable local anesthetic is given as soon as the infant is asleep, followed by ocular massage through the closed lid to reduce the intraocular pressure. Salivation increases, so atropine is given preoperatively. Apnea may occur if the drug is administered rapidly intravenously. Uncommonly, the gastric contents may be aspirated. Nightmarish dreams and emergent hallucinations may follow ketamine administration, particularly in older children.

Method of Administration

1. The patient should fast according to the following rules: no solid food for 6 hours, no breast milk for 4 hours, and no clear fluids for 2 hours preoperatively.

2. Give oral ketamine 0.5 to 1.0 mg/kg body weight 30 minutes preoperatively. This smoothes the induction and reduces the anesthetic dose needed.

3. Give atropine either 40 μg/kg by mouth or 20 μg/kg by intramuscular injection 30 minutes preoperatively, or 20 μg/kg intravenously on induction.

4. Ideally, attach an oximeter to a digit such as the big toe to follow the heart beat and the oxygen saturation.

5. If an oximeter is not available, then attach a precordial stethescope to the chest over the heart with some adhesive tape to monitor the heart rate. Observe skin and mucous membrane color while the patient is anesthetized to ensure there is no cyanosis.

6. Diazepam 0.15 mg/kg or promethazine 0.5 mg/kg can be given intramuscularly to older children weighing more than 15 kg to prevent hallucinations and bad dreams postoperatively.

---

* Gerard A. R. O'Connor, M.B., F.R.C.P.C. Pediatric Anesthesiologist, British Columbia's Children's Hospital, University of British Columbia, Vancouver, British Columbia, Canada.

7.   Ketamine anesthesia now begins with the administration of ketamine 5 to 7 mg/kg intramuscularly. This takes about 5 minutes to work and lasts 20 to 30 minutes. If more time is required, 3 to 5 mg/kg may be given intramuscularly after this interval.

The ketamine can also be administered intravenously 1 to 2 mg/kg, given slowly to prevent apnea. This lasts 10 to 15 minutes. Further doses of 0.5 mg/kg can be given if the anesthesia lightens, but not more than 5 mg/kg in total.

Instead of giving boluses, maintenance can be achieved by using an infusion of ketamine, the dose depending on the availability of nitrous oxide (15–45 μg/kg/min intravenously with nitrous oxide and oxygen, 30–90 μg/kg/min intravenously without nitrous oxide).

8.   The jaw needs to be supported by an assistant who is not going to be involved with the surgical procedure.

9.   As soon as the infant is asleep, a retrobulbar injection of local anesthetic such as xylocaine 1% should be given to the affected eye and some gentle massage performed through the closed lids.

10.   The older the child, the less likely the child is to have airway problems. Therefore, young infants should weigh more than 5.0 kg, which should correspond to approximately 2 months of age.

Ketamine is used as the only anesthetic agent in many developing countries. There are no perfect formulas for its use-much depends on the equipment available and the expertise of the nonmedical assistants. Therefore, every center should make guidelines that suit their particular location.

Summary

Sequence of a Ketamine Anesthetic

1.   Assess the patient for major problems that would cause the postponement or cancellation of the case; for example, severe chest infection, an abnormal airway, or an untreated heart condition.

2.   Food and fluid fasting according to the rules stated.

3.   Premedication by mouth: ketamine and atropine. Diazepam may be given to children who weigh more than 15.0 kg.

4.   To monitor the child, place the oximeter probe on the big toe, and tape the stethescope onto the chest.

5.   Induction: Ketamine given intramuscularly or intravenously.

6.   Maintenance: Either intramuscular or intravenous injections or continuous infusion of ketamine.

7.   Assistance: Continual support of the jaw and observation of the patient throughout the procedure and until the patient has fully recovered from the anesthesia.

8.   Conclusion of procedure: Observe for excitation and leave on oxygen until the child is fully awake.

Telemedicine and Treatment of Strabismus and Amblyopia

Many hospitals in developing countries have a computer. Currently the minimum requirement for telemedicine as it relates to the management of strabismus and amblyopia is a computer that can run Microsoft Windows 95 or its equivalent and has access to the Internet. In addition, the gift or acquisition of a digital camera with the specifications listed below will enable the hospital to contact and establish a consultation service with other larger institutions in that country, as well as consultants anywhere in the world that have agreed to provide such a service.

THE MINIMUM SPECIFICATIONS OF THE DIGITAL CAMERA

1. A liquid crystal display (LCD) screen
2. Resolution: 240 × 320 dpi
3. Charged coupled device (CCD) $\frac{1}{4}$-inch 350 k (gross), 330 k (effec)
4. Optical zoom lens (10×)
5. Flash
6. Image recorded on a 3.5-inch floppy disc in the body of the camera

INFORMATION THAT IS HELPFUL TO SEND TO THE CONSULTANT

1. Summary of the history and findings and diagnosis.
2. Photographic recording of the eyes in the nine diagnostic positions of gaze. Care must be taken to keep the patient's head straight so that the plane of the camera lens is parallel to the plane of the eyes. The advantage of the zoom is that photographs of the eye positions can be taken from several feet away from the patient. Available light in many surroundings is sufficient to give good enough clear photographs to record the eye positions. This method is least likely to disturb a child.
3. Photograph the eyes in the primary position with the head tilted to the right and then to the left.
4. Photograph the Hess charts and possibly the record of the Lancaster Red-Green Test or any other test results with the digital camera. Note that all photographs and records can be viewed on the LCD screen and if some are not satisfactory, they can be deleted and the photographs repeated until a satisfactory recording is obtained.

TRANSMISSION OF THE PHOTOGRAPHS RECORDED ON THE DISC

The 3.5-inch floppy disc is removed from the camera and inserted into the computer that has a connection to the Internet. A full history and details of the clinical examination are sent by e-mail to the consultant; the information on the floppy disc is sent as an attachment.

Suggested Consultant's Disclaimer (Courtesy of Dr. E.M. Helveston)

It is essential to emphasize that the ultimate responsibility for the treatment must rest with the patient's ophthalmologist who has performed the examination and who will perform the surgery.

Disclaimer: The opinions given in this report are based on the interpretation of photographs received and do not constitute a valid opinion on which to base treatment. Treatment undertaken by any physician should be based on personal observation of the patient.

Orbis E-Consultation

Dr. Eugene M. Helveston in cooperation with Orbis International has initiated The Orbis E-Consultation Program following Helveston's pilot project connecting ophthalmologists in Cuba with his home base in Indiana. His advice and experience helped us link ophthalmologists in Nepal with us in Canada. Contact Orbis International at 330 West 42nd Street, Suite 1900, New York, NY 10036, or by e-mail at executive@ny.orbis.org for more details concerning their e-consultation program.

Table 22–1.   Classification of Visual Impairment Based on WHO Standards

Classification of Visual Impairment		Visual Acuity of Better Eye with Refractive Error Corrected
Category 1	Visual impairment	<6/18–6/60
Category 2	Severe visual impairment	<6/60–3/60
Category 3	Blind	<3/60–1/60
Category 4	Blind	<1/60–Light perception
Category 5	Blind	No light perception

References

1. Givens, T.G., Lee, D.A., Jones, T., Ilstrup, D.M.: Congenital rubella syndrome: Ophthalmic manifestations and associated systemic disorders. Br J Ophthalmol 77:258–363, 1993.
2. Gregg, N. McA.: Congenital cataracts following German measles in the mother. Trans Ophthalmol Soc Aust 3:35, 1941.
3. Poudyal, B.: Roles of traditional healers in paediatric eyecare in Nepal. Proceedings of the National Conference on Children's Eyesight in Nepal. Kathmandu, 1998.
4. Schwab, L.: Eye Care in Developing Nations, 3rd ed. San Francisco: Foundation of The American Academy of Ophthalmology, 1999:69.
5. Sears, M.L.: Congenital glaucoma in neonatal rubella. Br J Ophthalmol 51:744, 1967.
6. Steinkuller, P.G., Du,.L., Gilbert, C., Foster, A., Collins, M.L., Coats, D.K.: Childhood blindness. J AAPOS 3:26–32, 1999 .
7. Wolff, S.M.: The ocular manifestations of congenital rubella. J Pediatr Ophthalmol Strabismus 10:101–141, 1973.

Glossary

Glossary of some terms used in this book, placed in the following categories: anatomy; binocular vision, fusion, and suppression; amblyopia; ocular movements; strabismus; refraction; and miscellaneous terms.

Anatomy

Fovea (fovea centralis): This is a depression in the inner retinal surface in the center of the macula. It measures 1.5 mm, about equal to one optic disc diameter.

Macula (macula lutea): It is that portion of the central retina surrounding the fovea containing xanthophilic pigment and two or more layers of ganglion cells. It is approximately 5.5 mm in diameter.

Positions of Gaze

Primary position: The position of one or both eyes looking straight ahead with the body and head erect.

Secondary position: The up, down, or side gaze positions of one or both eyes.

Tertiary position: The oblique position of one or both eyes.

Diagnostic positions: The primary, secondary, and tertiary positions of gaze.

Cardinal positions of gaze: Up, down, and side gaze.

Binocular Vision, Fusion, and Suppression

Binocular Vision

Binocular vision: The ability to use vision from both eyes simultaneously.

Binocular visual field (field of binocular vision): The total area seen with both eyes open fixing a target in the primary position.

Binocular single vision (single binocular vision): The ability to use both eyes simultaneously to obtain fusion.

Binocular single visual field (field of single binocular vision): The total area in which fusion is present without moving the head.

Corresponding points (areas): The points (areas) in the retina of each eye that localize to the same point in space.

Diplopia (Double Vision)

Binocular diplopia: Two images of the object of regard are seen only when both eyes are open.

Monocular diplopia: Two images of the object of regard are seen by one eye alone.

Crossed diplopia (heteronymous diplopia): Binocular diplopia associated with an exotropia. The image of the fixation object falls on the temporal retina of the deviating eye and is projected nasally.

Uncrossed diplopia (homonymous diplopia): Binocular diplopia associated with an esotropia in which the image of the fixation object falls on the nasal retina of the deviating eye and is projected temporally.

Incongruous diplopia: Occurs in some patients with abnormal retinal correspondence. The subjective separation of the diplopic images is less than expected from the objective angle of deviation.

Paradoxical diplopia: Binocular diplopia occurring in patients with abnormal retinal correspondence in which crossed diplopia occurs in esotropia and uncrossed diplopia occurs in exotropia.

Dissociation: The disruption of fusion causing a change in the alignment of both eyes.

Fusion

Sensory fusion: Images from corresponding retinal points from each eye come together in the visual cortex and are perceived as one.

Motor fusion: The ability to maintain sensory fusion with vergences (fusional convergence/divergence amplitude).

Central fusion (bifoveal fusion): The fusion of images from the fovea of each eye.

Peripheral fusion: Fusion of images from each eye from retinal areas outside the fovea and probably outside the macula area of each eye, the fovea of one eye being suppressed.

Central fusion disruption (horror fusionis, intractable diplopia): The disruption of motor fusion in a visual adult resulting in diplopia without suppression.

Retinal Correspondence

Normal retinal correspondence: The localization to the same point in space by corresponding points of the retina in each eye.

Abnormal retinal correspondence: A binocular condition in which there is a change of visual direction of the retina of the deviating eye such that an extrafoveal area in this eye corresponds with the fovea of the straight eye.

Retinal rivalry: The simultaneous stimulation of corresponding retinal points with dissimilar nonfusable targets in each eye that produces a rivalry for conscious attention of each nonfusable image.

Stereopsis (3D vision): The binocular appreciation of depth.

Suppression: The cortical inhibition of some part of the vision from one eye with both eyes open.

Visual adult (visual maturity): A patient who is over 8 years of age. This implies that the period for the cortical development of vision, fusion, and stereopsis or suppression has ended.

Visual immaturity: Pertaining to a child who is under 8 years of age.

Amblyopia

Amblyopia: A unilateral or bilateral decrease of visual acuity (form vision) for which no organic cause can be found in the eye.

Fix (fixate): To look directly at an object with one or both eyes.

Bifoveal fixation: To fix with the fovea of both eyes.

Central fixation: To fix with the fovea.

Eccentric fixation: A uniocular condition in which the patient fixes an object with a point on the retina other than the fovea.

Intractable amblyopia: Amblyopia resistant to treatment.

Occlusion (patching): The prevention or reduction of visual stimulation by covering eye.

Penalization: The artificial reduction of clear vision in one eye.

Ocular Movements

Active force generation: This is the active force generated by the contraction of one of the extraocular muscles.

Ductions: The movement of one eye from the primary straight ahead position with the other eye occluded.

Active duction: The duction movement produced by the patient's extraocular muscle action.

Forced duction test (passive duction test, traction test): The patient's eye is passively moved (without active muscle contraction) in a particular direction to test for mechanical restriction.

Paralysis: Complete loss of function of a muscle.

Paresis: Partial loss of function of a muscle.

Torsion: The rotation of the vertical meridian of one eye.

Incyclotorsion: The rotation of the upper end of the vertical corneal meridian inward toward the nose.

Excyclotorsion: The rotation of the upper end of the vertical corneal meridian outward away from the nose.

Version: The movement of both eyes together in the same direction from the primary position to another gaze position.

Vergence (disjunctive movement): The movement of both eyes in opposite directions.

Strabismus

AC:A ratio (accommodative convergence:accommodation ratio:) The ratio between the alignment of the visual axes when accommodation is used and the alignment when accommodation is not used. In this book it is measured by comparing the alignment present at 6 m or beyond with the full optical correction for distance in place and the alignment at 1/3 m with the same correction in place.

High AC:A ratio: The alignment is relatively more convergent at near than at distance.

Low AC:A ratio: The alignment is relatively less convergent at near than at distance.

Angle kappa: The angle between the line joining the fovea with the object of regard (visual axis) and a mid-pupillary line.

Positive angle kappa: The visual axis crosses the cornea on the nasal side of the mid-pupillary line giving the appearance of a divergent strabismus (pseudo-divergence).

Negative angle kappa: The visual axis crosses the cornea on the temporal side of the mid-pupillary line giving the appearance of a convergent strabismus (pseudoconvergence).

Bouncing end point: The involuntary movement of the deviating eye back and forth behind the prism as the neutralization point is approached with the prism cover test.

Deviation: The turn of an eye away from the axis needed to fix an object of regard.

Primary deviation: The deviation produced when the normal eye is fixing, the other eye being the site of a paretic or paralyzed muscle or a mechanical restriction or other cause of strabismus.

Secondary deviation: The deviation of the normal eye resulting from the other eye fixing when this eye has a paretic or paralyzed muscle or a mechanical restriction.

Dissociated vertical divergence (DVD): A vertical deviation of unknown etiology associated with the congenital strabismus syndrome and characterized by an upward drift and excyclorotation of the affected eye. If it is bilateral, it is sometimes referred to as alternating sursumduction or alternating hyperphoria.

Intermittent exotropia: Semantically this means that one eye is sometimes exotropic and sometimes straight, but always implied is the fact that the exotropia is accompanied by suppression. When the eyes are straight there is bifoveal fusion. This implication of suppression is exceptional in strabismologic terminology.

Monofixation: The term applies to fixing with both eyes open, but using the fovea of one eye while the fovea of the other eye is suppressed.

Muscle imbalance: The presence of any phoria (latent) or tropia (manifest) strabismus.

Orthophoria: Absence of any muscle imbalance in the fusion free position.

Orthotropia: Absence of any tropia (manifest strabismus) in the fusion free position.

Strabismus: The visual axes of the two eyes are not both aligned on the fixation object.

Concomitant strabismus: Strabismus in which the angle of deviation remains the same in all directions of gaze, whichever eye is fixing.

Consecutive strabismus: A reversal of the direction of the strabismus, eso to exo or exo to eso.

Incomitant strabismus: Strabismus in which the angle of deviation differs depending on the direction of gaze or which eye is fixing.

Microstrabismus (microtropia): A small angle manifest strabismus.

Cosmetic strabismus result: A strabismus in which the result of treatment is only the improvement of the patient's appearance.

Functional strabismus result: A result which is concerned with obtaining fusion.

Virgin muscle: Extraocular muscle on which surgery has not been performed.

Refraction

Anisometropia: Unequal refractive error in the two eyes.

Anisophoria: Unequal or different muscle balance in different directions of gaze, which results from corrected anisometropia.

Monovision: The correction of the refractive error of one eye for distance and the other for near vision.

Presbyopia: Difficulty in accommodating the eye to near vision associated with aging. It is caused by the crystalline lens being unable to modify its shape sufficiently.

Refractive surgery: Surgery that alters the refraction of an eye. This is usually accompanied by modifying the shape and thereby the power of the cornea, or much less commonly by the introduction of an intraocular lens.

Miscellaneous Terms

Asthenopia: Eye discomfort from malfunctioning extraocular or intraocular muscles or optical errors.

Digital camera: Camera recording images as electronic bits, stored on a disc.

Objective: Observable by people other than the patient.

Subjective: Only observable by the patient.

Ocular torticollis: Head tilt to improve visual acuity (to utilize a nystagmus null zone) or to maintain fusion.

Syndrome: A group of symptoms and signs that characterize a distinct entity.

Telemedicine: Medicine employing the use of a digital camera and computers linked by the Internet for electronic communication and consultation.

Traditional healer: A person without conventional medical training who treats various maladies, often with herbal and other remedies. In some cultures, synonymous with *herbalist* and in others with *witch doctor.*

Index

Page numbers followed by f indicate figures. Page numbers followed by t indicate tables.